Standard Haematology Practice/2

Standard Haematology Practice/2
Edited by Keith Wood
on behalf of the British Committee
for Standards in Haematology

FOREWORD BY BRYON ROBERTS
President, British Society for Haematology

Blackwell
Science

© 1994 by
Blackwell Science Ltd
Editorial Offices:
Osney Mead, Oxford OX2 0EL
25 John Street, London WC1N 2BL
23 Ainslie Place, Edinburgh EH3 6AJ
238 Main Street, Cambridge
  Massachusetts 02142, USA
54 University Street, Carlton
  Victoria 3053, Australia

Other Editorial Offices:
Arnette Blackwell SA
1, rue de Lille
75007 Paris
France

Blackwell Wissenschafts-Verlag GmbH
Kurfürstendamm 57
10707 Berlin
Germany

Blackwell MZV
Feldgasse 13
A-1238 Wien
Austria

First published 1994

Set by Excel Typesetters Co., Hong Kong
Printed and bound in Great Britain
at the University Press, Cambridge

DISTRIBUTORS

Marston Book Services Ltd
PO Box 87, Oxford OX2 0DT
(*Orders*: Tel: 01865 791155
        Fax: 01865 791927
        Telex: 837515)

USA
Blackwell Science, Inc.
238 Main Street
Cambridge, MA 02142
(*Orders*: Tel: 800 759-6102
        617 876-7000)

Canada
Times Mirror Professional Publishing, Ltd
130 Flaska Drive
Markham, Ontario L6G 1B8
(*Orders*: Tel: 800 268-4178
        416 470-6739)

Australia
Blackwell Science Pty Ltd
54 University Street
Carlton, Victoria 3053
(*Orders*: Tel: 03 347-5552)

A catalogue record for this title
is available from the British Library

ISBN 0-632-03739-3

Library of Congress
Cataloging in Publication Data

Standard haematology practice 2/
  edited by Keith Wood on behalf of
  the British Committee for Standards in Haematology;
  foreword by B.E. Roberts.
      p.   cm.
  Includes bibliographical references and index.
  ISBN 0-632-03739-3
  1. Hematology—Standards—Great Britain.
  I. Wood, Keith (J. Keith)
  II. British Committee for Standards in Haematology.
  III. Title: Standard haematology practice two.
  [DNLM: 1. Hematology—standards.
  2. Diagnosis, Laboratory—standards.
  3. Hematologic Tests—standards.
  WH 100 S785 1994]
  RB45.S75 1994
  616.07'561'021841—dc20

Contents

Contents

List of Contributors

British Committee for Standards in Haematology

J.K. Wood (*Chairman*); M.F. Murphy (*Secretary*); T.W. Barrowcliffe; B.T. Colvin; J.K.M. Duguid; P. Garwood; J.C. Giddings; D.A. Kennedy; A.S.J. Rejman; B.E. Roberts; R.M. Rowan; J.G. Smith; D. Voak; J.A. Whittaker.

Past Members
A.J. Bellingham; M. Brozović; M. Bruce; J.F. Davidson; W. Muir; A.H. Waters.

General Haematology Task Force

R.M. Rowan (*Chairman*); B.J. Bain (*Secretary*); J.M. England; K. Hyde; S.M. Lewis; E. Matutes; J.T. Reilly; A.D. Stephens.

Past Members and Contributors
R.J. Amos; M. Bhavnani; M. Brozović; D.W. Dawson; D.I. Fish; R.J. Leeming; J.C. Linnell; J.M. Old; C. Poynton; N.K. Shinton; J.G. Smith.

Haemostasis and Thrombosis Task Force

B.T. Colvin (*Chairman*); S.J. Machin (*Secretary*); T.W. Barrowcliffe; M. Greaves; C.A. Ludlam; I.J. Mackie; F.E. Preston; P.E. Rose; I.D. Walker.

Past Members and Contributors
M.P. Colvin; J.F. Davidson; J.C. Giddings; R.A. Hutton; P.B.A. Kernoff; E.A. Letsky; R.G. Malia; M. Raftery; R. Rivers; R.F. Stevens; D.A. Taberner; J.J. Walker.

Blood Transfusion Task Force

D. Voak (*Chairman*); J.A.F. Napier (*Secretary*); R.D. Finney; K. Forman; P. Kelsey; S. Knowles; R. Mitchell; P. Phillips; A.H. Waters.

Past Members and Contributors
F.A. Ala; A.J. Bell; B. Brozović; R. Cann; C. Chapman; M. Contreras; M. de Silva; J.K.M. Duguid; I.D. Fraser; B.E.S. Gibson; J. Gillon; M. Greaves; I.M. Hann; B. Holland; J.M. Hows; R.M. Hutchinson; K. Jestice; J. Jones; L.A. Kay; D. Lee; E.A. Letsky; M. Levin; H.L. Lloyd; S.J. Machin; C. Morgan; M.F. Murphy; W. Murphy; W. Ouwehand; D.E. Pegg; N.G. Testa; A.R. Thomson; W. Wagstaff; C.A.J. Wardrop; M.S.C. Webb; F.G. Williams; J.K. Wood.

Clinical Haematology Task Force

J.A. Whittaker (*Chairman*); G.P. Summerfield (*Secretary*); J.V. Clough; I.M. Franklin; B.E.S. Gibson; D.W. Gorst; J.G. Smith.

Past Members and Contributors
N.C. Allan; A.J. Bellingham; M. Brozović; B.T. Colvin; S.C. Davies; J. Gabbay; G.D.O. Lowe; Physicians' Group Central Middlesex Hospital; J.K. Wood.

Foreword

In the foreword to *Standard Haematology Practice*, Volume 1, Professor Waters wrote that the object of the British Committee for Standards in Haematology, a sub-committee of the British Society for Haematology, is to maintain standards in all branches of haematology in the UK, linked with parallel work at international level. One of the ways this is achieved is through the production of guidelines prepared by its expert Task Forces in general haematology, clinical haematology, blood transfusion and haemostasis and thrombosis.

Standard Haematology Practice, Volume 1, was a compendium of 20 guidelines and it was appreciated that at the time of publication there were significant gaps that needed to be filled. The second volume to a very large extent remedies this deficiency due to the hard work of the Task Forces and their associated Working Parties and as many as 22 guidelines have been produced in a short time.

These guidelines, representing the best of British haematological practice, are a considerable achievement for which the British Committee for Standards in Haematology can be justifiably proud.

Bryon Roberts
President
British Society for Haematology

Editor's Comments

This second volume of *Standard Haematology Practice* brings together 21 further guidelines written by the various Task Forces of the British Committee for Standards in Haematology on behalf of the British Society for Haematology. In addition there is a chapter relating to medical audit in haematology and an appendix concerning near-patient testing prepared by the Joint Working Group on Quality Assurance.

A majority of these new guidelines has been drafted by expert Working Parties co-opted by and from the Task Force concerned and in some cases include colleagues from outside haematology. Members of sister societies, in particular the British Blood Transfusion Society, the British Society for Haemostasis and Thrombosis and the Institute for Medical Laboratory Sciences, have been involved where appropriate. The first seven chapters relate to the management of haematology departments prepared by the General Haematology Task Force. Chapter 21 was produced by a Working Party of the National Blood Transfusion Service.

That this large number of additional guidelines has been completed in the 3 years since the first volume, is testimony to the assiduous work of the Task Forces and their Working Parties. More than 80 haematologists are involved and I thank them all. I have tried to name all of them but in the relatively easy task of putting the book together any sins of omission or commission are mine.

Keith Wood
Royal Infirmary, Leicester

Disclaimer
Whilst the advice and information contained in this book is believed to be true and accurate at the time of going to press, neither the editor, the authors or the publisher can accept any legal responsibility or liability for any errors or omissions that may be made.

Part 1
Haematology Laboratory
Management Practice

Prepared by the
General Haematology Task Force

WITH CONTRIBUTIONS FROM
THE HAEMOSTASIS & THROMBOSIS
& BLOOD TRANSFUSION TASK FORCES
EDITED BY R. M. ROWAN
& N. K. SHINTON

1 General Management

1 Introduction

Modern laboratory practice requires planning and managerial skills in addition to the technical competence and scientific innovation which have hitherto been the hallmark of the diagnostic service unit. The work of the laboratory must be justified in terms of the applicability and practical relevance of the procedures performed, the ability to function within defined cost limits and the assurance that the laboratory is a safe place in which to work. Because of the rate at which management practice currently mutates, it is difficult to describe this in other than very general terms. For this reason most of the 'buzz words' presently in use have been omitted in favour of more traditional descriptors of management practice.

The function of management is to coordinate resources so that an efficient and effective service is provided. This management process includes planning, decision-making, organization, direction and control to achieve defined goals (Shinton, 1988a,b).

Clinical laboratories in the UK in the future will be within a number of locations:

1 Trust hospital with clinical directorate under a chief executive.
2 Directly managed unit of a health authority under a general manager.
3 Private hospital.
4 Private laboratory.

The haematology department may have satellite laboratories for extra-laboratory testing, which should be incorporated within the central laboratory structure. Such satellites will vary in size and activity but will be close to or in (Dybkaer *et al.*, 1992):

- operating theatres;
- intensive care units;
- accident and emergency departments;
- ward siderooms/bedside;

3

- outpatient clinics, e.g. anticoagulant or antenatal clinics;
- general practitioner offices.

2 Planning of resource

2.1 Definition of planning

When planning a service the capital and revenue implications of the location must be considered. Siting near a clinical activity such as an operating theatre or oncology ward will reduce the costs of specimen and blood product transportation and improve patient safety. It may be necessary to plan satellite laboratories close to operating theatres, intensive care units or outpatient clinics. The need for general practitioner testing must also be considered.

Sharing of accommodation with other clinical laboratories should be considered, i.e. specimen reception, staffrooms, patient waiting and sampling areas. Multidisciplinary laboratories for automated procedures and for use of shared equipment, e.g. flow cytometers, may also be considered.

2.2 Premises

These will normally be a building with equipment already available and financed by a health authority, hospital trust, private company or other funding body. Premises should be considered under the following headings:

- space;
- services, which will include power, lighting, temperature control, gases, water and drainage;
- fittings and furnishings;
- equipment;
- storage space for reagents and other consumables;
- staff facilities;
- specimen reception;
- information technology;
- where appropriate facilities for patients must be provided, including facilities for the disabled.

Building Note 15 (DOH/Welsh Office, 1990) is a useful source for reference.

For a haematology department, premises should be available for the following sets of laboratory procedures:

- blood counting;
- haemostasis tests;
- haematological biochemistry;
- haematological immunology;

- transfusion serology;
- research and development.

A work-flow plan must be designed for each activity with a room-by-room work schedule. The choice of methods to be used, especially for automated blood cell counting, where size and services required by instruments vary, must also be considered. Each room will require a detailed plan for water, electrical and gas supplies, lighting, temperature control, ventilation and drainage. Special areas must be set aside for 24-hour emergency work and procedures involving the use of radionuclides. The whole plan must ensure a safe and healthy working environment in accordance with current legislation. There must be facilities for dealing with category 3 specimens. It is not anticipated that category 4 work will be carried out in a haematology department.

An early decision must be made on the relative proportions of open-plan accommodation versus separate rooms. The former allows easy movement and flexibility to alter functions, whereas the latter reduces noise and gives privacy for work. Allowance must be made for circulation space; offices for senior staff with administrative duties and for secretaries; data storage, retrieval and transmission facilities. Data-processing facilities should be compatible with the hospital information system. In addition, there must be rooms or areas provided for washing up; stores for specimens, reagents and records; personal lockers, cloakrooms, toilets and a rest room for staff. When appropriate, there should be overnight accommodation for on-call staff. Where there is a clinical function added to the laboratory, consulting and examination rooms, phlebotomy cubicles, waiting and reception areas and patient toilets must be included in the plans. These clinical facilities may be shared with other laboratory or hospital departments.

2.3 Equipment

For a new building, an operational policy, including a costed equipment schedule, must be prepared, but in the case of transfer of an existing laboratory an inventory (assets register) should already be available, to which only new or replacement items need be added. The level of equipment must be commensurate with the service offered. Before selecting equipment, consideration must be given to methodology, particularly precision and accuracy requirements, safety and ability to deal with anticipated workload.

National evaluation reports must be studied and option appraisal may be required where major capital purchases are envisaged (see Chapter 4). All equipment must be registered as capital assets.

Provision for back-up to allow for mains electricity failure must be made. This particularly concerns blood bank refrigerators, with alarm systems linked to a 24-hour manned area, such as the hospital switchboard.

2.4 Staff

The number and grades of staff must be appropriate to the levels of responsibility and to the quantity and type of work to be undertaken. There requires to be a designated head of laboratory, who may decide that the appointment of a laboratory manager is necessary (see Sections 5.1 and 5.2).

2.4.1 Medical

Medically qualified staff are essential for interpretation of results for clinicians and for giving clinical advice on haematological problems (Royal College of Pathologists, 1992). These will be consultants, usually having associated patient-care responsibilities. A number of staff-grade and junior medical staff in training posts may also be employed.

2.4.2 Clinical scientists

Such staff in haematology are usually employed only by the larger laboratories of university hospitals and by the Blood Transfusion Service. They are mainly employed for research and development rather than for routine procedures.

2.4.3 Medical Laboratory Scientific Officers (MLSOs)

This is the largest group of staff performing laboratory work. The number in each grade will vary but the most senior will usually be the laboratory manager.

2.4.4 Medical laboratory assistants

A *Manual for Training and Competence Assessment of Medical Laboratory Assistants* (1992) has been prepared by the DOH, the Institute of Medical Laboratory Sciences, the Royal College of Pathologists and representatives from discipline societies and associations. Medical laboratory assistants generally perform repetitive work. Their training will be in service for the particular task they are undertaking. A special group may be employed as phlebotomists.

2.4.5 Secretarial, clerical and computer staff

A number of persons are necessary to handle patients' notes, arrange dispatch of specimens and type orders and letters. A managerial structure must be agreed and documented, perhaps with an appropriate supervisor. In many larger laboratories regular computer housekeeping and troubleshooting are necessary. Access to appropriate computer expertise is essential.

2.4.6 Department nurses

These may be attached to the department for specific duties such as assistance with clinical care of patients suffering from haemophilia or haemoglobinopathies or receiving cytotoxic drugs. They are professionally responsible to their State

Registration Board through the nursing administration, but should be accountable managerially to the head of department.

2.4.7 Ancillary staff

These are employed as porters and cleaners but may carry out other duties, such as glass-washing. In this respect they will be responsible to members of the senior laboratory staff, particularly for safety practices, quality and discipline.

2.4.8 Terms and conditions of service

These will vary with the grade and type of staff. Each staff member must have a job description on appointment, which includes detail of scale point and incremental date, hours of work, annual leave, etc. Laboratory heads are advised to consult with their personnel manager on local agreements.

2.4.9 Job description

This must be prepared for all members of staff. It must include the accountability of the employee and relationships with other members of staff. The line management for each post must be documented. Key duties and responsibilities must be specified. Each employee must have agreed to and be provided with a copy of his/her job description.

2.4.10 Staff rotas

Arrangements for handling the workload by rotation of staff should be posted in advance. This should include detail of its provision during annual leave and statutory holidays and in the event of emergencies.

2.4.11 Staff recruitment or replacement

The normal turnover of laboratory staff requires a mechanism for replacement. If turnover is excessive, a policy of exit interview may identify the factors responsible. Good recruitment is inevitably tied to good training, for which the laboratory is both officially recognized and considered reputable. It is necessary to advertise posts, usually in the press or in professional journals. School visits often yield a regular supply of trainees for technologist posts. In times of recruitment difficulty, an invitation to careers guidance teachers to visit the laboratory can be of great value. An appointment procedure must be documented, with a system for interviewing. The level of staff involved in the interview will vary with the grade of staff required. When a person is selected by the interviewing panel, the terms and conditions of service must be agreed verbally and subsequently in writing. Claimed qualifications should be checked at this time. An equal opportunity policy is important. Advertising and interviewing guidelines are of particular relevance to prevent disputes. Good record-keeping of appointments procedures is mandatory.

The chairperson of the appointments advisory committee must keep a record of the meeting. It is good practice to undertake some form of counselling for unsuccessful internal members of staff. All new staff must be given an orientation and induction programme, including the safety policy.

3 The management process

Modern management places great emphasis on relating available resources to outcome. This is referred to as resource management. It is also necessary to develop a long-term, e.g. 5-year, strategic plan (business plan) by which an agreed outcome, including development, can be achieved. This is referred to as strategic management and may involve change in the external environment of the department. The short-term means by which this can be achieved is called the operational policy, which may be changed from time to time.

The business plan details the way in which a particular department will achieve its sources of income to handle the proposed workload within the resources available. The formulation of a business plan requires seven phases:

1 description of aims and objectives (possession of necessary skills and experience);

2 validation of business idea (market research, using appropriate methods and data sources);

3 development of business strategy;

4 details of all activities/objectives required to make the business strategy happen;

5 forecast of results (likely sales volume and value, pro forma profit and loss, cash-flow forecast and balance sheet, break-even analysis);

6 description of business controls (book-keeping system, market planning trends, customer records, personnel file, production control information, etc.);

7 final write-up of business plan.

An example of the format for a business plan is given in Appendix 1.1. While much of business planning inevitably centres around income generation, corporate objectives, in which members of staff are taking the lead, and the target completion dates are important.

Ascertainment of the workload and of the finance required to handle it is determined by negotiation with those requiring the service – the process of contracting. Within the contracting process, consideration must be given to how effectively the available resources may be used – cost-effectiveness. In order to achieve this, pricing for each service is necessary, which will entail cost analysis.

Decision-making is a component of all aspects of the management process and depends on proper assessment of relevant information. All decisions involve value judgement of what is beneficial/non-beneficial, important/unimportant in forecasting possible outcomes. Once a policy decision has been made, it must be adhered to. The style of decision-making can vary but ultimately rests with the head of the department. The method will to some extent depend upon the procedures in vogue within the particular service to which the department belongs. The procedure may vary from one set of decisions to another, depending especially upon the time available.

The management process is therefore the way in which decisions are taken to prepare the long-term strategy, encompassing an operational policy within a business plan. In order to achieve this end, a management structure is required, which includes detail of the following:

- head of department;
- laboratory manager;
- line management;
- communications;
- record-keeping.

Once the management structure is established, information will be required on:

- resources: premises, equipment, staff;
- sources of income.

Based on this information, a budget can be prepared. If the department is within a pathology directorate, the overall budget may be held by a clinical director, in which case the management process must include discussion at this higher level. Formal agreement may have to be sought from a chief executive.

Once the operational policy has been agreed, the day-to-day operational management can be prepared.

It is essential that the management process operates within the legal requirements of its environment, including compliance with Health and Safety Regulations.

The whole process must be subject to continuing method evaluation, including quality assurance, quality of service to purchasers and financial audit. There is also the need for continuing development, which may involve research or pilot projects.

4 Financial management

4.1 Sources of income by contract

Sources of income by contract are as follows:

- District Health Authority-managed hospitals;
- clinical directorates of trust hospitals;
- Family Health Services Authorities (FHSA);
- general practitioner fund-holders;
- private hospitals;
- industry;

- screening tests for employees;
- drug trials by pharmaceutical companies;
- training grants;
- donations from patients and friends of the laboratory for specific purposes;
- research and development.

Research and development must be an item in the budget to allow for inevitable change, even in a contracting service. It is also essential to maintain staff interest in their work and to prevent declining morale. External funding for research is available and it is the duty of the laboratory director to know of the sources to which he/she can apply. Staff time should be allowed for research and development activities, e.g. for evaluation of new methods and equipment.

4.2 Contracting

There are different forms of contract, e.g.:

1 block contracts with District Health Authorities or FHSA;
2 contracts for a specific workload;
3 cost per patient or test (cost and volume).

To attract contracts it may be necessary to prepare specifications which detail the service offered, how the service will be provided and by whom, the quality of service and the ability to maintain that quality (Webster, 1991). These service specifications will be subjected to option appraisal by the customer.

In a competitive market, the lower the price of the contract, the more likely is the possibility of concluding a contract, thus producing income for the department. The contract must at the same time guarantee quality and this must be allowed for in the pricing. Unrealistically low pricing will jeopardize the venture.

In order to gain acceptance of proposed tenders, marketing procedures are necessary. Arrangements should be made by the head of department for visits by potential customers in order to describe and display the service on offer, with special emphasis on the clinical advisory service by consultants. Techniques of marketing require to be mastered, including that of effective advertising.

4.3 Pricing

Price-setting involves the process of cost analysis and must be applied to each test or test set. In addition to direct costs, indirect costs, such as those involved in maintaining the quality system, must be included, e.g. the education and training of doctors, clinical scientists and technologists, medical audit, health and safety and research, including epidemiology.

4.3.1 Cost analysis

The following specific items of information are necessary:

1 Labour costs (L). These can be calculated either as cost per test, e.g. haemo-

globin, or cost per specimen for a group of analyses, e.g. the components of the blood count, and will comprise:

(a) cost of performing the analysis or test, which will depend on the time taken and the salary rate per hour of the staff. Assessment of time taken can be determined from the WELCAN-UK (1993) tables, which provide standard times for the performance of specified tests or procedures. The grade of staff performing the tests will vary, as will the salary, according to local availability and agreements;

(b) cost of specimen collection (if appropriate), reception and preparation;

(c) data-processing and production of reports;

(d) medical staff cost component for interpretation of result and advice given to clinicians.

2 Throughput (T). This must be based on contract requirements.

3 Consumables, including kits and reagents (C). This cost will depend upon throughput but cost per specimen must be calculated. Kits are being used increasingly in modern laboratory practice.

4 Annual capital cost (A). This is the cost of leasing, renting or replacement by purchase and must be based on amortization, as well as initial outlay. Depreciation due to inflation must be included in the calculation and is usually based on the Treasury discount rate, available from any bank. Any development equipment must be included in the annual capital cost.

5 Capital charge levy (CCL). This is a proportion of the levy made for the capital site on which the laboratory is located.

6 Housekeeping and services (HS). This information may be obtained from the unit finance officer and should include heating, lighting, water and waste disposal.

7 Unit overheads (UO). This information may also be obtained from the unit finance officer and is based on the unit figures, determined as a proportion of running the organization in which the laboratory is situated, e.g. car parking, social services, etc.

8 Maintenance cost (M). There must be a programme of preventive maintenance for each item of equipment in the laboratory. A decision must be made on the method by which this is achieved, either by contract with the supplier or by an in-house system. The latter may be more economical for a laboratory with ready access to a department of biological engineering, provided the latter can carry sufficient spares to prevent undue disruption of the service in the event of breakdown.

The annual total cost is then the sum of:

$$(L \times T) + (C \times T) + A + M + CCL + HS + UO + M$$

A more complex system can be used but requires microcomputer software, as described by Stilwell and Woodford (1987). Commercial packages are available and the recommendations of the Audit Commission have been published (1991).

4.3.2 Pricing policy

Heads of department must follow the appropriate finance arrangements, which will be based on the *Directory of Guidance for Financial Managers* (DOH, 1990). Major items to be considered in calculating prices for National Health Service (NHS) and non-NHS customers are whether or not capital charges have been calculated correctly and the general hospital overheads, which must be borne by the constituent departments. This refers to the cost of structures applied to each item of costed work output. It may be fair to disregard those within an inter-authority charging system but clearly that should not be the case where charges to non-NHS customers are concerned.

4.3.3 Cost accounting

A system of commitment accounting should be agreed with the pathology directorate.

5 Management structure

5.1 Head of department (director)

Whatever the size of organization, there must be a head of department or director with clear lines of accountability and responsibility. The appointee should have the respect of colleagues. The director should be a sound leader and possess organizational skills, with the ability to motivate subordinates. This requires an appreciation of human behaviour in different circumstances. It is desirable that the appointee has received basic training in management and essential that he/she has received accredited training in haematology.

It is usual for the director to be medically qualified and have associated clinical responsibility.

The management duties of the head of department are to determine broad policies, establish priorities and set objectives but not necessarily to directly manage or supervise. The person must be the budget holder, although budget management may be delegated. The head of department is ultimately responsible for discipline of staff, with direct involvement in association with personnel staff at the dismissal stage. He/she must be responsible for training, maintenance of standards, research and development but may delegate as appropriate.

Directing the department requires leadership and involves the human element of management. The needs of members of staff have to be appreciated and seen to be understood for efficient management of the department.

The head of department must appoint a deputy to cover for absence.

5.2 Laboratory manager

If the head of department decides to appoint a laboratory manager, their relationship must be clearly documented and understood.

It is desirable for the manager of a haematology laboratory to be a scientist or MLSO appropriately trained in management. This officer may, with the agreement of the head of department, be responsible for ordering supplies, accounting and the appointment and training of non-medical junior staff. The function of the manager will be to achieve the objectives of the department within the resources available. The laboratory manager requires skill in organization, combined with the ability to motivate subordinates. This officer must be involved in disciplinary procedures (see Section 7.5).

5.3 Line management

A staffing structure with line management must be determined and documented, with staff number and gradings dependent on the nature and quantity of the workload. The level of delegation, with functional appropriateness, must be defined. It is usual for the manager to designate a number of section supervisors, who will oversee the activities of other staff to perform specific tasks efficiently, focusing attention on operational provision. The relationship of these staff with ancillary staff, e.g. cleaners and secretarial and clerical staff, must be organized and defined.

Areas of operational responsibility include:
- distribution of duties;
- supervision of work;
- supervision of quality assurance;
- supervision of reporting;
- supervision of records;
- ensuring compliance with standard operating procedures, statutory regulations and legal responsibilities;
- provision for maintenance of equipment;
- updating of procedures.

The relationship within line management of other medical consultant staff must be considered and understood. Apart from being clinically responsible for patients and being given specific responsibility for sections of the laboratory, including, perhaps, their budgets, they may have no involvement in department management other than that of a user. Alternatively, consultants may play a coordinating role, as defined in the Institute of Health Services Management booklet *Models of Clinical Management* (IHSM, 1992). This allows consultants to take responsibility for certain sections within departments, particularly when they involve diverse groups of staff for whom the consultant would not personally have line-management responsibility.

A particular relationship has to be established with the department's secretarial office. This will vary with the degree of involvement of the secretarial staff in handling laboratory reports. It is preferable for the secretarial and clerical staff to be managerially responsible to the head of department, but, if not, agreement on duties and disciplinary arrangements must be clearly and unambiguously defined with the appropriate administrative body.

6 Operational management

Based on information in the contracts, the financial resources required by the laboratory for its annual workload can be determined. Operational management will then depend on the anticipated daily workload, the range of investigations offered and the premises and staff available. It will be of value to calculate the workload in the following sections:

- general haematology laboratory – blood counts, erythrocyte sedimentation rate (ESR), etc.;
- haemostasis laboratory;
- blood transfusion laboratory;
- special tests;
- clinical service;
- emergency service (see Chapter 3).

Additional information of value could include origin of work, e.g. outpatient, inpatient, general practice, screening clinic, individual consultant.

The process for organizing the work and directing and controlling it, together with an evaluation of results, must be laid down (see Chapter 2). This work organization must be coordinated in order to achieve both long-term and short-term objectives. Regular review is essential to ensure that the planned policy has been achieved. An important aspect of such a review would be to consider ways and means by which workload could be arranged to fit with periods of high staff availability and lowest cost.

6.1 Communication within the department

The effective function of a department depends on good communication at all levels. Senior staff should meet regularly (e.g. monthly). Larger meetings of all staff may be required from time to time. At all meetings the objectives must be clearly set out and ways of carrying out the selected policy determined. Such meetings provide feedback on the day-to-day efficiency of communication within the department. Transmission of information, either written or oral, within the department is a function of good administration and must be documented in the appropriate standard operating procedures. Effective personal communication is essential to maintain good staff relationships.

Both the head of department and the manager must make themselves available to other members of staff to discuss individual and personal problems. This may be time-consuming but can, in the longer term, have a valuable effect on morale.

6.2 Communication between laboratories and clinicians

Appropriate clear communication between laboratory staff and clinicians is essential if the laboratory is to undertake a useful and efficient role in health care. Communication may be verbal (in person or by telephone), written or facsimile, or by computer link, e.g. the Hospital Information System. It is essential for the laboratory to understand what the clinician requires and to make sure that the information is returned to the clinician in a clear, unambiguous manner. The clinician may wish to discuss a particular investigation or its result with a senior member of the laboratory staff or, in turn, laboratory staff may need to discuss a patient's clinical condition or medication with the clinician, since these may affect specimen collection or the technique used for the analytical procedure. It is important that all laboratory staff communicate with clinical staff in a friendly and cooperative manner because it is only in this way that effective and continuing communication can be ensured.

6.2.1 Request form

It is helpful to both clinicians and laboratory staff if the formats of most, if not all, pathology request forms and reports (see Section 6.2.3) are similar. This makes it easier to locate patient identification data and it will be more likely that the clinicians will fill in the appropriate information. Colour coding is often useful to differentiate tests which are undertaken in different departments or geographical sites. Whether or not computerized requesting is available, it is helpful if self-adhesive labels are provided for the clinician which contain the patient identification details, and where possible the hospital record number should be bar-coded as well as being given in eye-readable numbers. Clinicians should give the date and time of specimen collection, with relevant clinical information. It is often helpful, and sometimes essential, for laboratory staff to know why a particular test is being requested – to make or exclude a particular diagnosis, to monitor treatment or because a relative has a particular inherited condition. Space must be provided to identify the nature of any potential hazard associated with the specimen.

6.2.2 Specimen container labels

These must be completed at the time of specimen collection, stating patient's name, case record number and date of birth, together with the date and time of collection.

6.2.3 Report forms

As stated in Section 6.2.1, it is helpful if the layout of patient identification details on these forms is similar for all pathology disciplines. This will reduce the chance of the report being filed in the wrong patient's case notes. The purpose of the laboratory report is to impart the correct information about an analytical result to the correct clinician unambiguously. Legibility is important, whether handwritten or computer-generated. Layout is important as this may make it easier to impart information to those reading the report. Reports should indicate who in the laboratory has authorized them, in case there is a query. This is especially important where a written comment is included. A record of validation prior to dispatch should be kept, together with means of identification of the person who performed the analysis. It may be useful for the clinician to have reference ranges quoted with each test result.

6.2.4 Urgent requests

Only tests which will affect the immediate management of the patient can be considered to be urgent.

6.2.5 Advice on appropriate tests and interpreted data

A major role for the medical haematologist is to give advice on the appropriate test to be undertaken in a particular clinical situation, and then to assist the clinician in interpretation of the analytical data obtained.

6.2.6 On-line data transfer to clinicians

This is especially helpful when dealing with data produced by modern fully automated analysers, because it both reduces clerical work and avoids transcription errors. On-line data transfer is provisional and must be followed by hard copy.

6.2.7 Between laboratory departments and senior management

Communication must be established between heads of laboratory departments, who may meet as a group or division. Liaison with other colleagues in the speciality, both regionally and nationally, is advantageous.

6.2.8 Record-keeping

Good record-keeping is central to the efficient practice of haematology. It is necessary to enable, control and rationalize all interactions and transactions: (i) between the laboratory and its users; and (ii) within the laboratory itself. It is necessary to optimize the use of resources in a quality-assured environment and to provide data against which laboratory performance can be compared with performance indicators. It is also required to maintain the financial equilibrium of the laboratory and to permit soundly based forward planning.

Microcomputers are often helpful in maintaining the records, which are detailed in Appendix 1.3.

7 Professional and legal requirements

7.1 Approval of medical staff training schemes
Approval of training for junior medical staff must be agreed with the regional postgraduate dean.

7.2 Laboratory accreditation
With the increase in bureaucratic control and litigation, voluntary laboratory accreditation has been introduced (CPA, 1991). Accreditation may be granted for a specified range of tests. Validation for contractual purposes may be necessary. Accreditation may also be required for training approval.

7.3 Legal liability
Private laboratories are always directly liable for the validity of their procedures and reporting. Health services employers carry vicarious responsibility for employees on behalf of their constituent departments; however, this responsibility is limited where employees do not carry out their duties in accordance with agreed protocols. Medical staff are always responsible in any circumstances for opinions given on reports. In a specific legal case, any member of a laboratory may be called as a witness to fact or as an expert.

Management must be aware of relevant statutory regulations, including the Health and Safety at Work Act (1974) (Health and Safety Commission, 1975), Product Liability (Department of Trade and Industry, 1987) and Control of Substances Hazardous to Health (1988). Ignorance of these is never an acceptable plea in mitigation in a court of law.

7.4 Confidentiality
Laboratory reports on patients are confidential documents, the contents of which should ideally only be disclosed to the doctor making the request (Knox, 1984). All laboratories must be registered under the Data Protection Act (1984). Where information is stored on computer, the data are also available to the specific patient concerned on written application. Inappropriate disclosure of information is a disciplinary matter. Blood samples that have been provided for diagnostic purposes must always be handed to police officers (on formal request) with the identity label of the patient.

7.5 Discipline/grievance
In a well-run laboratory this will be conducted by the example set by senior staff,

but a disciplinary procedure is essential to deal with breaches of procedure, including those involving safety. All hospitals have a code of practice which defines which officer is responsible for each group of staff and the degree of disciplinary authority delegated before reference to a higher authority. Most codes stratify disciplinary procedures as early warning, final warning and dismissal. These policies are usually determined by the health authority, to whom reference may be made when necessary. It is essential for these codes of disciplinary practice to be understood and agreed by the appropriate trade unions.

7.6 Labour relations

Laboratory staff may belong to a trade union or similar organization. The head of department and the manager must have knowledge of the organizations involved and of the officially appointed officers in the laboratory. When necessary, arrangements for meetings of staff either within or outside the confines of the building must be agreed. Joint staff consultative committees, which involve both management and trade unions, provide the formal forum for involving staff in the management of change and problems within the department.

7.7 Staff records

A confidential file must be kept by either the head of department or the laboratory manager regarding personal details of each member of staff. This information should include curriculum vitae, record of training, annual leave, study leave and sick leave. Notes should be kept of grievances declared and the managerial response. Any reports on individual staff objectives and appraisal should be kept, along with medical records. Details of registration should also be included. These records require to be updated in respect of training and qualifications following individual performance review.

8 Training

In addition to formal academic training organized by an institute of higher education, medical, scientific and MLSO staff require in-service training. This should be a development of the scientific basis obtained during their initial formal degree training, but now applied to haematology. Prior to apprenticeship in a laboratory, a period of induction training is essential. Following completion of apprenticeship education, training should continue.

8.1 Induction training

The new entrant must be told how the laboratory is organized and given documents on general procedures, particularly those relating to safety of laboratory workers. As an aid to communication it is useful to standardize definitions (see Appendix 1.2). These documents should include national codes of health and safety practice. Before this period of training, trainees must be introduced to the personnel department of the institution and the occupational health department relevant to the laboratory.

8.2 In-service training

A period for in-service training should be allotted for tests routinely carried out in the laboratory. Training must include use of equipment, performance of analytical procedures and relevance of results for each test. These techniques must be practised under supervision. Appropriate procedures to be taught and practised are listed in Appendix 1.4. Because of advancing technology and methods of practice, these need to be reviewed regularly. Medical staff should be taught how to correlate the results of tests with the clinical state of the patient, with the aim of providing a clinically relevant opinion based on clinical and laboratory information.

8.3 Continuing education

For those who aspire to management posts in a laboratory, a period of formal training, followed by apprenticeship in management, is necessary. The current structure of clinical laboratories must be understood, as well as the prevailing terms and conditions of service for staff. Training in management should include resource allocation, budget control, audit, quality assurance and data-handling. Codes of safety practice must be studied in detail, including microbiological hazards, risk of chemical carcinogenesis, toxicity, flammability, explosion and radiation hazard.

9 Evaluation

9.1 Evaluation of methodology

All procedures must be subject to evaluation, the methods of which should be agreed and recorded.

9.2 Quality assurance (see Chapter 5)

Quality assurance consists of:
1 internal procedure proficiency;
2 internal quality control;
3 external quality assessment.

Arrangements for review of results from these procedures should be formally carried out and documented.

9.3 Evaluation of the service

Regular evaluation of the service provided to clinicians should be carried out in order to establish customer satisfaction.

9.4 Appraisal

A system of staff appraisal should be in place in each department. Each interview outcome should be fully documented and agreed with the interviewee. Staff undertaking appraisal should be trained for this purpose. Staff should have the opportunity of appeal, bypassing their immediate senior manager, if they feel the appraisal process has been unfair.

9.5 Audit

Audit in the NHS is defined as 'the systematic critical analysis of medical care including the procedures used for diagnosis and treatment, the use of resources and quality of life of the patient'. It is recommended that audit be professionally led and supported by appropriate postgraduate and continuing medical education programmes.

For the haematologist, audit has a variety of aspects:
1 Personal proficiency:
   (a) medical audit;
   (b) competence to practice.
2 Laboratory audit:
   (a) analytical;
   (b) non-analytical.
3 Financial audit.

The haematologist is also required to conduct clinical audit similar to that for other medical specialities. While many aspects of clinical audit can be organized locally in hospital units, speciality audit will have to be regional, e.g. haemophilia care, anticoagulant therapy (see Chapter 22).

Laboratory audit includes all aspects of laboratory function, resources and practice, commencing with the collection of specimens and ending with the reporting of results. This audit could include:
1 Specimens – details on report form:
   (a) patient identification;
   (b) clinical details.
2 Quality of material submitted for examination.
3 Laboratory turnaround time.
4 Specimen-handling procedure.
5 Accuracy of comments or interpretation of results.
6 Range of tests available, including emergency testing.
7 Availability of consultant advice.
8 Use of laboratory by clinicians.
9 Use of blood components by clinicians.

Financial audit is carried out in conjunction with finance officers and is an integral part of laboratory management. Details are given in the report of the Audit Commission (1991).

10 Health and safety

This is an important aspect of present-day laboratory practice. The subject is described in detail in Chapter 6.

Appendix 1.1: Example of the content of a corporate business plan suitable for laboratory medicine

1 Corporate management arrangements
2 Executive summary – corporate mission statement
3 Corporate vision
4 Key objectives
5 Major capital requirements
   5.1 Information technology
   5.2 Equipment
6 Finance
   6.1 Financial summary
   6.2 Financial pressures
   6.3 Implications of clinical changes in laboratory medicine
   6.4 Cost improvement programmes
   6.5 Future financial pressures
      6.5.1 Laboratories
      6.5.2 Blood products
7 Corporate objectives
   7.1 Service delivery
   7.2 Financial
   7.3 Business
   7.4 Management
   7.5 Research and development
   7.6 Personnel
   7.7 Estates
   7.8 Corporate safety
   7.9 Information management
8 Corporate SWOT summary
   8.1 Strengths
   8.2 Weaknesses
   8.3 Opportunities
   8.4 Threats
9 Teaching, research and quality
10 Personnel and communications

10.1 Manpower
10.2 Key staff retirement/changes
10.3 Individual performance management/staff appraisal
10.4 Training initiatives
10.5 Communications and team building
11 Corporate sickness and absence levels

Appendix 1.2: International Council for Standardization in Haematology definitions (ICSH, 1991)

1 Standards
1.1 Reference standard
A substance or device, one or more properties of which are sufficiently well established to be used for the calibration of an apparatus, for the assessment of a measurement method or for assigning values to a material. Where possible it must be based on or traceable to exactly defined physical or chemical measurement.

1.2 International biological standards
These are reference standards which cannot be determined by exactly defined physical or chemical measurement methods, but to which have been assigned international units of activity as defined by the World Health Organization. These materials are not intended to be used in the laboratory working procedures but serve as the means by which national and commercial reference materials and calibrators can be controlled.

2 Materials and methods
2.1 Reference method
A clearly and exactly described technique for a particular determination which, in the opinion of a defined authority, provides sufficiently accurate and precise laboratory data for it to be used to assess the validity of other laboratory methods for this determination. The accuracy of the reference method must be established by comparison with a definitive method, where one exists, and the degree of inaccuracy must be stated. The degree of imprecision must also be stated.

2.2 Calibrator
A substance or device used to calibrate, graduate or adjust a measurement. It must be traceable to a reference standard (see 1.1).

2.3 Diagnostic kit
A package containing two or more reagents and/or other material and a method protocol designed for performance of a specified analytical procedure.

2.4 Calibration
The determination of a bias conversion factor of an analytical process under specified conditions, in order to obtain accurate measurement results. The accuracy over the operating range must be established by appropriate use of reference methods, reference materials and/or calibrators.

2.5 Accuracy

A measure of agreement between the estimate of a value and the true value. Accuracy has no numerical value; it is measured as the amount of (degree of) inaccuracy.

2.6 Inaccuracy

Numerical difference between the mean of a set of replicate measurements and the true value. This difference (positive or negative) may be expressed in the units in which the quantity is measured, or as a percentage of the true value.

2.7 Bias

Systematic factor resulting in inaccuracy.

2.8 Precision

Agreement between replicate measurements. It has no numerical value but it is recognized in terms of imprecision.

2.9 Imprecision

Standard deviation or coefficient of variation of the results in a set of replicate measurements.

2.10 Quality control material

A substance used in routine practice for checking the concurrent performance of an analytical process (or instrument). It must be similar in properties to and be analysed along with patient specimens. It may or may not have a preassigned value.

3 Quality assurance

3.1 Quality assurance programme

All steps to be taken by the director of a laboratory to ensure reliability of laboratory results and to increase accuracy, reproducibility and between-laboratory comparability. This includes proficiency surveillance (3.4), the constant use of internal quality control and participation in an external quality assessment scheme. It also includes participation in training courses, conferences, collaborative studies of instruments and the improvement of laboratory performance. A quality assurance programme in haematology must also be concerned with clinical aspects of haematology.

3.2 Internal quality control

Internal quality control is the set of procedures undertaken in a laboratory for the continual assessment of work carried out within the laboratory and evaluation of the results of tests to decide whether the latter are reliable enough to be released to the requesting clinician. The procedures should include tests on control material and statistical analysis of patients' data. The main object is to ensure day-to-day consistency of measurement or observation, if possible in agreement with an agreed indicator of truth such as a control material with assigned values.

3.3 External quality assessment

External quality assessment refers to a system of retrospectively and objectively comparing results from different laboratories by means of surveys organized by an external agency. The main objective is to establish between-laboratory and between-instrument comparability, if possible in agreement with a reference standard, where one exists. External quality assessment schemes may be regional, national or international. They may also be limited to the users of a particular instrument.

3.4 Proficiency surveillance

This involves supervision and action to ensure good laboratory practice. An important aspect is internal quality control and participation in an external quality assessment scheme, but it also includes attention to proficiency in specimen collection and labelling, delivery of specimens to the laboratory, record-keeping and reporting environmental and storage effects on specimens, interpretation of test results and relevance of various tests for the clinical information required. It also includes maintenance and control of equipment and apparatus, staff training and protection of staff health and safety.

Appendix 1.3: Record-keeping

1 Management policies and procedures

1 The organization and scope of the department, including line of managerial accountability, with arrangements for regular meetings both with staff and with institutional management representatives for review of the service offered, setting of objectives and financial arrangements. These meetings must be documented.
2 Job descriptions.
3 Contracts of employment.
4 Staff reviews.
5 Training programme.

2 Equipment, kit and reagent maintenance records

1 Servicing, including contracts (technical details, frequency and costs), contact names and telephone/fax numbers.
2 In-house preventive maintenance.
3 Change of component parts.
4 Introduction of upgrades.
5 Introduction of kits or batch replacements.
6 Introduction of new reagents/reagent lots.
7 Calibration records.
8 Downtime records.
9 Specific accident records: in all cases the date and the individual worker undertaking the procedure must be recorded.

3 Quality assurance data

1 Clear and up-to-date compilation of internal quality control (IQC) data.
2 External quality assessment (EQA) survey data over several years:
    (a) regional;
    (b) national.
3 Record of corrective action.

4 Accident/incident records

Health and Safety Regulations require accurate written records of all such incidents, and this will often enable managers to minimize recurrences.

5 Inventory records

Maintenance of an accurate inventory of instruments and stock, i.e. glassware, kits, reagents, etc., is essential in order to assist planned servicing and replacement. It will often assist managers in making the best use of the available equipment. The following information should be recorded:

- name of item;
- model number;
- serial number;
- manufacturer;
- supplier;
- supplier's telephone number;
- purchased;
- price paid;
- replacement due;
- replacement cost.

6 Standard operating procedures

Standard operating procedures (SOPs) must be maintained for all procedures undertaken in the laboratory. It is helpful to staff if SOPs are written in a standard format and they should contain information on the following aspects of each procedure:

- A brief description of the purpose of the procedure and its scientific basis.
- Any safety precautions required.
- Details of the specimen (type and quantity) required together with details of any anticoagulant or storage restrictions (time/temperature).
- A list of reagents (including chemical purity) and how to prepare and store them.
- A list of consumables required.
- Brief information on particular instrumentation.
- Stepwise technique given in sufficient detail for it to be undertaken without supervision by a qualified analyst who has not previously undertaken that particular procedure.
- Any calculations required.
- IQC interpretation.
- The 'reference' range for healthy subjects together with any variation for age or sex.
- Validation procedure, including that for rapid reporting of results that require prompt clinical attention.
- Comments on interpretation.
- Specimen disposal.
- Literature referenced for the SOP.

7 Laboratory handbook for clinical staff

This must include procedures for specimen collection, transport and specimen-handling, and details of out-of-hours services, dealing with urgent tests and with high-risk specimens.

8 Major disaster procedure
This must be clearly and unambiguously documented and include names of individuals to be contacted (see Chapter 3, Section 12).

Appendix 1.4: Procedures for which training must be given

1 Specimens
Collection of blood specimen, transport and storage requirements.

2 General haematology
1 Morphology of blood cells and marrow aspirates, including cytochemistry and immunological techniques.
2 Haemoglobin estimation in whole blood and plasma and recognition of its catabolic products.
3 Haemoglobin electrophoresis and measurement of fetal haemoglobin (HbF) and HbA_2. Additional tests should be specified.
4 Blood cell counting (and sizing) by both manual and automated methods.
5 Erythrocyte sedimentation rate and plasma viscosity.
6 Erythrocyte osmotic fragility or autohaemolysis and detection of paroxysmal nocturnal haemoglobinuria.
7 Erythrocyte enzyme determinations.

3 Haemostasis
1 Screening tests: platelet count, bleeding time, prothrombin time, activated partial thromboplastin time, thrombin time, estimation of international normalized ratio (INR).
2 Factor assays: automated and manual coagulation, chromogenic and immunological assays.
3 Platelet function studies.
4 Control of: antithrombotic prophylaxis and therapy; heparin, oral anticoagulants; thrombolytic assays.

4 Radionuclide studies
Use of radionuclides for blood volume, red cell mass, erythrokinetics, vitamin B_{12}, folate and ferritin measurement (if appropriate).

5 Transfusion serology
1 Identification of blood group antigens and antibodies.
2 Testing compatibility of blood for transfusion.
3 Investigation of blood transfusion reactions.
4 Autoimmune antibody testing of erythrocytes.

6 Quality assurance
Quality assurance methods for all investigations should be studied.

References

Audit Commission (1991) *The Pathology Services: a Managerial Review*. HMSO, London.

Control of Substances Hazardous to Health Regulations (1988) S.I. 1988 No. 1657. HMSO, London.

CPA (1991) *Accreditation Handbooks*. Clinical Pathology Accreditation (UK) Ltd, Sheffield.

Data Protection Act (1984) HMSO, London.

Department of Trade and Industry (1987) *Guide to the Consumer Protection Act 1987: Product Liability and Safety Provision*. HMSO, London.

DOH (1990) *Working for Patients: Directory of Guidance for Finance Managers*. HMSO, London.

DOH (1992) *Manual for Training and Competence Assessment of Medical Laboratory Assistants*, 2nd edn. Distributed by the Institute of Medical Laboratory Sciences, London.

DOH/Welsh Office (1990) *Building Note 15: Accommodation for Pathology Services*. HMSO, London.

Dybkaer R., Martin D.V. & Rowan R.M. (1992) Good practice in decentralised analytical clinical measurement. *Scandinavian Journal of Clinical and Laboratory Investigation* **52**, Supplement 209, 1–116.

Health and Safety Commission (1975) *Health and Safety at Work Act 1974. Advice to Employees (HSC3)*. HMSO, London.

ICSH (1991) *Rules and Operating Procedures*. Leuven, Belgium.

IHSM (1992) *Models of Clinical Management*. Institute of Health Services Management, London.

Knox E.G. (1984) *The Confidentiality of Medical Records. The Principle and Practice of Protection in a Research-dependent Environment*, p. 176. Commission of the European Countries, Luxemburg.

Royal College of Pathologists (1992) *Medical and Scientific Staffing of National Health Service Pathology Departments*.

Shinton N.K. (1988a) Choice of analytical methods. In Verwilghen R.L. & Lewis S.M. (eds) *Quality Assurance in Haematology*, 177–192. Baillière Tindall, London.

Shinton N.K. (1988b) Organisation and management of the laboratory. In Verwilghen R.L. & Lewis S.M. (eds) *Quality Assurance in Haematology*, 213–228. Baillière Tindall, London.

Stilwell J.A. & Woodford F.P. (1987) Computer software to facilitate pathology laboratory costing. *Journal of Clinical Pathology* **40**, 817–825.

Webster D. (1991) How to do it – produce a service specification. *British Medical Journal* **302**, 1450–1451.

WELCAN-UK (1993) *Workload Measurement System for Pathology Manual with Schedule of Unit Values*. Welsh Office, Cardiff.

2 Work Organization

1 Introduction

Work organization within a haematology department depends on the size of department, daily volume of work, range of investigations performed, consumer needs and expectations, staff numbers and structure, and teaching and academic commitments, as well as on financial and managerial considerations.

It is probably most convenient to consider the organizational aspects of the laboratory separately from other functions, such as administration, accounting, personnel and teaching.

2 Laboratory

Most laboratories contain a general haematology module (that part of the laboratory concerned with performance of full blood counts, blood films, differential white cell counts, erythrocyte sedimentation rate (ESR), reticulocyte count, sickle solubility test, infectious mononucleosis screening test and many others), a haemostasis module, a blood bank module and a special tests module. In general, the organization of modules depends on geographical considerations, volume of work and staff structure.

Geographical considerations may dictate that an off-site haematology laboratory with some or many of the modules mentioned above is required in order to provide immediate laboratory services at a distant acute site.

Volume of work is by far the most important factor affecting laboratory organization. It influences the choice of equipment, the repertoire of tests and the back-up provisions for each module.

Staffing structure affects the organization by influencing the repertoire of tests and the triage, verification and authorization functions (see also Section 2.1). A laboratory with few qualified Medical Laboratory Scientific Officer (MLSO) staff can easily perform automated tests but may find it difficult to provide special tests requiring manual techniques and technical expertise. The functions of triage, verification and authorization can only be performed by highly trained staff, whose working time must be planned to allow for these functions. Quality control, troubleshooting and many administrative and managerial functions also depend on the presence or absence of trained staff and a pyramidal structure within the department.

2.1 General haematology module

The effect of workload on the repertoire of tests and on the choice of equipment in the general haematology module is shown in Table 2.1.

Reception/registration, sample identification and communication are covered briefly in Chapter 1 and quality control in Chapter 5. The function of the triage, verification and authorization is allocated to a senior MLSO and to medical staff, depending on local arrangements and the characteristics of work (e.g. leukaemia centre, acquired immune deficiency syndrome (AIDS) patients, radiotherapy, etc.).

Table 2.1 Effect of workload on the choice of tests and equipment

Workload size in FBC		Tests performed	Automation	Back-up
Per day	Per annum			
<100	<50 000	FBC, film, diff., sickle test, ESR, malaria	FBC/platelet counter	S/A counter
100–250	<100 000	As above with special tests* as required locally	FBC/platelet counter with 3-part diff.	S/A counter
250–500	<200 000	As above with selection of special tests	FBC/platelet counter with 5-part diff.	S/A counter
>500	>200 000	As above with many special tests	2 FBC/platelet counters with 5-part diff.	None

* For description of special tests see Section 2.4.
One staining machine should be sufficient for Romanowsky staining of blood films even in the largest laboratory. FBC, full blood counts; diff., differential leucocyte count; S/A, semi-automated.

Table 2.2 Erythrocyte sedimentation rate and viscometry according to workload

Workload (tests per day)	Method	Back-up
<80	Manual ESR	None
>80	Automated plasma viscometry	Manual ESR
>120	Automated plasma viscometry or automated ESR	Manual ESR

Erythrocyte sedimentation rate and/or viscosity measurements are large-volume tests traditionally performed by the general haematology module. The suggested equipment and back-up for different workloads are shown in Table 2.2.

2.2 Haemostasis module

Most laboratories have a haemostasis module concerned with performing tests which include the laboratory monitoring of oral anticoagulant and heparin therapy and the use of fibrinolytic drugs. The effect of the workload on the type of test and equipment is shown in Table 2.3.

Special tests include coagulation and inhibitor assays, platelet aggregometry and tests for the presence of lupus inhibitor. In the largest units full investigations of bleeding and thrombosis should be possible. The scope of tests is also dictated by the presence or absence of a haemophilia centre on site or by other special interests and whether or not the haemophilia centre is a designated comprehensive care centre. Semiautomated coagulometers are devices which automatically record the end point; fully automated coagulometers also dispense reagents, have a variable degree of automated sample-handling and possess computer interfacing capability.

Decision on the investigation of bleeding and hypercoagulable states are based on local factors; however, every laboratory should have access to a full range of coagulation, platelet function, fibrinolytic and inhibitor assays. Whether such assays are performed locally, regionally or supraregionally, or by the haemophilia comprehensive care centre depends on the size of population, the number of known patients resident in the area and the expertise of on-site medical and scientific staff.

Table 2.3 Effect of workload on selection of tests and equipment in haemostasis

Workload as clotting tests		Tests performed	Equipment
Per day	Per annum		
<10	<2000	PT, APTT, TT, bleeding time	Manual techniques or S/A coagulometer
<30	<5000	As above with some special tests	S/A coagulometer
<70	<10 000	As above with most special assays	Fully automated coagulometer
>100	>20 000	As above with selection of investigations	Fully automated coagulometer and chromogenic assays

APTT, activated partial thromboplastin time; PT, prothrombin time; TT, thrombin time; S/A, semi-automated.

Facilities for plasma storage at temperatures below −40°C, transport and availability of testing facilities by a reference laboratory must be ensured. If patients are required to travel for special investigations, transport and outpatient arrangements should be established.

Efficient anticoagulant clinics, tight control of heparinization and prompt diagnosis of acute haemostatic failure must be available on all acute sites.

Quality control and computerization are considered separately.

2.3 Blood transfusion module

The hospital transfusion module or blood bank is an essential part of all haematology laboratories serving an acute site. The minimum test repertoire consists of blood grouping, antibody screening, compatibility testing and investigation of transfusion reactions. In addition, receipt, storage and issue of blood, blood components and products are carried out. Many departments have additional functions, such as antenatal serology, investigation of haemolytic disease of the newborn (HDN), various immunological tests and investigation of haemolytic anaemia.

Equipment varies according to the size of the workload and the tests performed. Work can conveniently be considered under three headings:

1 Collection and reception of patient samples and of the requests for blood, blood components or products. Strict rules on sample identification and requesting policy must be in operation in each blood bank.

2 Reception of blood products and components from the transfusion centre, storage, stock-keeping and issue. This is an integral part of blood bank function and must be organized in accordance with the local rules and guidelines. Low-temperature and refrigerated storage of blood and blood products is central to the safe operation of a blood bank. Standard operation procedures must be available

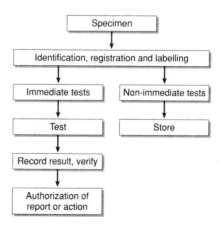

Fig. 2.1 Algorithm of blood bank functions.

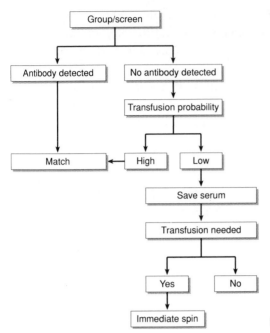

Fig. 2.2 Group, screen and save procedure.

to describe policy, particularly for monitoring refrigerators, assessing satellite refrigerators and the maintenance of freezers.

3   Laboratory functions are shown in Fig. 2.1. The procedure for operating a 'group, screen and save' policy is shown in Fig. 2.2.

2.4 Special tests

These may include a small repertoire only (e.g. haematinic assays and/or haemoglobin electrophoresis) or a variety of different tests requiring special facilities (e.g. radionuclide studies, cell markers, red cell enzyme assays, tissue typing, rheological measurements). Equipment needs vary according to the test repertoire. Spectrophotometers and counters are essential, but other, often automated, equipment, such as flow cytometers, microplate readers and filtrometers, may be required. Maintenance and regular calibration are essential for such apparatus.

Some special tests are costly if performed in small numbers. Adequate quality control and the technical experience necessary may in some instances only be possible if a large number of tests is handled. Because many special tests are not of an immediate nature, they may be suitable for processing at a central facility. If this is the case, communications with a central laboratory must be clearly defined and easy in order to avoid unnecessary delays.

2.5 Near-patient testing (see Appendix, p. 278)

This may be considered by the haematology department in special circumstances, such as providing a limited laboratory facility on site for acute services, for example, an intensive care unit. The equipment used in such a situation and the selection of tests must be carefully scrutinized and only used according to strict protocols. Quality assurance, staff training and maintenance of equipment must remain part of the central laboratory activities. Examples of possible patient facilities are: use of dry prothrombin time (PT) or activated partial thromboplastin time (APTT) for satellite anticoagulant control, use of particle counters in casualty.

3 Office

The office houses the administrative functions of the department and may also deal with the dispatch of reports. The office provides information to the users from within the hospital and to those from outside, such as general practitioners, private hospitals, clinics, occupational health units and others. It also serves as a reception point for patients, visitors and commercial representatives, deals with departmental and in some instances clinical correspondence, sends bills and carries out various other duties, including the ordering of office consumables, as well as the coordination of outpatients and medical records. Collection of statistics may also be a function of the office if the department is not computerized.

The staffing of the office depends on the profile of the work and the workload, as well as on the availability of computerized records and the need for filing. In general, an office manager supervises the work, assisted by secretarial, clerical and/or, visual display unit (VDU) operator staff.

Where information technology is used, the exact scope of the office work depends on the characteristics of the laboratory computer.

4 Other functions

Other functions relating to the work organization of the haematology department are the clinical care of haematology patients, clinical consultative service, training of departmental and non-departmental staff, teaching, research and development. Training is considered separately (see Chapter 1).

4.1 Clinical care of haematology patients

Clinical haematologists are often the largest users of the haematology laboratory, in particular of the special tests, and may influence or even dictate the profile and size of the workload. It is essential that the clinical commitments of medical staff and the dictates of busy in- and outpatient services are identified and the overall organization of the departmental work arranged to maximize the resources available. At the simplest level, conducting a leukaemia outpatient clinic and the anticoagulant clinic simultaneously is not possible for most, except the largest, haematology departments. Special laboratory arrangements may be required, for example, for day-ward transfusions and chemotherapy patients or for assaying factor VIIIC to assess therapeutic response to factor VIII concentrate.

4.2 Clinical consultation

This is an important function of the haematology department and represents a joint laboratory and clinical effort to provide the most appropriate advice on diagnosis and management of acute or complex haematological problems for inpatients, outpatients and general practitioners. The intensive therapy unit (ITU), accident and emergency, maternity, special care baby unit (SCBU) and acute surgery are the most frequent users of this service.

4.3 Research and development

These are carried out in most departments. Activities vary from simple evaluation of new equipment, through projects for technical staff taking their special examination, to clinical or basic research performed by doctors or specially appointed scientists. This enables forward planning, serves an important teaching and training function, attracts 'new blood' and ensures continuing staff interest and good morale. It may also help to retain high-quality staff within the department.

3 Emergency Service

The following guidelines for the provision of emergency services apply to the current style of normal working-day practice, and changes such as extended working hours or the introduction of shift working will create a service intermediate between one that is routine and one that is for emergencies only.

1 Definition of emergency service

This is the laboratory service required to undertake urgent requests which may arise both during and outside the routine working hours of the department.

1.1 The out-of-hours service

This is the service provided outside those hours when the staffing of the department permits the provision of a complete routine service. These times vary from one laboratory to another and within one department from one day to another, e.g. the service on a Saturday will differ from that available on other days. The role of the emergency service is to provide laboratory tests, the results of which are needed before the next routine work session. This implies a degree of urgency in the request, in the performance of the test by laboratory staff and in the issue of the report.

1.2 Urgent requests received during routine hours

In this situation limitations imposed by staffing do not apply, but written procedures for the recognition and handling of urgent specimens are required and in some situations it has been recognized that the arrival of specimens needing priority processing may have a potentially harmful effect on the routine work. It is important that clinicians are aware of this.

1.3 Service in response to a major disaster

This applies to departments of hospitals designated to receive casualties from a major disaster, either within or outside normal working hours.

2 Test repertoire

Tests available should be limited to those which will have a direct influence on the immediate management of the patient. Both normal and abnormal results may be of importance.

A list of the tests available should be drawn up by the haematologist after discussion with the appropriate clinicians before issue to all clinical staff. This list should be included in the laboratory handbook. The list should also be entered in the department's emergency or out-of-hours manual. The list may vary from hospital to hospital depending on the particular kind of clinical workload, but it would be unusual if the list did not contain haemoglobin estimation, total leucocyte count, band cell count for the neonatologist, platelet count, sickle-cell testing, identification of malarial parasites, haemostasis screening and provision of blood for transfusion. Some tests may be on the list but limited in application to certain clinical situations, e.g. plasma viscosity or erythrocyte sedimentation rate (ESR) for patients suspected or known to be suffering from temporal arteritis. An extended repertoire, to include, for example, bone marrow aspiration, will be necessary at times of statutory holiday when the routine service may be unavailable for up to 4 days.

The list of tests which may be done urgently during routine hours is likely to be more extensive and will depend on the nature of the clinical workload and departmental practice.

A clinician requesting a test not on the emergency list should be asked to discuss its need with the medical haematologist on call or in charge of the service during routine hours. No test request should be refused without this consultation taking place.

3 Transport of specimens to department

Although the transport of specimens to the department may not be within the control of the haematologist, he/she should ensure that the appropriate managers have made satisfactory arrangements for the swift delivery of specimens to the department. These arrangements must be documented and the appropriate staff (transport, portering, nursing) be made familiar with them.

The clinician must activate the transport of the specimen in an emergency situation.

4 Collection of specimens

The Medical Laboratory Scientific Officer (MLSO) on call cannot be expected to collect specimens from the clinical area out of hours. It is most efficient when the medical officer requiring the test takes the specimen at the time of examining the patient, but it may be practicable for the phlebotomy service to respond to urgent requests during routine hours.

The clinician initiating a test request should inform the MLSO on call out of hours or the department during routine hours of its imminent dispatch.

5 Identification of urgent specimens

A unique request card to accompany urgent samples may help the ready recognition of the urgent specimen and so assist in its transport and processing. Alternatively, the request card accompanying urgent specimens should have a box for ticking to indicate the urgency or have a specimen sticker securely attached to it.

6 Specimen reception

The reception point for urgent specimens should be identified. During routine hours this would probably be the same area as for routine specimens. Staff involved in the transport of specimens should be informed of this site. The staff of the reception area should be given written instructions in respect of the recognition and further transmission of the specimens. Depending upon the site of the reception area in relation to the department and on the frequency of urgent specimens, it may be advantageous, during routine hours, for the person receiving the urgent call to notify the reception staff of its expected arrival.

Blood banks should only accept inadequately labelled specimens in exceptional circumstances, i.e. unconscious patients when a hospital/casualty number and the sex of the patient may be the only information available.

Outside routine hours, if the reception area is closed, the point for delivery of specimens needs to be clearly labelled 'for urgent out-of-hours specimens only', together with instructions for handling particular specimens.

7 Staff

The MLSO staff participating in the service should be state-registered and preferably working in the same department during routine hours. In some laboratories, junior medical staff (MRCPath trainees) and scientific staff provide emergency cover. It is important that their competence is confirmed.

Staff trained in the techniques to be applied to the listed tests should be certified as competent to work without supervision, by the head of department.

There should be a medically qualified haematologist available by telephone or radiopager for consultation by the MLSO and the requesting clinician.

It would be expected that the provision of an out-of-hours service would involve residence of the on-call MLSO on the same site as the department, particularly when a blood transfusion service is included. Alternatively, residence within 15 minutes' journey time is acceptable. Appropriate secure accommodation including bedroom and toilet facilities, should be provided for the MLSO on call.

The head of department should consider whether, when the on-call commitment has been very demanding, a rest period should be allowed to the MLSO before resuming routine duties in order to reduce the chance of error by tired staff. This would normally be a half-day.

8 Test procedures

Techniques to be used should be recorded in the emergency or out-of-hours manual. The MLSOs on call should be specifically trained in these procedures and the manual should be signed by the trainer and trainee to indicate this. Any variation in a method should also be drawn to the attention of all the on-call staff and the variation signed by the MLSOs. Changes in storage methods should likewise be indicated to the staff; this is particularly important for those engaged in a multidisciplinary service.

When equipment with automated sample handling is in use, staff should be made aware of any potential danger in the introduction of 'one-off' samples.

The philosophy of 'universal precautions' is being adopted in most laboratories. This specifies that all specimens must be handled with care and treated as though they were high-risk. The use of automated instruments with closed-vial sampling capability makes it possible to handle the majority of haematology specimens with safety. Some laboratories where high-risk specimens are regularly tested allot equipment specifically for this purpose. Clearly the decision will depend on the methodology used for specific tests. Whichever route is chosen, the method detail must be unambiguously documented in the procedures manual and staff appropriately trained.

9 Reporting the test result

On completion of the test the MLSO must record the result in the same way as a routine result, if possible, or make a permanent record in some form. He/she must transmit the result to the clinician or to the person deputed by the clinician to receive the result. If this is done by telephone it is essential that the result be repeated back to the MLSO. The name of the person accepting the result should be recorded by the MLSO at the time at which it is reported.

10 Quality control

Quality control should apply to emergency tests to the same degree as to routine tests; indeed, with some operators doing some tests infrequently, the need for quality control materials becomes more imperative. Their frequency of use will depend upon how often the test is carried out and the susceptibility of the test to error. For example, a haemoglobin standard may only be needed once during an out-of-hours session, whereas a double-check of the ABO and rhesus group controls must be undertaken on each occasion blood is matched.

Quality assurance should be applied to the emergency service, though external monitoring may be more difficult to apply than to the routine service. However, the method of analysis, when it differs from the routine, should be included in an external quality assessment scheme (see Chapter 5).

11 Audit

It may be appropriate to use a different request card for out-of-hours or urgent tests. This could facilitate collection of workload figures. The card should be a common one for all the laboratory departments. Alternatively, emergency requests in or out of hours may be given an accession number with a unique initial digit.

When the request is recorded for this purpose, the unit and consultant making the request need to be recorded.

Computer facilities should be provided for the compilation of these statistics.

12 Major disasters

All hospitals designated to receive the victims of a major disaster must have a carefully prepared and comprehensive plan to deal with the event and a haematologist will have been involved in its definition. One haematologist should be made responsible for producing the plan of the departmental response to a disaster.

The consultant in overall charge of the department must know which member of the department is to be alerted first. The haematologist must know with whom he/she is to liaise, particularly in respect of provision of blood products. A list of persons to be subsequently called (with alternate names to cover those who may be absent) and the order in which this is to be done, and by whom, must be drawn up. The list should not be excessive and other members of the department should be advised to respond only to a call from one of the listed staff.

The details of the plan will depend upon local circumstances, but those persons in the department who may be involved must be made familiar with their roles. The listed staff should be made familiar with the labels and documentation which are to be used to identify and to accompany laboratory specimens.

The plan should indicate whether it is local policy for the police or ambulance service to notify the regional Blood Transfusion Service (BTS) of the incident, or if this function is to be carried out by a member of the department. The haematologist, who, from the information given and his/her knowledge of the hospital's blood bank stocks, should be in a position to warn the regional BTS of further likely demands. A direct telephone line between the department and the regional BTS is required for this purpose. Additionally, a direct telephone line independent of the hospital switchboard may prove invaluable.

4 Selection of Instruments and Kits

1 Introduction

When selecting instruments and kits, account must be taken of:
1 compatibility with existing instruments;
2 general factors, such as satisfactory accuracy and precision.

An important way of assessing whether the instrument or kit will satisfy all or most of the requirements is to look at published evaluations which have been done in accordance with nationally or internationally accepted protocols (Shinton *et al.*, 1981; ICSH, 1984). If the potential purchaser has not read such evaluations, the manufacturer may be able to provide literature references for study. Care should be taken before purchasing equipment or kits which have not been evaluated in accordance with accepted protocols, and the potential purchaser should resist the temptation to do a 'quick' evaluation. Full evaluations require considerable time and skill, although potential purchasers should always satisfy themselves of fitness for purpose of equipment (Rowan & England, 1992).

Additional points to consider are the various financial implications, i.e. the capital costs of the equipment and the revenue costs for equipment and kits.

A decision should be taken as to whether the method to be used is of appropriate clinical utility or whether an option appraisal might dictate the use of an alternative method or even a completely different test. Cost will be an important aspect of this. These aspects will now be considered in more detail.

2 Option appraisal

Before any decision is made to purchase particular equipment or kits, all alternative options should be explored with particular reference as to whether:
1 the test should be done at all;
2 the measurement is of maximal clinical utility or whether an alternative measurement would be better, e.g. should one automate the erythrocyte sedimentation rate (ESR) or measure plasma viscosity instead?

41

3 the method of measurement is the best one for the particular analyte, e.g. would a coagulometer working by clot detection be preferable to one using chromogenic substrates?

Prior to purchase of a specific instrument or kit, a limited evaluation should be undertaken.

3 Evaluation

As explained in the Introduction, potential purchasers should only rely on evaluations done in accordance with nationally or internationally accepted evaluation protocols (ICSH, 1984). These are designed by experts, who try to ensure that the protocol includes all important aspects to be considered and specifies how the more quantitative aspects, e.g. precision, comparability, etc., are to be measured. Unless such protocols are followed, it is likely that there will be serious omissions from evaluations and results may be presented in a misleading way, e.g. reliance on correlation coefficients in comparability studies may create a false 'good impression'. Some consideration should be given to performance in the appropriate National External Quality Assessment Scheme (NEQAS) survey. A list of evaluation protocols is given in the references.

4 Selection criteria

4.1 Selection of instruments

This will depend on whether local clinical requirements are such as to merit automation of either the analysis or the sample-handling. For example, blood counters are now widely available with the ability to process specimens of whole blood so that instruments requiring predilution would not be used in most laboratories. However, it may not always be necessary to have automated sample-handling, especially if the workload is small. Similar considerations also apply to coagulometers and it is probably only the large reference centres which are able to justify instruments with automated sample-handling. Indeed, many hospitals still find it preferable not even to automate the clotting tests of their coagulation services, since these can easily be done manually.

The throughput of any instrument being purchased must be suitable for the existing workload and for any anticipated increases over the likely working life of the instrument.

Back-up facilities will also need to the considered since the workload in automated laboratories will often exceed the level which can be dealt with manually in the event of instrument failure. The purchaser must decide whether it is better to have two medium-sized instruments which can operate simultaneously and provide back-up, or whether it is better to have one large instrument and a smaller one for back-up, e.g. for use on call. The problem with this latter approach is that the two instruments may produce results which differ significantly and the clinical users will be confused.

Safety is of crucial importance (see Chapter 6) and one important item to be considered is whether or not the instrument offers a closed-tube facility, so obviating the need for the operator to open specimens.

Finally, it is necessary to assess scientific factors, such as accuracy, precision, comparability, carry-over, whether satisfactory controls and calibrators are available and performance in NEQAS exercises. Practical factors to consider include reliability, ease of maintenance, safety, computer interfacing, the quality of the instruction manual and any training courses provided by the manufacturers.

4.2 Selection of kits

This will depend on many of the scientific and practical factors outlined above, as well as on factors specific to kits. These include whether the kit size is suitable for the local workload, the shelf-life of the kit and the frequency with which it is desired to perform the assay, e.g. a kit designed to perform 20 assays may not be cost-effective if the assay needs to be run weekly and only 10 specimens accumulate during this period. Another factor to be considered with certain kits is whether the spectrum of analytes conforms to the locally required testing profiles (ECCLS, 1986).

5 Financial aspects

The financial aspects which are of importance vary between different health-care systems from time to time. In the UK National Health Service, for example, capital had been considered a 'free good' until capital charging was recently introduced. However, even in the private sector, the treatment of depreciation may vary widely. The easiest area to assess is the cost of reagents and controls and equipment servicing. It may be more difficult to cost staff time and here too practices may vary between health-care systems from time to time.

Another problem is amortization, particularly in relation to the discounting of suppliers. In some instances, 'packages' may be sold in which leasing and maintenance are differentiated from the cost of consumables. In other instances, the equipment may be supplied and maintained gratis provided that a certain level of consumables is purchased.

References

ECCLS (1986) *Guidelines for the User Laboratory to Evaluate and Select a Kit for its Own Use. Part 1: Quantitative Tests.* ECCLS Document Vol. 3. Beuth Verlag, Berlin.

ICSH (1984) Protocol for evaluation of automated blood cell counters. *Clinical and Laboratory Haematology* **6**, 69–84.

Rowan R.M. & England J.M. (1992) Special aspects in haematology. In Haeckel R. (ed.) *Evaluation Methods in Laboratory Medicine*, pp. 141–151. VCH, Weinheim and New York.

Shinton N.K., Bloom A.L., Colvin B.T., Flute P.T., Preston F.E. & Kennedy D.A. (1981) Tentative protocol for the evaluation of coagulometers based on the one-stage prothrombin time. *Clinical and Laboratory Haematology* **3**, 71–76.

5 Quality Control
of the Test Procedure

This is a set of procedures and practices for assuring that reliable results of laboratory tests are received by the clinician. There are three components:

1 proficiency surveillance;
2 internal quality control (IQC);
3 external quality assessment (EQA).

1 Proficiency surveillance

This requires direct checking of the following items by laboratory staff. Where appropriate this will be in collaboration with the stores department, ward staff and porter and messenger administration.

1 Blood collection tubes must have the correct anticoagulant, conform to a specified standard and be used within a stated shelf-life.

2 Phlebotomy is carried out by a standardized procedure.

3 All specimens (and request forms) must be adequately identified at the time of collection; potentially hazardous specimens are appropriately marked.

4 All specimens must be placed in separate plastic bags, each with its own request form in a separate pocket of the bag to avoid contamination, but arranged so as not to be separated from the specimen until it is registered in the laboratory.

5 Specimens must be transported to the laboratory without delay, generally within 1 hour after phlebotomy, and they must be maintained at appropriate ambient temperature before analysis.

6 On arrival in the laboratory, specimens must be checked for the correct type of container, for the correct amount of blood in relation to anticoagulant and for the condition of the specimen. Leaking specimens must normally be discarded but if of critical importance require special handling. Unreasonable delays between collection of specimens and their receipt in the laboratory must always be investigated.

7 Request forms and specimen containers must have adequate identification; if any specimen is inadequately labelled, to ensure correct identification that

specimen should not be analysed. Specimens should be given a laboratory number and details should be entered into a current paper file or computer by a Medical Laboratory Scientific Officer (MLSO) or by clerical staff, who will at this stage identify potentially hazardous specimens in accordance with a list of high-risk conditions or by the presence of a warning label on the specimens and request forms. Such specimens and any leaking specimens (see above) must be brought to the attention of a senior technical or medical member of the laboratory staff and will require special handling. Similarly, urgent specimens should be identified and dealt with separately to ensure rapid analysis.

8 After analysis has been performed, results must be transcribed on to report forms or to computer-generated result sheets. Staff performing this work should ensure that the results are technically valid and that an appropriate quality control programme has been used. All reports should be scrutinized and validated by senior MLSOs in accordance with a protocol which has been laid down by the head of department. Urgent results should be scrutinized by a senior MLSO and reported as 'provisional'. If a report has been telephoned, this should be noted in the laboratory record.

9 Reports should be sent to the location indicated on the request form at appropriate intervals during the day. Unreasonable delay in reports reaching their destination must be investigated.

2 Internal quality control

2.1 Control material

At appropriate intervals (e.g. for blood cell counters not less than twice each day; for less frequently performed tests with each batch), control material must be included as samples in the analytical run. Results for patient samples should not be issued until it is clear, by analysis of the data (see below), that no significant change in the process has occurred. Once this has been demonstrated, results may be issued with confidence.

Control materials may be prepared in the laboratory or obtained commercially. During their preparation they must undergo testing in accordance with established health safety practice. When human blood is used, it should, as far as possible, be prepared from donations which have been tested individually for human immunodeficiency virus (HIV) antibody and for hepatitis B surface antigen, and shown to be negative. When it is necessary to use untested blood, this fact should be indicated on the label and the sample should be regarded as potentially infectious and treated with the same precautions as patients' specimens. The essential requirements for control materials are:

1 sterility;

2 stability for an identifiable period during which it can be used;

3 representative distribution from stock;

4 comparability to blood behaviour in the test procedure, at least within identified limits;

5 lot precision established under standard conditions (by at least 10 replicate measurements).

Some commercial control materials are supplied with assigned values. This is intended only as an indication of the level of analyte present; neither this material nor EQA samples should be used for instrument calibration.

The data obtained from the repeated measurements of the control materials must be analysed so that any consistent trend can be detected before it becomes clinically significant. Sequential results should be plotted as a control chart on linear graph paper and inspected regularly by the head of department and the most senior technical member of staff.

As an alternative, results can be subjected to cusum analysis. The presentation of the analysis can be graphical or numerical. The latter is generally more appropriate and can be carried out by personal computer. The size of the change that is to be detected must be set by the head of department on the basis of the level of sensitivity that is required.

2.2 Monitoring drift

In laboratories with computer facilities, when the population of patients from whom the laboratory's samples are drawn remains stable, it may be possible to use the estimate of the total daily or weekly patient mean of absolute values, mean corpuscular volume (MCV), mean corpuscular haemoglobin (MCH), mean corpuscular haemoglobin concentration (MCHC), for monitoring the occurrence of drift. However, before patient data are used, it is essential to establish the stability of the patient population from day to day and within any sub-batches that may be analysed. Laboratories which cannot demonstrate the stability of the sample populations must not use this procedure for quality control.

2.3 Changes in value

A change of value in the subsequent tests ('delta-check') which does not correspond to a recognizable clinical cause must be checked to ensure that it has not been due to an incorrectly identified sample, other clerical error or specimen collection fault. When necessary, a repeat sample must be measured before the result is validated.

2.4 Correlation of results

Correlation of results of related investigations (e.g. blood count and blood film) should also be used as a check of test performance. Laboratory work flow should be organized and results presented in an appropriate manner (e.g. in a cumulative report) to allow this correlation assessment to be carried out without unnecessary delay in validating test results.

2.5 Performance in duplicate

All tests should be performed in duplicate unless it has been shown that the method precision would permit single-form assay. Even then, some assays should be carried out in duplicate to check on the current precision. These measurements should be performed on a few specimens in a test batch taken randomly from the batch, or from a previous batch, provided that the specimens have been stored in an appropriate way so as to avoid deterioration of the analytes, and also on control samples.

2.6 Serological tests

Special IQC requirements for blood transfusion serological tests must always be accompanied by positive and negative controls. When serological reagents are made by individual laboratories, their potency and efficiency should be assessed by use of reagents obtained from commercial suppliers or a reference laboratory. Manufacturers' instructions regarding storage and use of reagents must be rigorously observed. Sera should be kept at $-25°C$ or below when not in use, unless the instructions issued with a particular serum state that it should not be frozen. All methods should be standardized and results should be expressed in international units, where these have been established. Emergency tests should be defined in the laboratory manual, with an indication of their reliability and the conditions under which they may be performed.

2.7 Special aspects of internal quality control for haemostasis

Blood specimens must be collected in such a manner that the integrity of the platelets and/or coagulation factors to be analysed is preserved. Only blood drawn rapidly and without difficulty by an experienced person should be used. If the blood is collected by means of a syringe, this must be made of plastic or siliconized glass and the blood must be collected into an appropriate anticoagulant, preferably in a plastic container. If the blood is collected directly into an evacuated glass container, this must be siliconized. Evacuated samples are only suitable for coagulation screening tests and anticoagulant control. In many hospitals evacuated samples are not used for any tests of coagulation, and phlebotomists and others are taught this. Otherwise, for example, it is not possible to undertake coagulation factor assays on the same sample used for coagulation screening without bringing the patient back for resampling. Additionally, they are not suitable for more detailed tests of platelet function or coagulation factor assays. The blood must be mixed with the anticoagulant by gentle inversion and frothing must be avoided. Blood must be kept under specified conditions before testing.

Whole blood and plasma must be kept stored in closed plastic containers at room temperature. These must be clean and free from any surface reactant substances. If all tests cannot be completed within 4 hours, plasma must be stored frozen ($-25°C$ or below) as soon as possible after centrifugation and then thawed rapidly at 37°C immediately before being tested. Manual end-point detection of clotting requires a temperature-controlled water-bath and stop-watch or foot-timer. The water-bath must be checked for maintenance of temperature at 37°C $\pm$ 1°C. An illuminated water-bath facilitates reading the end point. The reproducibility of the end-point detection must be checked and compared with the standardized method used in the laboratory. Generally, the clotting-time results obtained with optical devices are shorter than those obtained with mechanical devices. Alternating between types of end-point detection device is inadvisable. The main coagulation instrument should be periodically controlled by a back-up instrument of the same type. If more than one instrument is in daily use, they should be checked against each other at least once a week. If different systems are used, each should have its own reference intervals established.

Minor variations in technique, reagents, temperature or pH produce constant variation in test results. The incubation time and temperature are critical parameters of control in the one-stage prothrombin-time test. The plasma must be maintained at 37°C for no longer than 10 minutes and the thromboplastin for not longer than the manufacturer recommends.

All samples must be measured in duplicate. If results differ by more than 5% a further sample or pair of samples must be tested. Normal and, where possible, abnormal controls must be included in each assay. Lyophilized controls in both the normal and abnormal range are commercially available. Commercial firms maintain that these controls usually work best when they are prepared by the manufacturer who made the relevant thromboplastin and activated partial thromboplastin reagents. Controls made in the laboratory may be fresh, deep-frozen or lyophilized. The fresh plasma must be tested as soon as possible; the fresh-frozen plasma controls can be stored for up to 3–4 months before use, and lyophilized plasma controls for at least a year. Normal controls should be made from a minimum of 20 normal men and/or women who are not taking oral contraceptives.

3 External quality assessment

In the UK it is essential that the laboratory be registered with EQA schemes which are approved by the National External Quality Assessment Scheme (NEQAS) Advisory Panel for Haematology and participates in all the tests covered by these schemes. The head of the laboratory has ultimate responsibility for performance by the laboratory and to ensure that the laboratory returns results in each survey.

The head of laboratory may elect to nominate an individual contact to receive the survey samples and the subsequent reports and performance analyses. In this case the head must review results with the named contact regularly and must ensure that any correspondence from the scheme organizer (e.g. concerning unsatisfactory performance) is brought to his/her attention. Conversely, when the head is the contact, he/she must review the results with the most senior MLSO. The EQA reports should also be seen regularly by other medical and technical staff in the laboratory.

6 Health and Safety in Laboratories

1 Introduction

The Health and Safety at Work Act (1974) (Health and Safety Commission, 1975) specifies a requirement for all laboratories to create and enforce a safety code of practice. This must cover all activities and provide for the safety of employees and any persons visiting the laboratory, including patients and their escorts, nurses, porters, hospital tradesmen and industrial service engineers. Different codes should be written for each category of employee. Failure to produce and enforce such a code of practice or failure of employees to cooperate in maintaining it renders those concerned liable in law. Specific sections of the Act define responsibilities of management, employees and industrial and commercial suppliers of equipment and reagents, and the interrelationships of these.

The head of the laboratory is ultimately responsible for the definition, written description and regular revision of health and safety policies and procedures and for the education of staff in these. However, all employees are responsible for their own safety and for that of colleagues and any third parties present in the laboratory (duty of care). The safety policy is designed to ensure an environment in which laboratory workers can operate without risk or, alternatively, where hazards are identified and unambiguous procedures for their prevention and for accident management are defined.

The Act specifies the appointment of a laboratory safety officer by the head of laboratory to ensure that safe practices operate. Safety representatives, on the other hand, are elected by laboratory staff to protect their interests and have the right in law to approach the head of laboratory on perceived hazards but have no legal responsibility for defining corrective action.

Subsequent legislation builds on the Health and Safety at Work Act and includes:
- Ionising Radiations Regulations 1985, SI 1985 No. 1333 (International Commission on Radiological Protection, 1991);
- Acquired Immune Deficiency Syndrome (AIDS) (Control) Act, 1987 (DHSS/ACDP, 1990);

51

- Consumer Protection Act, 1987 (Product Liability and Consumer Safety) (Department of Trade and Industry, 1987);
- Control of Substances Hazardous to Health Regulations, 1988 (COSHH, 1988);
- Electricity at Work Regulations, 1989 (HSE, 1989).

A series of documents follows legislation to aid its interpretation. These documents are of three types. First are regulations, which carry the force of law and if broken can result in prosecution. Codes of practice and guidelines (guidance notes) are advisory but, may be admissible in evidence. In giving judgement, a court of law will almost certainly view such documents as representing exemplary practice.

All laboratory activities, not only analytical methods, must be described in standard operating procedures (SOPs). Where relevant, safety rules and procedures must be included in each. If described only in summary, there must be clear reference to the primary safety document. These documents form the basis for employee training. Staff should sign to indicate that they have read and understood these.

2 Staff welfare

2.1 Employee health programme

Routine pre-employment medical examination is not deemed necessary. Health status should be assessed by questionnaire and only those whose responses suggest a medical problem need be examined.

Accurate health records must be kept for all members of staff. Where hazards exist, employers must be able to monitor staff and to note and act on work-related illness or injury.

Baseline observations, including an assessment of immunization status, should be made by the local Occupational Health Service and recorded. All staff working in haematology laboratories should be offered hepatitis B vaccination.

All laboratory workers must be issued with medical contact cards bearing the following: the name, address and contact telephone number of general practitioner, the nature of the individual's employment and the names of a senior medically qualified person and the safety officer at the place of work.

2.2 Record of illness, accident and dangerous occurrence

Accidents or incidents affecting the health and safety of laboratory employees must be recorded in a book kept solely for that purpose. This must be reviewed regularly and revised where appropriate and any necessary action must be taken to prevent recurrence. Certain dangerous occurrences and illnesses must be reported directly to the Health and Safety Executive (HSE). Reportable incidents include fatal or major injuries or any injuries that result in incapacity for more than 3 days.

2.3 First aid

There are two complementary requirements: (i) several staff members must be trained in first aid, including artificial respiration, and must be re-examined at appropriate intervals; and (ii) a first-aid box must be provided, the contents of which are restricted to:

- instruction sheet giving general guidance;
- individually wrapped sterile adhesive dressings in a variety of sizes;
- sterile eye-pads with attachment bandages;
- triangular bandages;
- sterile coverings for serious wounds;
- safety-pins;
- selection of sterile unmedicated dressings.

Eye-irrigation equipment must be available, either the wash-bottle type or a system connected to the mains water supply. First-aiders must be trained to perform eye-irrigation procedures.

Antidotes to poisonous chemicals used in the laboratory must be available and protocols for their use clearly displayed.

Protective clothing and safety equipment must be provided for the person rendering first aid.

Finally, all first-aid equipment must be stored correctly and checked regularly to ensure that it is in good condition. The contents of the first-aid box must be replenished immediately after use.

A list of staff members trained in first aid should be prominently displayed in the laboratory.

3 Safety code of practice

This should list those procedures which are basic to safe laboratory practice (Health Services Advisory Committee, 1991). New staff must not be permitted to work independently until they have received this basic safety training and have demonstrated competence. Periodic training is advisable for all staff. A safety manual that identifies known or potential hazards and that specifies safe practices and procedures must be created and adopted. Personnel must be advised of hazards and required to read and follow standard procedures. All employees should become familiar with relevant international hazard symbols and indications of danger, as well as risk and safety phrases.

The following are basic general rules:

1 Only persons who are aware of the hazards and meet any specific entry

requirements are permitted access to the laboratory work area. Laboratory doors should be closed when work is in progress. Children and pets are forbidden. Restricted access should be clearly indicated by appropriate signposting.

2 Eating, drinking, smoking and the application of cosmetics in the laboratory are forbidden.

3 Regular hand-washing before leaving the laboratory or immediately after contamination by a chemical agent or biological material must be encouraged.

4 Suitable protective clothing, of approved design, must be worn, fastened, in laboratories and when venesecting patients. When not in use, laboratory coats must be hung on pegs located near the laboratory and not kept in personal lockers. The pegs must be located outside the laboratory area and the coats must be worn when leaving the laboratory to visit wards or outpatient clinics. Visitors to the laboratory area, e.g. service engineers and medical students, must be provided with suitable protective clothing.

Laboratory coats must not be taken home for washing but must be laundered through the hospital service. Laboratory protective clothing must be sent to the laundry in special bags and washed in these bags. When this is not possible, disposable protective clothing must be used and treated as contaminated waste after use.

5 Protection for existing wounds or skin lesions with a suitable dressing is mandatory.

6 Gloves should be used in the following situations:
   (a) all procedures where contamination by blood is probable;
   (b) venepuncture, especially when the venepuncturist is inexperienced or the patient is restless or in a high-risk category;
   (c) when cleaning equipment prior to sterilization or disinfection;
   (d) when handling chemical disinfectants;
   (e) when cleaning spoilages.
The type of glove used will depend on the task (non-sterile latex examination gloves – plastic or vinyl are alternatives; heavy-duty domestic gloves).

7 Protection of eyes, mouth and nose from blood splashes and droplet spread can be achieved by the correct use of goggles and visors. Various forms of combined eye and face protection are available.

8 Fenestrated footwear must not be worn in locations where sharps are handled. For procedures involving possible dissemination of blood or other biological materials, calf-length plastic overboots must be worn. Footwear may require decontamination following the treatment of spills.

9 Mouth-pipetting must be completely prohibited. Staff, therefore, require training in the use of bulb- or hand-pipetting devices.

10 A policy for the prevention of puncture wounds, cuts and abrasions by sharps must exist. Sharps include needles, edged instruments, broken glassware or other items which may cause laceration or puncture wounds. All sharps must be promptly placed in a secure puncture-resistant bin for incineration. Such bins must not be overfilled.

11 The laboratory must be kept neat and free from all materials not pertinent to work.

12 Work surfaces must be decontaminated at least once per day or after any spill of dangerous material (Appendix 6.2).

13 Centrifuges must be of a design which prevents opening of the lid during operation. Ideally, sealed buckets should be used. Alternatively, tubes containing blood or other fluids must be closed with shouldered caps before being placed in the centrifuge. Careful balancing of tubes within the centrifuge will minimize the risk of breakage. Sealed buckets or tubes containing infective samples must be opened in an exhaust-protected cabinet.

14 The following rules apply to handling specimens. Risk occurs at three times: (i) during specimen collection; (ii) during specimen reception; and (iii) during the measuring process. Therefore:

(a) do not contaminate the outside of the container;

(b) do not contaminate any part of the environment;

(c) decontaminate any spills immediately;

(d) when necessary, use high-risk labels both on the specimen container and on the request form;

(e) the request form must not come into contact with the specimen container;

(f) containers must be kept firmly stoppered;

(g) containers should be transported and stored in the vertical position;

(h) if sending specimens by mail, the General Post Office (GPO) rules must be followed;

(i) leaking specimens should generally be discarded unless there are compelling reasons for not doing so.

15 All biological waste is potentially infective and must be treated as clinical waste. All blood specimen containers, erythrocyte sedimentation rate (ESR) tubes, syringes and contaminated swabs must be placed in plastic bags and incinerated. The plastic bags must be sealed and labelled 'Infective – Risk of Infection – For Incineration' before leaving the laboratory. If facilities for incineration are not available, bags must be autoclaved before disposal. All waste should be removed at least once a day.

16 All technical procedures should be carried out in a way which minimizes the creation of aerosol or droplet formation. All instruments should be tested, during normal operation for the production of aerosol or droplet. An estimate of the degree of microbiological risk can be obtained by adding fluorescent chemical markers, such as fluorescein, to specimens, placing clean white absorbent paper over areas of possible contamination and then running the instrument.

Contamination is indicated by the presence of fluorescence under ultraviolet light. This is particularly useful when serum or plasma samples are being processed. A more sensitive method involves the use of bacterial spores, such as suspensions of *Bacillus subtilis* var. *globigii*, but for this method the services of a microbiologist are required.

17 All instruments should be checked for hazards which might injure the operator, such as sharp edges or unguarded moving parts. Staff must not wear pendant jewellery in the laboratory, since it may become entrapped in machinery. Ideally, watches and rings should be removed and long hair contained. Personal clothing must not protrude beyond the sleeves of protective clothing. Lifting heavy equipment often causes back injury and staff should receive training in this manœuvre.

18 A rest room must be provided where staff can eat and drink. Under no circumstances must laboratory coats, blood specimens or reagents be taken into the rest room. Hands must be washed before entering.

19 All spills involving exposure to potentially dangerous materials must be reported immediately to the laboratory supervisor. Special situations in the haematology laboratory include:

    (a) contamination of instruments;
    (b) breakage and spillage of specimens;
    (c) breakage within the centrifuge;
    (d) chemical spillage;
    (e) radioactive spills.

Management of these is detailed in Appendix 6.1.

4 Basic laboratory design features to ensure safety

The layout of the laboratory must be such that separate administrative, specimen collection and analytical areas exist. If patients attend for any reason, there must be a patient waiting area and a separate, private specimen collection area. Staff and patient toilets must be provided. There should be staff changing accommodation and living-in accommodation for staff on call.

Overcrowding is a common cause of laboratory accidents. Ample space must be provided for the safe performance of each laboratory procedure. Having determined the critical space dimensions for a procedure, in the interests of safety no other activity should be superimposed on this area.

In the analytical area, walls, ceilings and floors should be smooth, easily cleaned, impermeable to liquids and resistant to the chemicals and disinfectants in everyday use. Cavity ceilings must be avoided or sealed. Floors should be slip-resistant. With modern materials, slip hazard is low when floors are dry, but high when wet. The floor should be mopped immediately following any liquid spill and dried thoroughly. Floor tiles should be sealed at all joins and where they meet the wall. Sloping floors and steps should be avoided if possible.

Benches should be of solid construction with a sealed surface which is impervious to water and resistant to disinfectants, acids, alkalis, organic solvents and moderate heat.

Doors should have appropriate fire ratings, be self-closing and have vision panels.

Laboratory furniture should be sturdy and free from sharp edges and projections. Open spaces between and under benches, cabinets and equipment should be accessible for cleaning. All fittings should be of ergonometrically correct design for height and reach. Work surfaces should not cause glare.

There must be adequate lighting to perform all activities. Natural lighting is preferred when possible. Task lighting requires an intensity of approximately 23 lumen/m^2 with low-contrast glare-free background illumination. Fluorescent ceiling lights should be installed directly above and parallel to benches to avoid shadow.

Natural ventilation should be provided where possible, particularly in the staffroom, patient areas and office. Windows should be openable, preferably having fly-proof screens. Where mechanical ventilation is necessary, 6–10 air changes per hour are recommended. A higher exchange rate is necessary where unpleasant fumes are generated. Alternatively, the use of fume-cupboards prevents dissemination of unpleasant odours and is necessary to remove noxious and flammable fumes. A mechanical exhaust system should provide inward air flow and exhaust without recirculation. The exhaust system must be sited in such a way that fumes are not drawn back into the building at a different level or drawn into an adjacent building.

A dependable mains water supply must be guaranteed. Cross-connection of laboratory analytical area supply and drinking water is avoided by installing a back-flow preventer. A wash-hand basin separate from laboratory sinks must be provided in each laboratory room, preferably close to the exit. Taps must be capable of elbow, wrist or foot operation.

A reliable electricity supply with adequate capacity should be available. There should be emergency lighting to assist safe exit in the event of failure of the mains power supply.

A reliable supply of town, natural or bottled gas should be available where required. Good maintenance of the installations is mandatory. Bottled gases should be avoided where possible. If their use is unavoidable, the smallest available cylinder should be used. Inspection and approval by a Health and Safety Authority are necessary before use. Compressed-gas cylinders must not be incinerated.

Storage space must be adequate to hold supplies for immediate use. Poisonous substances must be kept in a locked cupboard. Flammable solvents must be kept on spill trays inside a metal flame-proof cabinet. A deep-freeze may be necessary for patient samples, labile reagents or reference materials. This should be lockable. Thermal protective gloves must be provided for temperatures below $-20°C$.

Bulk stores, preferably located outside work areas, must also be provided. For the latter, the specific requirements are:

1 the bulk store must be lockable;
2 portable step-ladders must be provided if high shelving is used;
3 toxic laboratory chemicals must be kept in a separate part of the bulk store;
4 strong acids and alkalis must not be kept on high shelves;
5 chemicals which react together must be stored apart;
6 bulk flammable liquids require a separate external flammable store (vented-brick building with metal shelving and gas-proof light fittings).

Where flammable laboratory gases are not in use or are stored, the site should be so located that in the event of fire there is no danger to non-laboratory staff, patients or third parties.

Procedures for the safe disposal of waste must be documented according to national guidelines and adhered to. This must include effete specimens and other waste. Solid waste should be placed in containers or autoclavable bags which can be sealed. Arrangements must be made to ensure either that these sealed containers are incinerated or that they are autoclaved before disposal. Containers must be opened before autoclaving. Ideally, the autoclave should be available on the same premises as the laboratory. This will require specially designed accommodation and services. If autoclaving cannot take place on the premises, a specialist disposal company should be employed. In this event, special care must be taken to ensure that containers are appropriately labelled and well sealed before leaving the laboratory.

The range of chemical waste is potentially very large. Many water-soluble materials can be disposed of through the bench drain. Waste-pipes must be constructed of resistant materials, such as polypropylene. Copper must not be used as it may cause explosion if azides or picrates are discharged. Waste traps should be readily accessible. Flammable solvents are particularly hazardous and their removal, burning or recovery requires a specialist service. Laboratory drains should be piped directly into the main sewer. This is mandatory on sites where low-activity radionuclides are used.

Laboratories are occasionally the target of vandals. In addition, assaults on staff and theft of expensive technical and office equipment are recognized problems. There is a danger that unauthorized persons may become exposed to potential biological or chemical hazard. For these reasons the laboratory should be designed as an integrally secure area with entrances which can be controlled. Security may be augmented by strong doors, screened windows and restricted issue of keys. Since the requirements for fire safety and security may conflict, experts in both should be consulted at the design stage.

5 Fire hazard

5.1 Cooperation (DHSS/Welsh Office, 1982a,b; DHSS/Welsh Office, 1987)

Close cooperation between the laboratory safety officer and the local fire prevention officer is essential. Fire prevention is subject to statutory requirements and guidelines. Training of laboratory staff in fire prevention, immediate action in case of fire and the use of fire-fighting equipment is necessary. Fire warnings, instructions and escape routes must be displayed prominently in each room and in corridors. Fire-fighting equipment must be placed near to the doors of rooms and at strategic points in corridors.

5.2 Causes of fires

Common causes of laboratory fires include:
- electrical overloading;
- poor electrical maintenance;
- excessively long electrical leads;
- electrical equipment left on unnecessarily;
- excessively long gas tubing;
- perished gas tubing;
- misuse of matches and ignition devices;
- naked flames;
- carelessness with flammable substances;
- flammables and explosives storage in domestic refrigerator.

5.3 Fire-fighting equipment

This consists of:
- fire-hoses;
- water and sand buckets for use against burning paper, wood and fabrics, but not against electrical fires;
- fire-extinguishers (see below);
- fire blankets.

5.4 Fire-extinguishers

There are various kinds of extinguisher:
- carbon dioxide (CO_2) for use against electrical fires, flammable liquids and gases, but not in the presence of alkali, metals or paper;
- dry powder which has the same uses and contraindications as CO_2;
- foam for use against flammable liquids but not electrical fires;
- bromochloridifluoromethane (BCF) for use against both flammable liquids and electrical fires.

The shelf-life of fire-extinguishers must be ascertained and arrangements made for their regular inspection and maintenance. Water extinguishers are CO_2-driven;

care is necessary with CO_2 extinguishers as the force of the jet may spread burning materials; rooms must be well-ventilated after use of BCF extinguishers.

5.5 Fire detection and alarm systems

These should be installed in all laboratories. In laboratory work areas, heat detection systems are preferable. Fire detection systems must be connected to the hospital switchboard, provided this is manned 24 hours per day. In addition, break-glass call-points should be installed which are capable of triggering the alarm system. Audible alarms must be capable of being heard in all areas of the laboratory suite.

6 Chemical hazard

6.1 Regulations

The emergence of the Control of Substances Hazardous to Health (COSHH) Regulations (1988) has made laboratory workers aware of the dangers of chemical substances. The regulations require that exposure to substances hazardous to health must be kept below a level that can actually cause harm. This entails:
- identifying all chemical substances used in work activity;
- assessing a substance's potential for causing harm;
- assessing the chance of exposure actually causing harm to or in the body;
- assessing how much the individual is exposed to the substance and for how long.

The regulations cover all toxic (poisonous) chemical substances in the form of solids, liquid and gases, as well as micro-organisms. Employers are required to assess the risks created by work which is liable to expose workers to hazardous substances and take steps to protect them from such hazardous substances. Employers must provide appropriate control measures and ensure that they are kept in good working order. Employees must comply with these safeguards conscientiously. Non-laboratory workers, including outside contractors, students, nursing staff and secretarial and clerical staff, may all need information, instruction and training to ensure that they are aware of any health risks and the measures required to avoid these.

6.2 General chemical safety requirements

These include:
- correct storage of chemicals (immediate use, bulk);
- adequate separation of incompatible chemicals;
- all large containers to be at floor level with siphoning for filling bottles from bulk;
- strong acids/alkalis and corrosives to be stored at floor level;

- bulk stores should have concrete floors with sills to contain spillage;
- separate flammable store, suitably vented and with sealed electrical fittings;
- written procedures for dealing with chemical spills;
- adequate materials for dealing with spills;
- written procedure for use of antidotes to chemical poisons;
- adequate containment facilities for handling solvent vapours and carcinogenic and teratogenic substances;
- adequate protective clothing;
- adequate control procedures for dealing with potential carcinogens, explosive substances, dusts (including asbestos), organic solvents, acids, alkalis, corrosives and cyanide solutions.

7 Electrical safety

7.1 Regulations
Familiarity with the Electricity at Work Regulations (1989) is now mandatory. The head of the laboratory must take measures to ensure that all electrical equipment is safe and that all relevant persons are made aware of the associated hazards and of the requirement to adopt safe working practices. Regular safety inspections must be carried out.

7.2 Hazards
The hazards of electricity include:
- electric shock;
- burns;
- risk of fire;
- risk of explosion.

7.3 Safety
General safety precautions are as follows:
- All installations, maintenance and repairs must be carried out by qualified electricians.
- All electrically operated equipment should carry manufacturer certification of electrical safety.
- Always use correctly fused plugs with flat pins.
- Cables must be of correct rating to carry the current which will flow through them in both normal and abnormal conditions; they must be adequately insulated and must be no longer than necessary.
- Adaptors must not be used.
- The external metal casing of electrical equipment must be earthed.
- Double-wound transformers provide a means of isolating equipment from the

mains supply and are a valuable aid to safety when employed to supply mains to hazardous areas.

7.4 Laboratory rules

Laboratory rules in addition to the general rules defined in Section 7.3 include:
- Know where the main isolators in the laboratory are situated.
- Ensure regular inspection and maintenance of all electrical equipment.
- Never use equipment which you consider to be faulty.
- Inspection covers must never be moved from electrical devices other than by a qualified person.
- In the event of fire, use only CO_2 or BCF extinguishers.
- Always follow the manufacturers' operating instructions.
- Remember that in hazardous areas (in the presence of wet or flammable substances) electrical appliances require to be specially designed; always seek expert advice.
- Never use equipment with exposed live terminals.
- Special attention should be paid to earth connections.

8 Microbiological safety

All blood specimens should be considered potentially infective and should be handled in accordance with established infection-control precautions.

Micro-organisms are classified into four hazard groups on the basis of: (i) pathogenicity for man; (ii) hazard to laboratory personnel; (iii) transmissibility in the community; and (iv) the availability of effective prophylaxis and treatment (ACDP, 1984).

The four hazard categories are numbered 1, 2, 3 and 4. The hazard category of a particular organism matches the containment level under which it must be handled. The term 'containment' describes safe methods for handling infectious agents in the laboratory environment. General microbiological safety measures are described in Section 3.

In the haematology laboratory in areas where there is risk of exposure to the viruses causing the various forms of hepatitis and AIDS, all laboratory work must be carried out under not less than containment level 2, upgraded as follows:
1 There must be limited access to the laboratory.
2 Each member of staff requires $24\,m^3$ space.
3 Procedures must be performed only by state-registered staff.
4 Work may be conducted on a specially selected area of open bench, with no other activities being carried out in the area.
5 Bench tops must be disinfected immediately on completion of the procedure.
6 An autoclave for waste sterilization must be available, preferably in the same building.

Where there is risk of droplet spread, a microbiology safety cabinet (class 1: British Standard (BS) 5726 (British Standards Institution, 1979) or equivalent) must be used.

9 Radiation hazard

Although only small quantities of radionuclides of low activity are handled in haematology laboratories for diagnostic purposes, their use is governed by stringent codes of practice. Radionuclides can only be used in a designated laboratory under the direction of an authorized person. Doses administered must not exceed those specified by the International Commission on Radiological Protection (ICRP, 1991).

An appropriately trained and qualified radiation protection adviser must be appointed by the employer. This individual should be available for consultation whenever required and is responsible for advising on all aspects of radiation practice. A radiation protection supervisor (RPS), on the other hand, assists the employer to comply with radiation protection requirements. The RPS is a laboratory employee directly involved in the work with ionizing radiation, preferably in a line management position.

Premises in which low-activity radionuclides are used must meet certain specifications:

1   Wall and ceilings must be painted with good-quality high-gloss paint.
2   Woodwork must be sealed and varnished by suitably durable material.
3   Floors must be covered with vinyl or linoleum sheet (not tiles) with joins sealed or welded; linoleum must be polished.
4   Bench tops should be constructed from resin plastic laminates carried over on to the front edge of the bench, with a small upstand; the rear edge must be curved and properly sealed to the wall; there must be no gaps or overhangs around sinks.
5   A wash-hand basin must be provided, with elbow- or foot-operated taps. A separate laboratory sink with similar taps must be provided for disposing of liquid contaminated waste and for decontaminating equipment; an integrated sink with an upstand all round is recommended; this sink must be clearly marked with the international radiation symbol. A second laboratory sink must be available for non-radioactive waste.
6   Good ventilation is necessary; for most radionuclides used in haematology, it is unnecessary to have a fume-cupboard.
7   A simple lockable cupboard with a high-gloss interior paint finish is necessary.

All staff working in the radionuclide designated area must be provided with personal dosimeters, usually of the film type, which should be worn on the trunk at chest or waist level underneath any protective clothing.

The consultant haematologist must hold a licence issued by the Administration of Radioactive Substances Advisory Committee to be able to administer radioactive substances to patients. If members of laboratory staff administer radioactive substances on behalf of the licence-holder, they must have a letter of authorization from the holder, as well as the knowledge necessary to deal with a spill of radioactive substance. They must hold an appropriate Ionising Regulations (1988) POPUMET (protection of persons undergoing medical examination or treatment) certificate or equivalent.

Appendix 6.1: Decontamination procedures

Training must be provided in all relevant decontamination procedures (Health Services Advisory Committee, 1991). Five principal situations arise in haematology.

1 Breakage/spillage of specimens

The area of spillage, including any broken container should be flooded with appropriate disinfectant. The area is left undisturbed for 10 minutes prior to mopping with excess cotton wool or absorbent paper. Appropriate protective clothing should be worn during the procedure. If a dustpan, brush or forceps is used, it will require disinfection.

2 Breakage within centrifuge

If breakage is suspected during centrifuge operation, the motor must be switched off and the lid kept closed for 30 minutes. If breakage is discovered on opening the lid, it should be closed immediately and left for 30 minutes. Disposable gloves must be worn. Forceps or cotton wool held in forceps must be used to pick up glass debris. All broken tubes, glass fragments, buckets, trunnions and the rotor must be placed overnight in disinfectant. The centrifuge bowl must then be swabbed with disinfectant, left for 30 minutes and then reswabbed, washed with water and dried. Swabs must be dealt with appropriately.

3 Chemical spillage

To deal with chemical spills two considerations apply. The first is to contain the spills safely and the second is to employ methods and precautions to deal with the specific hazard generated. Hazards generated may include explosion, fire or toxicity. A wall chart showing how to manage chemical spillage should be prominently displayed. Protective clothing (gloves, apron, boots and safety goggles) must be worn. If the amount spilled is small, dilution with water or a dispersing agent, e.g. detergent, will suffice. Spill control bags should be available for larger spills. These are effective for general chemicals, including corrosives. They can then be swept into a plastic bag for disposal. No attempt must be made to wash down spills of carcinogenic material until the bulk of the chemical has been treated as above.

Many common laboratory chemicals interact when allowed to come into contact. Such incompatibilities must be documented, e.g. cyanides with acids or alkalis, or sodium azide with lead, copper or other metals. The preparation of documentation following COSHH Regulations will be of assistance. The toxic effects of organic solvents represent a special case. In some instances these effects may have no obvious detrimental effect, but may cause lack of coordination or drowsiness leading to increased accident-proneness.

4 Decontamination of instruments

In the first instance, a local risk assessment must be made. Certain items of equipment can cause splashing or spillage during normal operation (e.g. centrifuges and certain types of analyser). These must be decontaminated after each period of routine use, according to a written protocol. Instrument manufacturers have a responsibility under the Health and Safety Act (1974) to provide detailed instruction for the safe use, decontamination and cleaning of their equipment. Where splashing or droplet dispersion cannot be avoided, effective barriers must be provided to safeguard the operator. The surrounding area must be regularly disinfected and cleaned.

Service staff must be fully aware of all risks associated with working in the laboratory and any equipment which they have to work on. Guidance is given in *Decontamination of Equipment Prior to Inspection, Service or Repair* (HSG(93)26) (HSG, 1993).

Care must be taken not to mix instrument diluents with hypochlorite, since they may react together to produce chlorine gas. This reaction inactivates the disinfectant, rendering it ineffective. Any instrument effluent must either be trapped in bottles containing a suitable disinfectant or discharged directly into the waste-water plumbing system. The discharge must flow freely through the waste-pipe whilst the instrument is working. At the end of the day, the drain should be flushed with disinfectant so that the trap retains an effective concentration overnight.

5 Radioactive spills

The RPS must be informed immediately. Procedural priorities are as follows:

1   protection of other personnel;
2   confinement of contamination;
3   decontamination of personnel;
4   decontamination of the area involved.

All non-contaminated staff must be evacuated and re-entry forbidden.

To decontaminate affected skin, the area must be washed thoroughly with soap and water, taking great care not to damage the skin. Detergents and abrasive materials must not be used.

To decontaminate cuts or eye splashes, irrigate with water, taking care to prevent spread of contamination from one area to another. Contaminated garments should be removed immediately and placed in a container and should not be removed from the room until the contamination has been monitored. Any surplus liquid must be mopped up with absorbent tissues and then the area washed with detergent and water. All contaminated materials must be placed in a separate, appropriately labelled container and retained until monitored. Entry to the area must be restricted until contamination monitoring has been carried out and the radiation level measured.

In the UK there is a statutory requirement that radionuclides only be used under the direction of an authorized person and that the doses must not exceed the limits defined by the ICRP (1991). The hazard for the external environment is negligible in view of the small quantities of isotope used. The greatest danger arises from accidental contamination of persons, work area or equipment. To obviate the danger of undetected contamination, monitoring devices and procedures capable of detecting contamination of work areas, sinks and drains must be available.

Appendix 6.2: Disinfection/disinfectants

In a microbiological context, decontamination is a general term for removal of microbial contamination, thus rendering an item safe, and includes methods of cleaning, disinfection and sterilization.

Disinfection is the process which reduces the number of micro-organisms on an item to a level which makes handling safe but does not destroy or remove all, e.g. bacterial spores. Sterilization is the complete destruction or removal of micro-organisms, including the most resistant bacterial endospores, to a particular level (sterility assurance level (SAL)). In all cases, thorough cleaning must precede disinfection. Laboratory workers undertaking the cleaning procedure must wear suitable protective clothing, including household-quality gloves. Where instruments are involved, manufacturers' instructions must be consulted on compatibility of construction materials with the method of disinfection. Chemical disinfection is the method most frequently employed in the haematology laboratory. The use of chemical agents is restricted by many factors, including:

1 variable effects on different micro-organisms;
2 incompatibility with various surface finishes, including corrosive properties;
3 reduced efficacy due to the presence of organic matter;
4 deterioration on storage post-activation;
5 toxicity to the operator.

Effective disinfection depends on three main factors:

1 activity, which refers to the range of micro-organisms against which the disinfectant is active;
2 adequate contact must be ensured to enable the disinfectant to be effective;
3 adequate time must be allowed for the disinfectant to perform its function.

Adequate labelling must be supplied by the manufacturer. Disinfectants must be used according to the manufacturer's instructions. Use of all disinfectants must be described in SOPs.

Types of disinfectants in use include:

1 Hypochlorites:
   (a) generally effective against vegetative bacteria, bacterial spores, lipid and non-lipid viruses;
   (b) may corrode metal and damage rubber;
   (c) compatible with ionic and non-ionic detergents;
   (d) in use dilutions: (i) 10 000 p.p.m. free chlorine – general cleaning of equipment and benches; (ii) 2500 p.p.m. free chlorine – discard containers; and (iii) 1000 p.p.m. free chlorine – spillages.
   NB Stability limited; working solutions must be changed frequently.
2 Clear soluble phenolics:
   (a) generally effective against vegetative bacteria, tubercle bacillus, fungi, lipid viruses and some non-lipid viruses;
   (b) inactivated by organic materials, rubber and certain plastics;
   (c) compatible with ionic and non-ionic detergents and metals;
   (d) in-use dilution: in accordance with the manufacturer's instructions; do not store diluted.

3   Alcohols:

(a) effective against bacteria, lipid and non-lipid viruses;

(b) ineffective in presence of organic material;

(c) flammable;

(d) in-use dilution: 70–80% v/v solution in water.

4   Aldehydes:

(a) effective against vegetative bacteria, bacterial spores, fungi, lipid and non-lipid viruses;

(b) formaldehyde is used to fumigate safety cabinets and rooms, while glutaraldehyde has been used widely for many years; occupational exposure limits have now been set for both (see HSE Guidance Note HE 40, *Occupational Exposure Limits*) (HSE, 1990).

5   Surface-active detergents: very limited use against vegetative bacteria.

The following precautions must be taken by persons handling disinfectants:

1   Heavy-duty domestic gloves must be worn.

2   Safety spectacles and disposable plastic aprons must be worn when handling strong disinfectants, especially when dilutions are being prepared from concentrated stock.

3   Some disinfectants emit corrosive and/or toxic vapours and are subject to occupational exposure limits; always check for this before introducing disinfectants into the laboratory.

References

ACDP (1984) *Categorization of Pathogens According to Hazard and Categories for Containment.* HMSO, London.

British Standards Institution (1979) *Specifications for Microbiological Safety Cabinets.* BS5726. HMSO, London.

Control of Substances Hazardous to Health Regulations (1988) SI 1988 No. 1657. HMSO, London.

Department of Trade and Industry (1987) *Guide to the Consumer's Protection Act 1987. Product Liability and Safety Provision.* HMSO, London.

DHSS/ACDP (1990) *HIV – the Causative Agent of AIDS and Related Conditions.* 2nd Revision of guidelines. HMSO, London.

DHSS/Welsh Office (1982a) *Fire Safety in Health Care Premises – Fire Alarms and Detection Systems.* HTM82. HMSO, London.

DHSS/Welsh Office (1982b) *Fire Safety in Health Care Premises – General Fire Precautions.* HTM83. HMSO, London.

DHSS/Welsh Office (1987) *Fire Precautions in New Hospitals.* HTM81. HMSO, London.

Health and Safety Commission (1975) *Health and Safety at Work Act 1974. Advice to Employees (HSC3).* HMSO, London.

Health Services Advisory Committee (1991) *Safe Working and the Prevention of Infection in Clinical Laboratories.* HMSO, London.

International Commission on Radiological Protection (1991) *Recommendations of ICRP – a Summary.* Publication No. 62. Pergamon Press, Oxford.

HSE (1989) *Memorandum of Guidance on the Electricity at Work Regulations.* HMSO, London.

HSE (1990) *Occupational Exposure Limits.* Guidance Note HE40. Revised annually. HMSO, London.

HSG (1993) *Health and Safety Guidance (HSG(93)26). Decontamination of Equipment Prior to Inspection, Service or Repair.* HSE Books, Sudbury, Suffolk.

Ionising Regulations (Protection of Persons Undergoing Medical Examination or Treatment) (1988) HMSO, London.

7 Protocol for Establishing Haematological Reference Values

1 Introduction

The traditional method for assessing the significance of a test result is by comparison with 'normal values'. This will, as a rule, take into account age and sex. In contrast, 'reference values' provide comparison between the individual patients and a population with essentially the same characteristics, e.g. a hospital patient population or a population living in a particular environment.

The principle is that reference individuals constitute the reference population, from which is selected a reference sample group (RSG), on which are determined reference values, which provide a reference distribution, from which are calculated reference limits, which define the reference interval.

The theory of reference values and the procedures for obtaining them have been described in a series of publications of recommendations by the International Council for Standardization in Haematology (ICSH), in collaboration with the International Federation of Clinical Chemistry (IFCC) (ICSH/IFCC, 1982, 1987a,b,c).

2 Selection of a reference sample group

2.1 Criteria for selection

Group 1 consists of a healthy population, e.g. first-time blood donors, students, industrial workers, infants, children, pregnant women or old people. For most of the subgroups, outpatient sessions or other arrangements are usually available at which blood collection is possible.

Group 2 consists of patients with specific diseases, e.g. sickle-cell anaemia, thalassaemia, hypertension or diabetes.

Group 3 consists of the total hospital-patient population. It may include a small proportion of patients with specific diseases, provided that they do not bias the overall distribution disproportionately.

2.2 Description of the reference sample group
It is essential to obtain sufficient data to have an accurate description of the RSG. For each subject, information must be given about age, sex, ethnic origin, geographical area, socio-economic status, and whether a smoker now or previously (give details).

2.3 State of health
Each 'known disease' must be specified. It is important to have information about the nutritional status (height, weight, serum protein concentration, if available), erythrocyte sedimentation rate (ESR) and serum ferritin.

2.4 Size of the reference sample group
The minimum number of individuals in a group depends on whether the data clearly fit a specified type of distribution (Gaussian or log-normal) or are non-parametric, when no *a priori* assumptions can be made about the type of distribution. In the former case, 40 measurements will suffice to determine the 95 percentile (2 standard deviations (SD)) reference interval. For calculation of the reference limits, a large number of measurements, at least 120, are necessary, but knowing the reference interval period from the smaller number will suffice for clinical use.

3 Specimen collection

Venous blood is normally required. If capillary blood is used, this must be noted. The procedure to be followed should conform to the ICSH recommendations with regard to type of container, anticoagulant, needle and use of tourniquet. The blood samples should be collected after a night's rest in a fasting subject, or after at least 15 minutes' rest in a fasting ambulant subject. When these criteria are not met, specification should be given to:
- hospitalization or ambulant status;
- food intake and alcohol during the 12 hours before collection;
- exercise previous to the venepuncture;
- time of collection.

4 Test procedure

The record should indicate:
- type of instrument or system used;
- time lapse and conditions of storage between sample collection and analysis;
- method of calibration and quality control procedures;

- deviation index in current National External Quality Assessment Scheme (NEQAS) surveys.

5 Analysis of results

Before carrying out the above analysis, it is necessary to check for any systematic difference between males and females and determine separate reference intervals, if necessary.

   If the data fit a Gaussian distribution, calculate the arithmetic mean (x) and SD. If there is any question about the Gaussian fit, plot a frequency histogram. Taking the modal value and the calculated SD as reference points, superimpose a Gaussian curve. From this curve, practical reference limits can be determined, even if the original histogram outlines results from some subjects not belonging to the normal population. Calculate limits representing the 95% range (reference interval) from the arithmetic mean $\pm 2\,SD$. Where there is a skewed (log-normal) distribution of measurements, the range of $-2\,SD$ may extend below zero. To avoid this, convert the data to their logarithms by means of log tables or a calculator with the appropriate facility. Calculate the mean and SD in the usual way; then convert the figures to their antilogs to express the data in the original scale.

References

ICSH/IFCC (1982) Standardisation of blood specimen collection procedure for reference values. *Clinical and Laboratory Haematology* **4**, 83–86.

ICSH/IFCC (1987a) The concept of reference values. *Journal of Clinical Chemistry and Clinical Biochemistry* **25**, 337–342.

ICSH/IFCC (1987b) Statistical treatment of collected reference values: determination of reference limits. *Journal of Clinical Chemistry and Clinical Biochemistry* **25**, 645–656.

ICSH/IFCC (1987c) Presentation of observed values related to reference values. *Journal of Clinical Chemistry and Clinical Biochemistry* **25**, 657–662.

Part 2
Guidelines

8 Investigation and Diagnosis of Cobalamin and Folate Deficiencies*
Prepared by the
General Haematology Task Force

1 Introduction

The investigation of a patient for cobalamin (cbl) or folate deficiency involves the demonstration of tissue deficiency, delineation of the particular deficiency and establishment of the cause of the deficiency. Tests should be undertaken with a clear objective, which is usually to determine whether clinical or laboratory features are due to deficiency of either vitamin† or, less frequently, to exclude deficiency as their cause. At one time, deficiency was synonymous with macrocytic anaemia, but it is now recognized that many patients with pernicious anaemia (PA), the best example of these deficiencies, may present without either anaemia or macrocytosis, which are late signs of the disease process. In most cases, however, the marrow will show megaloblastic change.

2 Indications for investigation

The tests need to be restricted to avoid unnecessary investigation of unaffected individuals but to be applied broadly enough to include all patients with a clinical state or laboratory abnormality which may be associated with vitamin deficiency. The clinical indications are of prime importance since routine screening tests, such as the blood count, are not always abnormal. The same criteria apply to both sexes and to all age-groups, including preterm infants and children.

2.1 Clinical criteria
The clinical features may indicate which vitamin deficiency is the more likely, although in most circumstances both will need to be assessed.

  1 Gastrointestinal disease, including glossitis, abnormalities of taste, previous surgery or radiotherapy to the stomach or small bowel, malabsorption or

* Reprinted with permission from *Clinical and Laboratory Haematology*, 1994, **16**, 101–115.
† In this chapter, the word 'vitamin' refers solely to cobalamins and folates.

unexplained diarrhoea. In infants, recurrent vomiting with failure to thrive.

2 Neurological disease, including peripheral neuropathy, evidence of possible demyelinating disease of the spinal cord and visual loss.

3 Psychiatric disorders, including dementia, mental impairment with decreased initiative and concentration, confusion and alterations in mood, depression.

4 Malnutrition, including growth impairment in children and those on restricted diets (e.g. vegans).

5 Alcohol abuse, which may be combined with dietary neglect and malnutrition.

6 Autoimmune disease of the thyroid, adrenal and parathyroid glands; hypogammaglobulinaemia.

7 Family history of PA or of inherited disorders of cbl and folate metabolism; the family history should include non-immediate relatives.

8 Infertility, when anatomical causes have been excluded.

9 Haematological disease known to be associated with vitamin deficiency — chronic haemolytic anaemias, myelofibrosis, myelomatosis.

10 Drug therapy known to interfere with vitamin absorption or metabolism, including nitrous oxide, phenytoin and other anticonvulsants, and dihydrofolate reductase inhibitors, e.g. methotrexate, trimethoprim and pyrimethamine.

11 In infants, a possibility of inherited metabolic disease.

The initial investigation of possible vitamin deficiency in these groups of patients should always include a blood count and blood film examination.

2.2 Laboratory criteria

1 Macrocytosis is the most common reason for initiating investigation, although vitamin deficiency is not the most common cause of a macrocytosis. Macrocytosis without known cause warrants a blood film examination.

2 Blood film abnormalities. The morphological features of vitamin deficiency, oval macrocytes and neutrophil hypersegmentation, are not always present or easy to detect. Vitamin deficiency may present without macrocytosis, particularly when there is concomitant iron deficiency or thalassaemia trait. There may be a dimorphic red cell population and macrocytosis may only become manifest when iron deficiency has been corrected. Neutrophil hypersegmentation is not specific for vitamin deficiency, being seen in renal failure, iron deficiency and myelodysplasia and as a congenital abnormality. In addition, it is not present in every patient with vitamin deficiency; its absence is especially to be noted in patients who are seriously ill and neutropenic.

3 Unexplained anaemia always demands a blood film examination. The blood film abnormalities mentioned above would be indications for further investigation.

4 Cytopenias. Severe megaloblastic anaemia, for whatever reason, may be associated with thrombocytopenia or neutropenia. Patients with acute folate deficiency may present with thrombocytopenia or pancytopenia. This may arise in late pregnancy or the puerperium, precipitated by an intercurrent infection, in critically ill patients and in patients with borderline folate stores treated with antifolate drugs. Failure of the platelet count to recover as expected following bone marrow transplantation may also be due to unsuspected vitamin deficiency. Neutropenia can be a dominant feature of cbl disorders in the neonate.

3 Investigations

Essential investigations are a blood count and blood film examination, serum cbl, serum and red cell folate assays and assessment of the response to treatment. Bone marrow aspiration is always of value.

Subsidiary investigations, which may be particularly useful in specific circumstances, include the deoxyuridine suppression test (DUST), estimation of methylmalonic acid (MMA) in serum or urine and of homocysteine (Hcy) in serum and assay of cbl and folate coenzymes.

3.1 Bone marrow examination

Bone marrow examination is always of value to confirm tissue deficiency or to indicate an alternative diagnosis. It is essential when the results of other tests are equivocal, e.g. borderline mean corpuscular volume (MCV) or assays. The recognition of mild megaloblastic change is critically dependent on having well-spread films with good-quality fixation and staining. Megaloblastic change may be completely or partially masked by concomitant iron deficiency.

3.2 The assay of cobalamin and folate

The assay of the vitamins in blood is the current routine procedure for determining the patient's vitamin status (Dawson *et al.*, 1991). Microbiological assays remain the yardstick against which alternative methods should be compared. Although perhaps more technically demanding, they are particularly suitable for the economic processing of large numbers of samples, especially by automated and microplate techniques (O'Broin & Kelleher, 1992). The use of β-lactamase (Kelleher *et al.*, 1990) overcomes some of the difficulties created by antibiotic therapy but not those due to antifolates.

Radioisotope dilution assays (RDAs) are in common use and commercial kits have made the assays available to all laboratories with access to the appropriate equipment. They are generally satisfactory. Radioimmune and enzyme-linked immunosorbent assay (ELISA) methods have been described but have not yet been subjected to an assessment which would allow recommendation for routine use at present. Failure to follow the manufacturer's instructions, when a laboratory uses a commercial kit, may absolve the manufacturer of any product liability.

Whichever assay is used, the haematologist should follow the code of practice of the Royal College of Pathologists (1989) and the haematology laboratory management practice of the British Committee for Standards in Haematology (BCSH) (see pp. 41–50). The accuracy, precision, compatibility with other procedures, acceptability by the user and cost of the chosen method should be known. External quality assessment schemes give some guidance to the relative technical performance of the methods in current use. The accuracy of the assays can also be checked by means of cbl standards. The National Institute of Biological Standards and Control* (NIBSC) currently holds and will make available the World Health Organization (WHO) international standard for vitamin B_{12}. A secondary UK cbl standard is available from the same source. In regard to accuracy, the overall median or mean of cbl assays from a large number of participants in external quality assessment schemes is close to the true result. This is not the case with folate assays; kit results vary, particularly for red cell assays, although most give results of clinical value when compared against the appropriate reference interval for the particular kit.

Variations in the preparation and storage of the haemolysate for red cell folate assay are the main causes of different values obtained by different kits (Gilois *et al.*, 1990). It is important that any kit user follows the manufacturer's instructions exactly and has satisfied him/herself that the reference interval he/she uses is appropriate for that technique.

The precision of most RDAs at normal levels is good and the need for assay in duplicate should be considered. The code of practice (Royal College of Pathologists, 1989) indicates that singleton assays are permissible provided that some samples are done in duplicate to check on current precision. The in-batch precision quoted by most manufacturers is based, however, upon the repeated assay of samples at only a few concentrations. This does not guarantee that a similar precision is attainable for samples tested in duplicate over a wide range of concentrations. The duplicate results from a number of batches should be reviewed to see whether any fall outside a decision level, e.g. a coefficient of variation of 10% at the lower end of the reference interval, before contemplating the introduction of singleton assays.

To ensure satisfactory quality, a certain minimal number of control samples should be included – samples of known analyte concentration at a normal level, at the lower end of the reference interval and at a subnormal level – and three or more samples from the previous batch, which should, with the standards, always be done in duplicate.

Samples giving results within ±20% of the lower end of the reference interval,

---

*National Institute for Biological Standards and Control, Blanche Lane, South Mimms, Potter's Bar, Hertfordshire EN6 3QG, UK.

an 'indeterminate' level in regard to decision-making, should be repeated in the next batch.

The frequency of assay depends upon the number for suitable batching but should be at least weekly. Although some reagents in a kit may be stored after opening, it is generally better not to do this. A laboratory having few requests should consider sending specimens elsewhere. Such a practice could result in some delay in reporting, although this is unlikely to be clinically important.

Performance in the National External Quality Assessment Scheme (NEQAS) is deemed satisfactory when results fall within 20% of the method mean. The participant needs to check whether he/she is following the method protocol exactly when results fall regularly outside this limit. A laboratory may, when it differs from others using the same system, consider itself to be 'right' and the rest 'wrong' but in this situation its clinical interpretation of the results must be correct.

Kits do not differ greatly in regard to their cost. The larger ones are cheaper per patient sample, and dual systems, measuring serum cbl and serum folate at the same time, are even more cost-effective. The most useful pair of assays, the serum cbl and the red cell folate, cannot be carried out by a dual system.

3.2.1 Interpretation of assays – serum cobalamin

A result below the lower limit of the reference interval may be due to deficiency or to alterations in cbl metabolism or be normal. As reference intervals are usually based upon 2 standard deviations (SD) spread around the mean or median of the population, there will inevitably be some normal persons with a serum cbl outside the reference interval.

The serum level in deficiency is related to the degree of tissue depletion, with the lowest levels in the most severely affected. Very low levels are seen in some inherited disorders and in PA, although PA may present at any reduced level of serum cbl. The clinical significance of a mildly reduced serum cbl may be difficult to determine but, if the assay request is based upon sound clinical or laboratory grounds, any low level cannot be ignored and investigation to find a cause should be pursued.

Patients with cbl deficiency may occasionally present with a normal serum cbl. This may occur in the presence of liver disease or of myeloproliferative disorders, after nitrous oxide anaesthesia, with a marked neutrophil leucocytosis and, most importantly, in transcobalamin II (TCII) deficiency and in some other inherited disorders of cbl metabolism.

Disturbances in cbl metabolism, with a reduced serum cbl not associated with tissue cbl deficiency, occur commonly in folate deficiency and pregnancy and in myelomatosis and TCI deficiency.

3.2.2 Interpretation of assays – serum and red cell folate

A low serum folate may indicate deficiency, although a subnormal level is common in hospitalized patients due to negative folate balance. The lower the level, the more likely there is to be deficiency. A low level, without deficiency, may occur occasionally in cbl deficiency and with recent ethanol ingestion. Antibiotic therapy is a common cause of falsely low levels with microbiological assays.

A low red cell folate usually indicates tissue deficiency and is of greater significance than a low serum level in the diagnosis of depletion. A low red cell folate without deficiency is common in cbl deficiency. A normal level in the presence of deficiency can occur with acute folate deficiency, in patients with a reticulocytosis and following a blood transfusion.

In a small proportion of patients with vitamin deficiency, all assay results are low. This may be due to combined deficiency but more commonly to the metabolic effect of a lack of one vitamin upon the other. The degree of change of each assay result usually indicates the primary defect. With cbl deficiency the serum and red cell folate are not as low as in folate deficiency and with folate deficiency the cbl level is not as affected as the folate levels and infrequently reaches the very low levels which may be seen in PA.

3.3 Response to treatment

Not only does response to treatment confirm the diagnosis but failure to respond, partially or completely, may indicate the presence of complicating pathology, e.g. infection, hypothyroidism, iron deficiency or myelodysplasia. For this reason, only one haematinic should be given at any one time, except when the patient is seriously ill and the results of serum assays or a DUST are not available.

In severely anaemic patients, the clinical and reticulocyte responses confirm vitamin deficiency. Clinical response in the more difficult case is often subjective, and significant changes in the red cell count (an increase of 6% or more) and MCV (a decrease of at least 5 fl), together with correction of neutrophil hypersegmentation, are required. Such red cell changes may not occur if the initial blood count is normal or if the clinical picture is complicated by iron deficiency or thalassaemia trait.

Additional tests, such as the DUST, estimation of cbl and folate metabolites or TCII saturation, may be performed to confirm or indicate the likelihood of vitamin deficiency. The results may be abnormal when serum assays are normal. Assays of cbl and folate coenzymes, fibroblast culture and TC estimation are required in the investigation of the rare inherited disorders of cbl and folate metabolism.

3.4 The deoxyuridine suppression test

This test is a sensitive indicator that megaloblastosis is the result of impaired thymidine synthesis due to deficiency or metabolic inactivation of either cbl or folate (Wickramasinghe & Matthews, 1988). It is of use in confirming the presence of mild deficiency when morphological changes are equivocal, although the test is normal in a small proportion of patients with vitamin deficiency. The degree of abnormality correlates inversely with the patient's red cell count.

The addition of either folic acid or 5-formyltetrahydrofolic acid corrects the defect. The addition of cbl is less uniform; it sometimes fails to correct in cbl deficiency and may correct in folate deficiency.

The DUST should be carried out in a laboratory with experience in the technique and one which has determined its own reference range, because minor technical variations can affect the result. It should be carried out on marrow and not on peripheral blood lymphocytes. The test should be set up as soon as possible after bone marrow aspiration; even a short delay may lead to a reduction towards normal in an abnormal DUST value. It is an expensive and time-consuming test.

3.4.1 Interpretation of results
Despite variations in technique, most laboratories report normal results to be suppression of the incorporation of tritiated thymidine to less than 10% on the addition of deoxyuridine. The significance of correction with added vitamins depends upon the precision of the technique used; usually a correction of 15% or more of the initial DUST value is significant.

3.5 Methylmalonic acid and homocysteine
The serum levels of two metabolites, MMA and Hcy, are increased in patients with cbl deficiency, while in patients with folate deficiency Hcy alone is elevated. In cbl deficiency, serum Hcy rises before MMA and provides a more sensitive though less specific index of deficiency. The serum level of MMA may rise dramatically in cbl deficiency and, when measured by a sensitive technique, is now considered by many to be a more reliable indicator of cbl status than the serum cbl assay.

Measurement of urinary MMA in a random sample is a useful screening test. Estimation of 24-hour urinary excretion of MMA (Norman *et al.*, 1982) is more sensitive and may be as valuable as a serum assay and possibly of greater specificity, since the serum MMA fluctuates in patients with renal failure. However, urinary MMA also rises in Fanconi's syndrome and other amino acidurias, and an advantage over urinary assays is that serum cbl and MMA, together with other metabolites if appropriate, can be measured on the one sample.

The preferred method depends on the purpose of the assay, whether for diagnosis or for monitoring progress. Cost and availability of equipment will also influence choice. Capillary gas chromatography–mass spectrometry (GC–MS) permits a definite identification of compounds but is an expensive technique unlikely to be available in any but specialist units. Thin-layer chromatography (TLC) is excellent for urinary MMA screening, is inexpensive yet sensitive and should be readily available to the haematologist in any district general hospital. A recommended method is given in the appendix.

3.5.1 Reference intervals (for most methods)
These are as follows: serum MMA, 100–750 nmol/l; urine MMA, 1.0–4.0 nmol/l (5 µg/mg creatinine); serum Hcy, 6–29 µmol/l.

3.6 Transcobalamin II saturation
The saturation of TCII with cbl decreases early in cbl deficiency. A cbl assay method of good sensitivity is required because of the small amounts of cbl which may be bound by TCII. As a diagnostic tool, this estimation is open to more error than a single cbl assay.

3.7 Cobalamin coenzymes
When inherited disorders are under consideration, assay of cbl coenzymes is essential. A specific radioisotopic assay for plasma adenosylcobalamin has been described which requires high-specific-activity ^{57}Co-adenosylcobalamin. Thin-layer chromatography, coupled with a microbiological plate assay (bioautography), has the advantage of estimating methylcobalamin at the same time. This method may also be used to confirm normal synthesis of cbl coenzymes by detecting the urinary excretion of both methylcobalamin and adenosylcobalamin following treatment with hydroxocobalamin in neonates and adults.

3.8 Folate coenzymes
Folate species can be measured semiquantitatively by bioautography or by differential microbiological assays, methods rarely applied today. 5-Methyl tetrahydrofolic acid in plasma and red cells can be measured fluorometrically or electrochemically after separation by high-performance liquid chromatography (HPLC), an estimation of value in the investigation of inherited disorders of folate metabolism when used in conjunction with measurement of total folate.

3.9 Fibroblast studies
Fibroblasts should be cultured in the investigation of any case in which a genetic error of cbl or folate metabolism is suspected. A sterile full-depth skin biopsy should be taken into a rich culture medium for urgent transport to an appropriate centre for specific enzyme and coenzyme analysis. Fibroblast complementation is required to establish the exact nature of the metabolic error.

3.10 Interpretation of results
The interpretation of each investigation has been considered individually above.

In practice, the results of all investigations should be considered together and in the light of the clinical picture. In this way, allowance is made for the relative significance and specificity of each finding, the quality control of each test is enhanced and there are potential benefits for both clinical and laboratory audit.

3.11 Megaloblastic anaemia in infancy

Severe megaloblastic anaemia in infancy demands urgent investigation and treatment (Cooper *et al.*, 1992). Prior to treatment, a blood count, blood film examination, serum cbl and serum and red cell folate assays should be performed in the mother and child, and the child's serum should be stored for later estimation of TCII if appropriate. A 24-hour collection of urine for MMA, Hcy and protein should be completed and marrow aspirated to confirm the diagnosis, with a DUST if possible (Chanarin, 1983).

4 Investigation of the cause of cobalamin deficiency

Pernicious anaemia is the most important disease to diagnose or exclude. The demonstration of serum intrinsic factor (IF) antibodies (IFAs) or malabsorption of free cbl which is improved or corrected by added IF is required to make the diagnosis.

4.1 Intrinsic factor antibodies

The presence of IFAs in the serum of a patient with evidence of cbl deficiency is indicative of PA, despite their occasional occurrence in other autoimmune disorders (e.g. thyroid disorders, diabetes mellitus, myasthenia gravis). They are found in 50–75% of patients with PA, the incidence depending upon the sensitivity of the test used and the duration of the disease. They are present in 90% of children with the juvenile form but are absent in the congenital type of the disease. Their detection obviates the need for an absorption test in nearly all patients.

Two types of IFA have been detected in the sera of patients with PA; type I prevents the attachment of cbl to IF and type II prevents the attachment of IF or the IF–cbl complex to ileal receptors.

The standard tests depend upon the inhibition by type I antibody of the attachment of isotope-labelled cbl to IF. The sensitivity of the technique depends upon the relative antigen and antibody concentrations and is limited by the effect of TCs in the test and control sera. It can be improved by prior treatment of the sera to remove TCII (Nimo & Carmel, 1987). Free cbl in the serum following a recent injection can give false positive results with some techniques and in general should be avoided. A method using ^{125}I-labelled IF (Conn, 1986) is more sensitive than the standard test. An advantage of this method and of ELISA methods is that they detect both types of antibody.

4.2 Cobalamin absorption

Cobalamin absorption is initially assessed using free cbl, repeating an abnormal test with added IF. Normal absorption of free cbl does not exclude cbl deficiency due to malabsorption and, if dietary intake is satisfactory, a food cbl absorption test should be considered.

It may be reasonable to delay testing until the patient has been treated, since cbl and folate deficiency can affect the bowel mucosa. Correction of the bowel lesion may take up to 2 months. However, if the patient is in hospital, it can be an advantage to proceed with the test during admission. Absorption tests involving the use of radioactive isotopes must not be carried out on women who are, or might be, pregnant.

Free cbl absorption can be assessed by a number of procedures.

4.2.1 The Schilling test

This is the most commonly used and the indirect one recommended by the International Council for Standardization in Haematology (ICSH, 1981). The urinary excretion of an oral dose of radioactive cbl is determined. Points to note are:

1 A preliminary 12-hour collection is advocated by ICSH so that other isotopes which the patient may have received can be detected and allowed for. This is unnecessary if the management of the patient is precisely known.

2 A standard oral dose of radioactive cbl should be used in adults. The conventional dose of labelled cyanocobalamin is 1 µg. For children, 0.5–1.0 µg is generally used.

3 The most usual cause of incorrect results is incomplete urine collection. This produces falsely low results. Because the test requires a cooperative and understanding patient, it is preferable for outpatients to attend the haematology department or a day ward so that the procedure may be explained by someone familiar with it.

4 For patients with renal failure, the urine collection should be extended to 48 hours and a second 'flushing' injection given at 24 hours. An alternative test, such as the plasma uptake test, is preferable.

5 The 'flushing' subcutaneous or intramuscular injection can be of hydroxocobalamin and this can be given at the same time as the test dose is drunk.

6 Patients on cbl therapy can have the test carried out 24 hours or more after the last injection.

7 Another test can be carried out 24 hours or more after the previous one.

8 The IF should be mixed vigorously with the aqueous cbl just before administration.

A 'dual' test, the simultaneous administration of ^{58}Co-cbl and ^{57}Co-cbl bound to IF, has the advantage that the ratio of the excretions shows the effect of IF on cbl absorption, regardless of the adequacy of urine collection. An abnormal result indicates a deficiency of IF. However, partly because there is interchange of the isotopes bound to IF, dual tests cannot be relied upon to give a true estimate of the absorption of free cbl.

Interpretation of results
Normal is >10% of a 1-µg dose excreted in the urine (>11% when the flushing injection is hydroxocobalamin). In PA or intestinal disease, it is usually <5%. The addition of IF in PA should correct the result, or at least improve the excretion by >25% of the original value. In atrophic gastritis with a low serum cbl, it is often 5–9% but may be normal.

4.2.2 Other free cobalamin absorption tests
Other tests of the absorption of free cbl are:
1 The whole-body retention test, which is the ICSH-recommended direct method (ICSH, 1981). It is sensitive and reproducible and the best absorption test if the equipment is available.
2 The plasma uptake test (McIntyre & Wagner, 1966), which should be performed with the Schilling test. The result is helpful when there is doubt about the completeness of the urine collection.
3 The spot-faeces test (Hjelt *et al.*, 1977), which overcomes the inconvenience of total stool collection.

An abnormal test by any method should be repeated with added IF. Failure to correct with IF may be due to ileal disease or resection, bacterial overgrowth (repeat after a 7-day course of an oral broad-spectrum antibiotic, e.g. oxytetracycline), pancreatic exocrine insufficiency (repeat with pancreatic enzymes), drugs (para-aminosalicylic acid, colchicine, neomycin, anticonvulsants, potassium salts, metformin, phenformin), Zollinger–Ellison syndrome (repeat with bicarbonate), TCII deficiency and inactive or inadequate amounts of IF (check activity of IF *in vitro*, repeat with increased amount of IF).

4.2.3 Food cobalamin absorption test
This test should be considered when the absorption of free cbl is normal and the dietary intake of cbl is satisfactory (Doscherholmen *et al.*, 1983).

The doses may be made individually or in batches and stored at −20°C. A single dose is prepared by taking 50 g dried powdered egg yolk and reconstituting it with water, adding a 1-µg radioactive dose of cbl, mixing well and cooking this as scrambled egg. This is eaten with tea and one or two rounds of buttered toast. Absorption has been determined from urinary excretion (as in the Schilling test), faecal excretion and whole-body counting. Chicken serum, the more commonly used binder in the UK, is no longer available commercially for human administration.

Interpretation of results
Normal is 4–7% of a 1-µg dose excreted in urine. It is usually <2% when gastric atrophy or resection is associated with cbl deficiency. Although low results have been described in a variety of conditions, and rarely without cause, defective food cbl absorption, with normal free cbl absorption, relates closely to reduced gastric acid secretion.

4.3 Tests of gastric function
Other tests connected with cbl absorption are:
1   Assay of intrinsic factor. This is a direct measurement of the defect in PA and is of value when other investigations have yielded equivocal results or there is a possibility of both a gastric and an intestinal lesion.
2   Parietal cell antibodies. The frequency of these in elderly individuals is such that their presence is of limited value in the differential diagnosis of cbl deficiency. Since they are found in about 90% of patients with PA, their absence would weigh against this diagnosis.
3   Marked changes in the serum gastrin and in the ratio of serum pepsinogen I to II are not specific for PA but at least direct attention to a gastric lesion as a probable factor in cbl deficiency.

4.4 Cobalamin intake
This can be assessed by a questionnaire from the hospital dietitian and by the patient recording his/her food intake over a period of at least 1 week. Particular importance should be given to milk intake. When the precise intake of cbl is in doubt, the patient should be referred to the dietitian. The Food and Agriculture Organization (FAO)/WHO have revised downward the recommended minimum level of cbl intake to 1 µg daily for adults.

4.5 Response to treatment
Patients with a negative IFA in whom an absorption test is not practicable cannot be given an absolute diagnosis. A response to oral cbl, 50 µg daily, including correction of the serum cbl, over a 2-month period, indicates normal absorption of free cbl. If the dietary intake is satisfactory, a presumptive diagnosis of food cbl malabsorption can be made.

4.6 Transcobalamin II deficiency
The diagnosis of this rare, congenital deficiency requires measurement of this

individual binder. This may be done by saturating the serum with ^{57}Co-cbl and separating the binders on a Sephracryl or Sephadex column.

When estimating TCs, collect blood (10 ml) into tubes containing 10 mg disodium ethylenediamine tetra-acetic acid (Na$_2$EDTA) + 20 mg sodium fluoride (NaF) to prevent release of R binders from granulocytes.

5 Investigation of the cause of folate deficiency

5.1 Folate intake
Although there are many causes for folate deficiency, malnutrition is nearly always a significant, if not the only, factor. When malnutrition has been determined to be responsible for the deficiency, the reason for this should be sought. The common causes are ignorance, apathy and poverty.

5.2 Folate absorption
The appropriate tests will depend upon the patient's history and clinical features, but would be expected to include tests of cbl and iron status. A cbl absorption test is usually required and, rarely, a folic acid absorption test in the neonate for congenital folate malabsorption. Radiological and special isotopic tests are often required.

It can be difficult to decide if a patient without intestinal symptoms should be investigated for malabsorption. Gluten enteropathy cannot be excluded without biopsy, may first present at any age and only comes under consideration when malnutrition is superimposed. The increased incidence of malignancy in untreated gluten enteropathy indicates that exclusion of this is necessary in most patients, except perhaps the elderly and those with increased folate requirements – although it is not uncommon for folate deficiency in pregnancy to be the first indication of an underlying enteropathy.

The decision to investigate for malabsorption will also depend upon the severity of malnutrition in the individual and in the local population.

5.3 Response to treatment
The same principles apply as for cbl therapy. Folate deficiency is a common cause of a low serum cbl. If the serum cbl, serum folate and red cell folate assays are all low, but the relative levels favour folate deficiency (see interpretation of assays) and a test to demonstrate metabolic cbl deficiency is not available, it is recommended that the folate deficiency is treated, provided that the patient has no neuropathy and the serum cbl is repeated in 4 weeks' time. A low serum cbl secondary to folate deficiency will rise to normal in this period and the former low level will require no further investigation. The patient will need to be investigated for cbl deficiency if the serum cbl remains low.

Table 8.1 Costs of cobalamin and folate tests in some hospitals, 1992

Test	Cost (£)
Serum cbl assay	7
Serum folate assay	7
Serum cbl and folate dual assay	7
Red cell folate assay	7
Urinary MMA (TLC)	5
Serum MMA (HPLC)	12–15
Serum MMA (gas chromatography/mass spectrometry)	16
Cbl coenzymes (TLC and bioautography)	25
Fibroblast culture and cbl coenzyme analysis	120
IFA	5
Schilling test, each part	27–45

6 Costings

Refer to haematology laboratory management practice (BCSH) (see pp. 41–50) for calculation of the cost of tests. This is a retrospective assessment. A laboratory considering setting up a particular test will obtain some idea of the potential cost from another laboratory, although the figures are affected by volume of work, staff mix, type of equipment, etc. The costs recorded in some hospitals in 1992 are given in Table 8.1.

Appendix 8.1: Screening test for methylmalonic acid in urine (Bhatt *et al.*, 1982)

1 Principle
Methylmalonic acid is separated from other substances by TLC on cellulose, followed by staining with a diazo reagent.

2 Samples
The urine may be from a random sample. It can be stored at $-20°C$ until testing, or merthiolate can be used as preservative.

3 Standards
Dilute a stock solution of 100 mg MMA (Sigma) per 100 ml in 0.5 mol/l hydrochloric acid (HCl) to give standards of 50, 100 and 500 ng/μl. The stock solution is kept at 4°C.

4 Diazo reagent
Dissolve 1 g tetrazotized *o*-dianisidine–zinc complex (Sigma) in 12 ml water (H_2O), mix thoroughly with 3 ml glacial acetic acid and make up to 45 ml with methanol. Prepare in a fume-cupboard and use immediately.

5 Chromatography

Apply samples in 1- and 5-µl and standards in 1.0-µl aliquots by syringe 1.5 cm from the longer edge of a 20 × 10 cm aluminium-backed cellulose thin-layer plate (Merck 5552). Keep the diameter of the point of application as small as possible. Develop by ascending chromatography in *n*-butanol/acetic acid/water (5:1:1, v/v). At 18°C, the solvent rises 8 cm in about 50 minutes, when the plate is removed, oven-dried at 50°C for 3 minutes and cooled in contact with a metal surface. Spray for 10 seconds from a distance of 50 cm with the diazo reagent and reheat at 100°C for 2 minutes.

6 Reading the plate

Only creatinine, malonic acid and authentic MMA are visible. Amounts of MMA greater than 100 mg are present as bright magenta spots within 5 minutes. Lesser amounts can be compared visually after leaving the plate face down on the bench overnight.

7 Interpretation

A 5-µl spot as large as the 50-µl standard is equivalent to 10 mg/l, approximately twice the upper limit of the reference interval. If the spot is of this size or greater, carry out full assay, relating excretion to that of creatinine.

References

Bhatt H.R., Green A. & Linnell J.C. (1982) A sensitive micromethod for the routine estimation of methylmalonic acid in body fluids and tissues using thin layer chromatography. *Clinica Chimica Acta* **118**, 311–321.

Chanarin I. (1983) Management of megaloblastic anaemia in the very young. *British Journal of Haematology* **53**, 1–3.

Conn D.A. (1986) Intrinsic factor antibody detection and quantitation. *Medical and Laboratory Science* **43**, 48–52.

Cooper B.A., Rosenblatt D.S. & Whitehead V.M. (1992) Megaloblastic anaemia. In Nathan D.G. & Oski F.A. (eds) *Haematology of Infancy and Childhood*, 4th edn, pp. 354–390. W.R. Saunders, Philadelphia.

Dawson D.W., Hoffbrand A.V. & Worwood M. (1991) Investigation of megaloblastic and iron-deficiency anaemias. In Dacie J.V. & Lewis S.M. (eds) *Practical Haematology*, 7th edn, pp. 397–420. Churchill Livingstone, Edinburgh.

Doscherholmen A., Silvius S. & McMahon J. (1983) Dual Schilling test for measuring absorption of food-bound and free vitamin B_{12} simultaneously. *American Journal of Clinical Pathology* **80**, 490–495.

Gilois C.R., Stone J., Lai A.P. & Wierbicki A.S. (1990) Effect of haemolysate preparation on measurement of red cell folate by a radioisotopic method. *Journal of Clinical Pathology* **43**, 160–162.

Hjelt K., Munck E., Hippe E. & Bärenholdt D. (1977) Vitamin B_{12} absorption determined with a double isotope technique employing incomplete stool collection. *Acta Medica Scandinavica* **202**, 419–422.

ICSH (1981) Recommended methods for the measurement of vitamin B_{12} absorption. *Journal of Nuclear Medicine* **22**, 1091–1093.

Kelleher B.P., Scott J.M. & O'Broin S.D. (1990) Use of beta-lactamase to hydrolyse interfering antibiotics in vitamin B_{12} microbiological assay using *Lactobacillus leichmanii*. *Clinical and Laboratory Haematology* **12**, 87–95.

McIntyre P.A. & Wagner H.N. (1966) Comparison of the urinary excretion and 6-hour plasma tests for vitamin B_{12} absorption. *Journal of Laboratory and Clinical Medicine* **68**, 966–971.

Nimo R.E. & Carmel R. (1987) Increased sensitivity of detection of the blocking (type 1) anti-intrinsic factor antibody. *American Journal of Clinical Pathology* **88**, 729–733.

Norman E.J., Martelo O.J. & Denton M.D. (1982) Cobalamin (vitamin B_{12}) deficiency detection by urinary methylmalonic acid quantitation. *Blood* **59**, 1128–1131.

O'Broin S.D. & Kelleher B.P. (1992) Microbiological assay on microtitre plates of folate in serum and red cells. *Journal of Clinical Pathology* **45**, 344–347.

Royal College of Pathologists (1989) *Codes of Practice for Pathology Departments*, pp. 4–5. The Chameleon Press Ltd, London.

Wickramasinghe S. & Matthews J.H. (1988) Deoxyuridine suppression: biochemical basis and diagnostic applications. *Blood Reviews* **2**, 168–177.

9 Investigation of the Alpha- and Beta-Thalassaemia Traits*

Prepared by the General Haematology Task Force

1 Introduction

The thalassaemia syndromes are inherited disorders of haemoglobin production, characterized by a reduction in globin chain synthesis, leading to an imbalance of the globin chains. There are many different deoxyribonucleic acid (DNA) mutations leading to these disorders (see Chapter 10), but it is helpful to subdivide them into two groups: α^o and β^o, where no globin is synthesized, and α^+ and β^+, where some, but a reduced amount, of globin is synthesized. Although most individuals have either α or β thalassaemia, these may interact with each other ($\alpha\beta$ thalassaemia), with δ thalassaemia ($\delta\beta$ thalassaemia) and with haemoglobin variants, such as haemoglobin S (HbS), HbE, HbO^{Arab} and Hb Lepore. Although most cases of hereditary persistence of fetal haemoglobin (HPFH) have no clinical or genetic implications, a few are associated with a β-thalassaemia-like phenotype and can occasionally interact with β-thalassaemia trait to produce a β thalassaemia intermedia phenotype. Cases with thalassaemic features may be genetically and phenotypically related to $\delta\beta$ thalassaemia.

Although the carrier states for these conditions are clinically silent, the homozygote and double heterozygote states may have major clinical implications and it is therefore essential to be able to detect and identify the carrier states (shown in Table 9.1). Knowledge of the carrier state can also be useful in explaining hypochromic, microcytic red cell indices.

The thalassaemia disorders are common in people of Mediterranean, Middle Eastern, African, Pakistani, Indian and South-east Asian ancestry, but occur sporadically in all populations. In our increasingly multicultural society, it is becoming important to consider the diagnosis of thalassaemia trait, regardless of the apparent ethnic origin. The universal availability of electronic cell counters provides the haematologist with a simple screening procedure which can be used to select patients for further investigation.

* Reprinted with permission from *Journal of Clinical Pathology*, 1994, **47**, 289–295.

Table 9.1 Alpha and beta thalassaemia

Phenotype	Genotype		MCV	MCH	HbA$_2$	HbH bodies
				Usual		
*Alpha thalassaemia**						
1 α-Thalassaemia trait	−α/αα	α$^+$/α	N	N	N	−
2 α-Thalassaemia trait	−α/−α or −−/αα	α$^+$/α$^+$ or α^o/α	↓	↓	N or ↓	±
3 HbH disease						
Mild	−−/α−	α^o/α$^+$	↓	↓	N or ↓	+++
Severe	−−/αα^T	α^o/α^T	↓	↓	N or ↓	+++
4 Hb Bart's hydrops (α thalassaemia major)	−−/−−	α^o/α^o	↓	↓	−	−
Beta thalassaemia†						
1 β-Thalassaemia trait	β^o/β or β$^+$/β		↓	↓	↑	−
2 δβ-Thalassaemia trait	δβ^o/β		↓	↓	N or ↓	−
3 β-Thalassaemia trait (normal HbA$_2$)	β$^+$/β		↓	↓	N	−
4 Hb Lepore trait	Hb Lepore/β		↓	↓	N	−
5 β-Thalassaemia intermedia	Heterogeneous		↓	↓	↓, N or ↑	−
6 β-Thalassaemia major	β^o/β^o, β^o/β$^+$, β$^+$/β$^+$		↓	↓	↓, N or ↑	−

* There are two pairs of allelic structural genes which code for the α-globin chains and 'classical' α-thalassaemia is due to gene deletion (α−), but non-delectional forms (αα^T) also occur, which may vary in severity, and more than 30 genotypes have been characterized. The following is a classification of α thalassaemia, which indicates two ways of expressing the genotype.
† There is only one pair of allelic genes which codes for the β-globin chains, but there are more than 100 DNA subtypes of β thalassaemia, most of which are non-deletional.
N, normal; −, absent; +, present.

The purpose of these guidelines is to:
1 advise on which people should be tested and on how the diagnosis should be established;
2 document the routine procedures available in most laboratories which are necessary to make the diagnosis (DNA analysis is covered in Chapter 10);
3 provide useful addresses for counselling, haemoglobinopathy cards, etc.

2 Selection of patients to be investigated

Investigation is usually carried out for genetic purposes, that is, to identify individuals at risk of producing offspring with a clinically significant form of thalassaemia (homozygous or doubly heterozygous), such as β thalassaemia major, Hb Bart's hydrops, or HbS β thalassaemia, or for clinical purposes, to establish the cause of microcytosis. The methods of selecting patients for investigation depend on which of these circumstances applies and on whether or not the patient is a pregnant woman.

2.1 Red cell indices and thalassaemia traits

The majority of individuals with thalassaemia traits have a reduced mean corpuscular volume (MCV) (microcytosis) and a reduced mean corpuscular haemoglobin (MCH) in the presence of a normal or near-normal mean corpuscular haemoglobin concentration (MCHC). The haemoglobin concentration is usually normal or only slightly reduced and the red cell count is often raised. Although many individuals with α^+-thalassaemia trait have normal red cell indices (Weatherall & Clegg, 1981; WHO, 1988), with information available at present, it is highly likely that individuals with α°-thalassaemia trait will have an MCH below 26 pg. Rare individuals with β-thalassaemia trait (silent β-thalassaemia trait) may also have normal red cell indices.

Haematologists rely heavily on their automated blood cell counters to select which patients require further investigation for these conditions. Careful attention must therefore be paid to the calibration of the cell counter, and its performance should be satisfactory both by local assessment and in the National External Quality Assessment Scheme. Each laboratory should establish its own reference range for the haemoglobin concentration and the red cell indices. Selection of patients for investigation may then be based on the MCH or the MCV or on various formulae. However, it is still necessary to undertake further testing to distinguish microcytosis due to thalassaemia trait from that associated with iron deficiency, the anaemia of chronic disorders or sideroblastic anaemia, and to identify which type of thalassaemia trait an individual has inherited.

2.2 Use of formulae based on red cell indices

A number of formulae can be used (England & Frazer, 1979; England, 1989) to determine whether the blood count is more suggestive of thalassaemia trait or iron deficiency, but these formulae are not applicable to children, pregnant women or polycythaemic patients with iron deficiency and will only predict the correct diagnosis in 80–90% of patients (d'Onofrio *et al.*, 1992). The following formula may be used, where each of the variables included makes a contribution and the overall function is better than any single measurement:

$$\text{MCV (fl)} - \text{RBC } (10^{12}/\text{l}) - 5\text{Hb (g/dl)} - K$$

where RBC is the red blood cell count and K is a constant factor dependent on the instrument calibration and is adjusted by each laboratory so that a negative result with this formula suggests a diagnosis of thalassaemia trait (England & Frazer, 1979) whereas a positive result suggests iron deficiency.

2.3 Thalassaemia trait without microcytosis

The red cell indices may also be affected by concomitant vitamin B_{12} or folate deficiency or liver abnormalities and in these situations people with thalassaemia trait may have normal red cell indices. Individuals with certain β-thalassaemia mutations may also have normal red cell indices (see Chapter 10).

2.4 Investigation for genetic purposes

This can be carried out preconceptually or during pregnancy. In either circumstance, it is essential that the great majority of cases of β-thalassaemia trait be detected (silent β-thalassaemia trait cannot be detected from red cell indices) and that α-thalassaemia trait be detected in those ethnic groups where the $--/\alpha\alpha$ (or $\alpha°$) genotype occurs and where the condition Hb Bart's hydrops fetalis is therefore possible. Patients may be selected for further testing on the basis of either the MCH or the MCV. Further testing may be carried out on all those who fall below the lower limit of the reference range for the selected parameter. Alternatively, a laboratory may investigate a large population of subjects with suspected thalassaemia trait in order to establish a satisfactory lower cut-off point, thus reducing unnecessary testing.

If the individual is not pregnant, formulae such as that given above may be applied to determine whether iron deficiency or thalassaemia trait is more likely. A provisional diagnosis of iron deficiency should be confirmed and treatment given. If the red cell indices do not return to normal after correction of the iron deficiency, investigation for thalassaemia trait is then indicated. When a patient is already pregnant, such formulae become invalid and either the MCH or the MCV should be used to select patients for further investigation. If the woman is pregnant, it may be necessary to test for thalassaemia even though she is known to be iron-deficient. This is because both thalassaemia and iron deficiency can occur in the same individual and undue delay may occur if thalassaemia testing is not undertaken until the iron deficiency is corrected; this is especially likely if the woman is of non-Northern European extraction. If the pregnant woman is thought to have β-thalassaemia trait or δβ-thalassaemia trait or has an interacting haemoglobin variant, such as HbS, HbC, HbE, HbO^{Arab} or Hb Lepore, the putative father should have similar investigations.

At the present time, it appears that Hb Bart's hydrops is extremely rare in individuals of ethnic origins other than those from South-east Asia (see Chapter 10) (Higgs *et al.*, 1989; Bowden *et al.*, 1992). If the woman is thought to have α-thalassaemia trait and originates from South-east Asia, she may have the $\alpha°$ genotype and the precise genetic diagnosis may therefore be important and the putative father should also be tested for α thalassaemia.

2.5 Investigation for clinical purposes

This is most commonly undertaken in people with microcytosis or a low MCH in the absence of iron deficiency or after correction of iron deficiency. Except in the special circumstances of pregnancy, it is not generally useful to investigate for thalassaemia trait in the presence of iron deficiency and moderately severe anaemia (Hb <8 g/dl).

2.6 Diagnosis in special groups

2.6.1 Infants less than one year old

The presence of Hb Bart's at birth indicates α-thalassaemia trait and, if it is markedly elevated, the baby may have HbH disease (British Committee for Standards in Haematology, 1988; International Committee for Standardization in Haematology (ICSH), 1988) and may need specialist follow-up. Beta-thalassaemia heterozygotes will develop thalassaemic indices and elevated levels of HbA_2 between 3 and 6 months of age. At present, the diagnosis of β-thalassaemia trait cannot be made reliably in the neonatal period, but, if clinically indicated, studies can be carried out when the baby is over 6 months old.

2.6.2 Thalassaemia interactions with structural variants

In families that carry certain structural haemoglobin variants (e.g. HbS, HbE, HbO^{Arab}, Hb Lepore and some unstable haemoglobins), it is necessary to investigate for the presence or absence of β-thalassaemia genes which may interact with these structural variants.

3 How to establish the diagnosis

In most clinical situations, the first step in the diagnosis of the thalassaemia traits and the phenotypically similar syndromes, such as Hb Lepore trait, is the measurement of the red cell indices (Fig. 9.1). If the red cells are normocytic, the diagnosis can be excluded with sufficient accuracy for clinical purposes, as long as there is no coexisting disorder, such as vitamin B_{12} or folate deficiency or liver disease, which may raise the MCV and MCH into the normal range. Once the possibility of thalassaemia trait has been identified, specific tests are required to confirm or exclude the diagnosis of thalassaemia and, if present, to determine whether it is α, β, or δβ thalassaemia, HbE trait or Hb Lepore trait. The general classification of the thalassaemia syndromes, together with the typical haematological features for individuals more than 1 year of age who have the common genotypes discussed in these guidelines, is summarized in Table 9.1. More precise diagnoses require the measurement of globin chain synthesis ratios and/or DNA analysis.

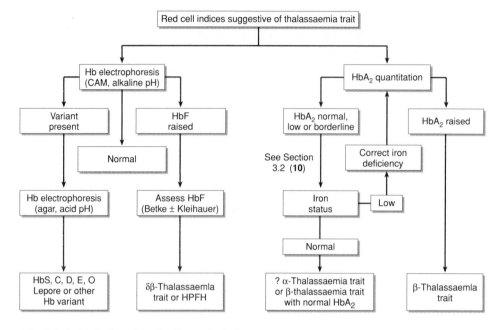

Fig. 9.1 A simple flow chart for diagnostic tests.

Specific tests are an essential step in the diagnosis of thalassaemia trait and include the following:

1   haemoglobin electrophoresis on cellulose acetate membrane (CAM) at alkaline pH;

2   quantitation of HbA_2;

3   assessment of fetal haemoglobin (HbF);

4   looking for HbH inclusion bodies;

5   assessment of iron status.

Additional tests are sometimes required, such as isoelectric focusing (IEF), globin chain synthesis or DNA analysis.

3.1 Haemoglobin electrophoresis

Haemoglobin electrophoresis at alkaline pH on CAM should be carried out on all samples tested for thalassaemia, since this procedure will detect the haemoglobin variants, Hb Lepore, HbS, HbC, HbE and HbO^{Arab}, together with HbH, Hb Bart's and most HbA_2 variants, all of which have medical implications when associated with thalassaemia trait. The technique used is based on that described by Schneider (1973) and given in detail by the ICSH (1988).

1   Tetrasodium ethylene diamine tetra-acetic acid (EDTA) (1 g/l in 100 mg/l potassium cyanide) should be used as the haemolysing reagent. The haemolysate is liable to oxidation and should be used within 7 days.

2 Strong detergents, such as Triton X-100, should not be used with adult specimens since they are likely to denature HbH and, if this happens, HbH disease may be missed; however, they do not seem to harm Hb Bart's and so can be used for neonatal specimens.

3 If a variant haemoglobin is detected, the sample should also be examined by haemoglobin electrophoresis on citrate agar at acid pH (ICSH, 1988) or by a similar technique on commercial precast agar or agarose gels. Some workers find commercial gels easier to use than gels prepared in house, but they are expensive and some agarose gels do not give as much information as a well-run citrate agar gel.

4 It is important to detect the presence of HbA_2 variants during the haemoglobin electrophoretic run since it is the sum of the 'normal' HbA_2 and the HbA_2 variant which must be assessed in the diagnosis of β-thalassaemia trait (see below). If the presence of an HbA_2 variant is missed, it may mean that any coexistent β-thalassaemia trait is also missed.

3.2 Estimation of haemoglobin A_2

A raised HbA_2 is the hallmark of classical β-thalassaemia trait. It should be quantitated whenever thalassaemia trait is suspected. Details of techniques are to be found in ICSH (1978) recommended methods, but the following points should be observed:

1 Preparation and storage of haemolysate: the haemolysate for HbA_2 and HbF determinations should be prepared by washing packed red cells with three volumes of isotonic saline (0.15 M). Mix the washed, packed red cells with an equal volume of distilled water and a half-volume of carbon tetrachloride and mix well for 10 minutes. Centrifuge and remove the supernatant haemoglobin solution, check the haemoglobin concentration and adjust to 10 ± 2 g/dl. The haemoglobin solution may then be stored in a stoppered tube at 4°C for up to 2 weeks.

2 Both electrophoresis and elution from cellulose acetate and microcolumn chromatography are recommended by ICSH (1978), but the precision and accuracy of automated scanning densitometry are inadequate for HbA_2 estimations (see **8** below). Routine techniques cannot be used for the determination of HbA_2 in the presence of HbC, HbE and HbO (and some other haemoglobins) because of their similar mobility to HbA_2 on cellulose acetate and microcolumns. Family studies and/or DNA analysis may be helpful in these situations.

3 When preparing tris(hydroxymethyl)aminomethane (TRIS) buffers, it is essential to use a pH electrode which is known to be suitable for use with TRIS, because TRIS interferes with the function of some electrodes. If an electrode can be calibrated with two standard buffers after immersion in TRIS buffer for at least 15 minutes, it may be considered suitable for use with TRIS.

4 Improved results may be obtained with microcolumn chromatography when a 10 mM rather than a 50 mM TRIS buffer is used (Efremov, 1986).

5 If a glycine 'developer' is used, the pH must be adjusted very slowly, since the molarity of the developer is an important factor in the elution of the haemoglobin fractions; if the developer is made too acidic, it must be discarded and not made alkaline again since this would increase the total ionic concentration and therefore alter the elution pattern.

6 Commercial microcolumn kits for the estimation of HbA_2 are available. It is important to follow the manufacturer's instructions carefully regarding the preparation, equilibration (especially temperature) and use of the columns.

7 Automated high-performance liquid chromatography (HPLC) can save time but is expensive in both capital and revenue costs. If used, it is important to examine the peak shape, baseline and resolution and to ensure that they are satisfactory before using the computed peak areas.

8 Reference materials have been developed by the ICSH for use in HbA_2 quantitation and will be available in 1994 from the National Institute of Biological Standards and Control* (NIBSC).

9 If an HbA_2 variant is present, it is essential to quantitate both the normal HbA_2 and the variant HbA_2 because it is the total HbA_2 which indicates whether or not a person has β-thalassaemia trait. If an HbA_2 variant is present, electrophoresis and elution of the HbA_2 and the HbA_2 variant bands are usually the best technique to use for quantitation.

10 Interpretation: values below 3.3% are usually normal and over 3.7% usually indicate β-thalassaemia trait. Some overlap in HbA_2 levels between normal and β-thalassaemia trait has been reported (Efremov, 1986) and levels between 3.3 and 3.7% need to be interpreted with care. Knowledge of the iron status of the individual is important since iron deficiency sufficient to cause moderately severe anaemia (Hb <8 g/dl) can reduce the HbA_2 level and lead to people with β-thalassaemia trait being classified as not having this condition (Wasi *et al.*, 1968; Kattamis *et al.*, 1972; Alperin *et al.*, 1977). Normal HbA_2 levels can be found in δβ-thalassaemia trait and in Hb Lepore trait (see Table 9.1), although both these conditions have the same clinical significance as β-thalassaemia trait. Raised levels have been described in the presence of some unstable haemoglobin β-globin variants and in some cases of pernicious anaemia. A level above 7% suggests either an analytical error or the presence of another haemoglobin that is not HbA_2.

If HbA_2 levels are found to be in the borderline area (3.3–3.7%) in the

---

*National Institute for Biological Standards and Control, Blanche Lane, South Mimms, Potter's Bar, Hertfordshire EN6 3QG, UK.

absence of HbS (see below), the estimation should be repeated on another blood sample and the iron status assessed. If the patient is iron-deficient, the iron deficiency should be corrected before the analysis is repeated. If repeat analysis again gives a borderline result, globin chain synthesis or DNA analysis should be considered if the diagnosis of β-thalassaemia trait, or its exclusion, would alter the clinical management of the patient or the genetic advice given to a couple. An example of such a situation would be if a pregnant woman had β-thalassaemia trait and her partner had borderline results.

If a person has both sickle-cell trait and α-thalassaemia trait, the HbA_2 may be slightly raised (3.5–4.0%), but this does not of itself indicate coexistent β-thalassaemia trait. The simplest way of obtaining a correct diagnosis in this situation is to quantitate the HbS. In uncomplicated sickle-cell trait (HbA + HbS), the HbS comprises less than 40% of the total haemoglobin. If α-thalassaemia trait is also present, the HbS will be lower (Serjeant, 1992), whereas the combination of sickle-cell trait and β-thalassaemia trait results in an HbS level of more than 60% and usually 80–90%.

3.3 Fetal haemoglobin

The HbF is raised (approximately 1–3%) in about one-third to half of the people with β-thalassaemia trait. However, a raised HbF (5–20%) in the presence of hypochromic, microcytic, red cell indices is the hallmark of δβ-thalassaemia trait, and it should be quantitated whenever HbF is detected on haemoglobin electrophoresis on CAM. It may also be raised in other conditions, such as in pregnancy and in the myeloproliferative disorders.

1 HbF should be quantitated by the 2-minute alkali denaturation technique described by Betke and colleagues (1959) and in detail by Pembrey and colleagues (1972). Attention to detail is extremely important when undertaking this assay. In particular, the concentration of the haemolysate (10 ± 2 g/dl), the temperature of the alkali denaturation mixture ($20 \pm 2°C$) and the time that the denaturation is allowed to proceed (2 minutes) must all be carefully controlled. If the HbF is above 50%, a more accurate result may be obtained, using the technique of Jonxis and Visser (1956), but the increased accuracy will rarely, if ever, alter the clinical management of the patient.

2 Reference materials have also been developed by ICSH for use in HbF quantitation and will be available in 1994 from NIBSC.

3 If the HbF is 5–20%, the individual may have δβ thalassaemia or HPFH. Marked microcytosis would favour the former diagnosis . If the HbF is more than 20%, it is likely that the patient has HPFH and in this condition the Kleihauer cytochemical test for HbF will show a pancellular distribution. If the patient is pregnant, the partner should be tested and if his tests are abnormal a definitive diagnosis by DNA analysis should be considered.

3.4 Haemoglobin H inclusions

1 Haemoglobin H inclusions are due to the oxidation and precipitation of HbH within the red cell and they can be generated *in vitro* by the redox action of certain dyes. They are found in some forms of α thalassaemia. Unfortunately, there is batch-to-batch variation with the dye and any new batch should be checked with a known positive sample.

2 Blood (preferably anticoagulated with EDTA and used within 24 hours of venesection) is incubated with 1% brilliant cresyl blue or new methylene blue at room temperature (18–25°C) for 4 hours; a normal control should always be included (C.S.R. Hatton & D.R. Higgs, personal communication). Blood films are made and examined. Haemoglobin H inclusions form a 'golf ball' appearance inside the cells.

3 In people with α-thalassaemia trait, there are usually a few red cells (1/1000–1/10 000) which contain typical inclusions (Weatherall, 1983; see Table 9.1), but in HbH disease they are found in 30–100% of the red cells. However, the absence of HbH inclusions does not exclude α-thalassaemia trait.

3.5 Isoelectric focusing

As a general rule, the separation of haemoglobins on IEF is similar to that obtained by electrophoresis on CAM, but the bands are sharper and the resolution of some haemoglobins is better. Isoelectric focusing is not usually indicated in district service laboratories but can be very useful in reference centres and also in regional laboratories where very large numbers of samples are processed. This is a useful technique to differentiate Hb Bart's from 'fast' variants, such as HbJ and HbN, in anticoagulated umbilical cord blood samples. It is also useful in laboratories undertaking neonatal screening on dried blood spots from Guthrie cards, because it reduces the interference from methaemoglobin, which usually prevents adequate resolution of haemoglobin bands when using electrophoresis to analyse haemoglobin eluted from such dried blood spots.

3.6 Globin chain synthesis

This technique is valuable in detecting the presence of α- or β-thalassaemia trait in couples considering prenatal diagnosis when the usual tests give equivocal results; it may sometimes also be useful in fetal diagnosis (see Chapter 10). The technique is very time-consuming and involves culturing the blood in the presence of tritiated leucine, and therefore facilities for the use and disposal of radioactive material must be available. For these reasons, this test is usually only undertaken in reference centres. If it is undertaken, it is essential that adequate numbers of normal and abnormal controls are analysed regularly.

3.7 Deoxyribonucleic acid analysis

Deoxyribonucleic acid can be analysed from white blood cells or from amniocytes or chorionic tissue obtained by the transabdominal or transvaginal sampling methods. These techniques are usually undertaken in specialist referral centres, and the laboratory techniques are discussed in Chapter 10.

3.8 Quality control

Since these procedures are all used to make, or exclude, the diagnosis of an inherited condition, it is essential to ensure that adequate quality control is undertaken for the determination of the red cell indices and all the other tests described in these guidelines. In-house protocols should clearly elucidate all aspects of the procedures to be undertaken. In particular, quantitative diagnostic analyses, such as HbA_2 and HbF, should be undertaken in such a way that duplicates agree to within 0.2% of each other (standard deviation (SD) <0.05%). All laboratories should check their reference ranges with each method they use to ensure that their results are accurate as well as precise. The haemoglobin concentration of the haemolysate used for the HbA_2 and HbF determinations should be recorded, as should the temperature of the reagents for the HbF. Laboratories should participate in the appropriate national and regional quality assessment schemes.

4 Interpretation of results

Although a definitive diagnosis of one of the thalassaemia traits requires detailed DNA analysis (see Chapter 10), a diagnosis which is accurate for most clinical purposes, except for fetal diagnosis, can usually be obtained by assessing the results of a group of laboratory tests. The presence of one of these traits or one of the phenotypically similar variant haemoglobins, such as Hb Lepore, Hb Constant Spring or HbE trait, may have been suspected because of the presence of red cells with reduced MCH and MCV, or the measurement of these indices may be used as the first of a series of investigations.

Beta-thalassaemia trait is typically associated with a raised HbA_2, but the HbA_2 is not raised in $\delta\beta$-thalassaemia trait and it may not be raised if there is coexistent severe iron deficiency anaemia. Haemoglobin Lepore, which is phenotypically similar to β-thalassaemia trait, can be detected by haemoglobin electrophoresis.

Alpha thalassaemia is not associated with a consistent marker, such as the raised HbA_2 in β-thalassaemia trait, but HbH bodies may sometimes be detected. The diagnosis of α-thalassaemia trait must usually be made by the exclusion of iron deficiency and other forms of thalassaemia in a person who has hypochromic, microcytic red cells. Haemoglobin Constant Spring (and other variant haemoglobins with globin chain elongation which are phenotypically similar to α thalassaemia) may be detected by haemoglobin electrophoresis, but may be confused with an HbA_2 variant or a carbonic anhydrase variant. Haemoglobin A_2 variants can be differentiated from carbonic anhydrase variants by haem staining with dyes such as *o*-dianisidine (ICSH, 1988).

The typical haematological features of the common thalassaemia traits are given below and in Table 9.1. The subtypes of α thalassaemia are classified according to the number of deleted genes which cause each type, since gene deletion is the cause of 'classical' α thalassaemia. However, non-deletional forms also occur and are clinically important in that they can cause a severe form of HbH disease.

4.1 Alpha-thalassaemia trait (one-gene deletion)

This can often be detected at birth by the presence of Hb Bart's. The condition is often haematologically silent in later life, although it may be associated with some of the changes found in the variety of α-thalassaemia trait caused by two-gene deletion (see below).

4.2 Alpha-thalassaemia trait (two-gene deletion)

This is characterized by red cells with a reduced MCH (usually less than 26 pg) and MCV in the absence of iron deficiency and no evidence of β- or δβ-thalassaemia trait (a normal or reduced $HbA_2 - <3.5\%$). Haemoglobin H bodies may be detected, but their absence does not exclude α thalassaemia. Haemoglobin electrophoresis will be normal unless a variant haemoglobin is also present.

4.3 Haemoglobin H disease (three-gene deletion)

This is characterized by anaemia and by red cells with a reduced MCH and MCV in the absence of iron deficiency and with no evidence of β- or δβ-thalassaemia trait (a normal or reduced $HbA_2 - <3.5\%$). Haemoglobin H bodies are found in 30–100% of the red cells. Haemoglobin electrophoresis shows the presence of an abnormal band anodal to HbA, comprising approximately 1–40% of the total haemoglobin.

4.4 Beta-thalassaemia trait

This is characterized by red cells with a reduced MCH and MCV in the absence of iron deficiency. The HbA_2 is raised (3.5–7.0%) and the haemoglobin electrophoresis is otherwise normal, unless a variant haemoglobin is also present.

4.5 Alpha-thalassaemia trait combined with beta-thalassaemia trait

This is characterized by red cells with a normal or reduced MCH and MCV in the absence of iron deficiency. The HbA_2 is usually raised and the haemoglobin electrophoresis is otherwise normal, unless a variant haemoglobin is also present.

4.6 Delta-beta-thalassaemia trait

This is characterized by red cells with a reduced MCH and MCV in the absence of iron deficiency. The HbA_2 is normal or slightly reduced and the HbF is raised (5–20%). Haemoglobin electrophoresis is otherwise normal, unless a variant haemoglobin is also present.

4.7 Haemoglobin E trait

This is characterized by red cells with a slightly reduced MCH and MCV in the absence of iron deficiency. Haemoglobin electrophoresis shows a variant band (usually 20–30%) in the position of HbA_2 on CAM at alkaline pH which does not separate from HbA on citrate agar at acid pH. The haemoglobin stability is usually slightly abnormal.

4.8 Haemoglobin Lepore trait

This is characterized by red cells with a reduced MCH and MCV in the absence of iron deficiency and a normal HbA_2 (less than 3.5%). Haemoglobin electrophoresis shows a variant band (7–15%) in the position of HbS on CAM at alkaline pH which does not separate from HbA on citrate agar at acid pH.

Note: Iron deficiency can occur in conjunction with any of these genotypes and, if it is moderately severe (Hb <8 g/dl), it may reduce the HbA_2. For this reason, it may be necessary to retest an individual after correction of any iron deficiency.

5 Conclusions

No guidelines can be all-inclusive – there will always be exceptions and cases must be considered individually. Individuals diagnosed as having one of the thalassaemia traits should be counselled and given an explanation of the results of the tests. A haemoglobinopathy card or other written record of the results should be made available to the patient and his/her doctor. Special counselling and follow-up arrangements must be established for couples considering prenatal diagnosis.

6 Useful addresses

1 Prenatal diagnosis by DNA analysis and other information on the thalassaemias is available as a national service from:

Dr John Old
National Haemoglobinopathy Reference Service
Institute of Molecular Medicine
John Radcliffe Hospital
Oxford OX3 9DU
UK
Tel: 0865 222449
Fax: 0865 222500

2 Haemoglobinopathy cards and leaflets can be obtained from:

HMSO
Broadway
Chadderton
Oldham OL9 9QH
UK
Tel: 061-681 1191

3 Multilingual explanatory booklets on some of these conditions are available from:

The UK Thalassaemia Society
107 Nightingale Lane
London N8 7QY
UK
Tel: 081-348 0437

4 The names and addresses of National Health Service (NHS) counselling centres can be obtained from the UK Thalassaemia Society.

References

Alperin J.B., Dow P.A. & Petteway M.B. (1977) Hemoglobin A_2 levels in health and various hematological disorders. *American Journal of Clinical Pathology* **67**, 219–226.

Betke K., Marti H.R. & Schlicht I. (1959) Estimation of small percentages of fetal haemoglobin. *Nature* **184**, 1877–1878.

Bowden D.K., Vickers M.A. & Higgs D.R. (1992) A PCR-based strategy to detect the common severe determinants of α thalassaemia. *British Journal of Haematology* **81**, 104–108.

British Committee for Standards in Haematology (1988) Guidelines for haemoglobinopathy screening. *Journal of Clinical and Laboratory Haematology* **10**, 87–94.

d'Onofrio G., Zini G., Ricerca B.M., Mancini S. & Mango G. (1992) Automated measurement of red blood cell microcytosis and hypochromia in iron deficiency and β-thalassaemia trait. *Archives of Pathological and Laboratory Medicine* **116**, 84–89.

Efremov G.D. (1986) Quantitation of haemoglobins by microchromatography. In Huisman T.H.J. (ed.) *Methods in Haematology No. 15: The Haemoglobinopathies*, pp. 72–90. Churchill Livingstone, Edinburgh.

England J.M. (1989) Discriminant functions. *Blood Cells* **15**, 463–473.

England J.M. & Frazer P.M. (1979) Discrimination between iron deficiency and heterozygous thalassaemia syndrome in differential diagnosis of microcytosis. *Lancet* **i**, 145–148.

Higgs D.R., Vickers M.A., Wilkie A.O.M., Pretorius I.M., Jarman A.P. & Weatherall D.J. (1989) A review of the molecular genetics of the human α-gene cluster. *Blood* **5**, 1081–1104.

International Committee for Standardization in Haematology (ICSH) (1978) Recommendations for selected methods for quantitative estimation of HbA_2 and for HbA_2 reference preparation. *British Journal of Haematology* **38**, 573–578.

International Committee for Standardization in Haematology (ICSH) (1988) Recommendations for neonatal screening for haemoglobinopathies. *Journal of Clinical and Laboratory Haematology* **10**, 335–345.

Jonxis J.H.P. & Visser H.K.A. (1956) Determination of low percentages of foetal haemoglobin in blood of normal children. *American Medical Association Journal of Diseases of Childhood* **92**, 588–591.

Kattamis C., Panayotis L., Metaxotou-Mavromati A. & Matsaniatis N.J. (1972) Serum iron and unsaturated iron-binding capacity in β thalassaemia trait: their relation to the levels of haemoglobins A, A_2 and F. *Medical Genetics* **9**, 154–159.

Pembrey M.E., McWade P. & Weatherall D.J. (1972) Reliable routine estimation of small amounts of fetal haemoglobin by alkali denaturation. *Journal of Clinical Pathology* **25**, 738–740.

Schneider R.G. (1973) Sickle cell disease. In Abramson H., Bertles J.F. & Wethers D.L. (eds) *Developments in Laboratory Diagnosis*, pp. 230–240. Mosby, St Louis.

Serjeant G.R. (1992) *Sickle Cell Disease*, 2nd edn. OUP, Oxford.

Wasi P., Disthasongchan P. & Na-Nakorn S. (1968) The effect of iron deficiency on the levels of haemoglobin A_2. *Journal of Laboratory and Clinical Medicine* **71**, 85–91.

Weatherall D.J. (1983) Haematologic methods. In Weatherall D.J. (ed.) *Methods in Haematology No. 6: The Thalassaemias*, pp. 27–30. Churchill Livingstone, Edinburgh.

Weatherall D.J. & Clegg J.B. (1981) *The Thalassaemia Syndromes*, 3rd edn. Blackwell Scientific Publications, Oxford.

WHO (1988) *The Report of the Fifth Annual Meeting of the WHO Working Group on Hereditary Anaemias: Alpha thalassaemia*. WHO unpublished report HDP/WG/HA/87.5. Available from Hereditary Disease Programme, WHO, Geneva.

10 Fetal Diagnosis of Globin Gene Disorders*
Prepared by the General Haematology Task Force

1 Introduction

The inherited disorders of haemoglobin are a vast group of disorders, which include the thalassaemias and sickle-cell disease (SCD) and which can involve complex interactions between several different mutant genes. The majority of these mutations can now be detected directly by deoxyribonucleic acid (DNA) analysis, enabling fetal diagnosis to be carried out for couples at risk of an affected fetus without the necessity for linkage studies on any children or relatives. Each mutation is detected by its own specific probes or primers and therefore it is vital to determine accurately the parental genotypes, preferably before fetal diagnosis, otherwise mistakes may occur if mutations are missed because of an incorrect diagnosis of the carrier state. It also means that a large number of probes and primers is required especially for the identification of β-thalassaemia mutations, and it is recommended that fetal diagnosis by DNA analysis is only undertaken in referral centres.

The aim of this chapter is to: (i) summarize the types of haemoglobin disorders for which fetal diagnosis may be indicated; (ii) review the current procedures that are used for fetal diagnosis; (iii) provide guidelines for clinicians requesting a fetal diagnosis test; and (iv) provide guidelines for clinicians and scientists carrying out a fetal diagnosis test.

2 Indications for prenatal diagnosis

The important haemoglobin disorders in the UK populations at risk are the thalassaemias, SCD and their interactions. These are summarized in Table 10.1. All the clinical details etc. of the thalassaemias and their interactions can be found in the authorative book by Weatherall and Clegg, *The Thalassaemia Syndromes* (1981).

* Reprinted with permission from *Journal of Clinical Pathology*, 1994, **47**, 199–204.

Table 10.1 Phenotypes of thalassaemias, sickle-cell disease (SCD) and various thalassaemia interactions

Type	Phenotype
Homozygous state	
α° Thalassaemia	Hb Bart's hydrops fetalis
β Thalassaemia:	
β° or severe β^+ mutation	Thalassaemia major
Mild β^+ mutation	Thalassaemia intermedia
$\delta\beta^\circ$ Thalassaemia	Thalassaemia intermedia
Hb Lepore	Variable: intermedia to major
HbS	SCD
HbC	No clinical problems
HbD	No clinical problems
HbE	No clinical problems
Compound heterozygous state	
β°/severe β^+	Thalassaemia major
Mild β^+/β° or severe β^+	Variable: intermedia to major
$\delta\beta^\circ$/β° or severe β^+	Variable: intermedia to major
$\delta\beta^\circ$/mild β^+	Mild thalassaemia intermedia
$\delta\beta^\circ$/Hb Lepore	Thalassaemia intermedia
Hb Lepore/β° or severe β^+	Thalassaemia major
HbC/β° or severe β^+	β-Thalassaemia trait $\rightarrow$ intermedia
HbD/β° or severe β^+	Variable: usually similar to β-thalassaemia trait
HbE/β° or severe β^+	Variable: intermedia to major
HbO^{Arab}/β°	Severe thalassaemia intermedia
HbS/β° or severe β^+	SCD
HbS/mild β^+	Usually mild SCD
HbS/HbC	SCD, variable severity
HbS/HbD^{Punjab}	SCD
HbS/HbO^{Arab}	SCD

2.1 Alpha° thalassaemia

The α thalassaemias are a group of disorders characterized by a reduction in α-globin synthesis. They can be divided into the severe types (α° thalassaemias), which have two α-globin genes deleted per chromosome, and the mild types (α^+ thalassaemias), which have one α-globin gene per chromosome either deleted or non-functional. Alpha thalassaemia is most frequently due to deletions although α^+ thalassaemia can also be caused by point mutations (Higgs, 1990). The homozygous state for α° thalassaemia results in haemoglobin Bart's (Hb Bart's) hydrops fetalis syndrome and is lethal, resulting in stillbirth or early neonatal death. Prenatal diagnosis for the homozygous state is normally required, as the mother of such an infant may suffer from toxaemia of pregnancy, obstructed labour and ante- or postpartum haemorrhage, as well as the psychological burden of carrying a non-viable fetus to term.

Alpha° thalassaemia is particularly common in South-east Asia (China,

Thailand, Vietnam, Malaysia, Philippines) and also occurs in the eastern Mediterranean countries (Greece, Cyprus). In contrast, it is extremely rare in Africa, the Caribbean and India, where α^+ thalassaemia predominates. The compound heterozygous condition of α^0/α^+ thalassaemia results in haemoglobin H (HbH) disease, in which three out of the four α-globin genes are deleted or non-functional. However, many patients with HbH disease lead a relatively normal life and thus fetal diagnosis is not normally requested. In the UK, there have been 28 prenatal diagnoses carried out for homozygous α^0 thalassaemia up to 1992. These were for couples mainly of Chinese, Vietnamese and Cypriot extraction (Petrou *et al.*, 1992).

2.2 Beta thalassaemia

Beta thalassaemia is now known to be caused by more than 100 different mutations (Kazazian, 1990), although, in each at-risk population, only a limited number of molecular defects are usually prevalent (Huisman, 1990). The mutations differ greatly in their phenotypic effect. At one end of the spectrum are a group of rare mutations involving exon 3 of the β-globin gene which are so severe that they behave in a dominant fashion and may produce thalassaemia intermedia in the heterozygous state (Thein *et al.*, 1990). At the other end are mild alleles which produce the phenotype of β thalassaemia intermedia in their homozygous state and, in just a few cases, are so mild in the heterozygous state that they are phenotypically silent, with normal mean corpuscular volume (MCV) and HbA_2 levels (Gonzalez-Redondo *et al.*, 1989). However, by far the majority of the β-thalassaemia mutations lie in between these two extremes. These are the β^+ and β^0 alleles which cause β thalassaemia major, either in the homozygous state for one allele or in the compound heterozygous state with two different alleles. By defining the mutations, it is now possible in many cases to predict whether a fetus is at risk for transfusion-dependent thalassaemia major or the milder non-transfusion-dependent thalassaemia intermedia.

The phenotype of thalassaemia intermedia is itself heterogeneous, with both mild and severe forms, because there are many different genetic determinants responsible for producing this phenotype (Wainscoat *et al.*, 1987). These include: (i) the homozygous state for a mild β^+ allele; (ii) the combination of a mild β^+ allele with a severe β^+, or β^0 in some cases (unfortunately, this situation is not very clear, as this combination sometimes results in β thalassaemia major); (iii) two severe β^+ or β^0 alleles in combination with either α thalassaemia or a raised fetal haemoglobin (HbF) determinant, such as the -158 $^G\gamma$-globin promoter mutation; (iv) one severe β^+ or β^0 allele in combination with a triplicated α-gene allele; (v) homozygous $\delta\beta^0$ thalassaemia; (vi) $\delta\beta^0$ thalassaemia in combination with β^+ thalassaemia or Hb Lepore; and (vii) a β^0 or severe β^+ allele in combination with Hb Lepore or HbO^{Arab}.

2.3 Haemoglobin S and its interactions

The SCD gene is caused by an adenine (A) → thymine (T) substitution in codon 6 of the β-globin gene. Beta-globin haplotype analysis has shown that the SCD gene has arisen at least three times in Africa and once in Asia. Sickle-cell anaemia patients bearing homozygous forms of the four most common African haplotypes (the Senegal, Benin, Bantu and Cameroon) exhibit a great variability in the phenotypic expression of this disease, and it is not possible to predict how severe the disease will be in any particular family, because there are a number of different factors (genetic, cellular and physiological) which can modify the course of SCD. However, recent evidence suggests that the Bantu (also known as Central African Republic (CAR)) is often associated with a clinically severe condition (Powars, 1991), while homozygotes for the Asian haplotype from Saudi Arabia and India have high levels of HbF, coupled with only a modest level of anaemia and a relatively mild course of the disease, although bone pathology (painful crises, avascular necrosis of the femoral head and osteomyelitis) remains common (Padmos *et al.*, 1991). The latter effects appear to be most marked in patients with homozygous α^+ thalassaemia.

The SCD gene also interacts with β-thalassaemia genes and several structural haemoglobins to produce sickling disorders of variable severity. The clinical course of SCD β thalassaemia is very variable, depending on the particular type of β-thalassaemia mutation that is coinherited. It tends to be particularly mild in African populations because of the likelihood of the coinheritance of a mild β^+ transcription mutation, although even here occasional severe interactions are encountered. A severe course, similar to that found in SCD, results from the interaction of the sickle gene with either a β°- or a severe β^+-thalassaemia allele. Haemoglobin S/C disease can be mild, though it may be associated with ocular, central nervous system (CNS) and bone complications, and thrombotic problems in pregnancy. However, the combination of HbS/D^{Punjab}, HbS/O^{Arab} and HbS/Lepore result in diseases similar in severity to homozygous SCD.

2.4 Haemoglobin E/β thalassaemia

This disorder is restricted mainly to individuals of oriental, Indian or Pakistani background. It shows remarkable clinical variability, ranging from a symptomless disorder to a condition as severe as homozygous β thalassaemia, which occurs when HbE interacts with a β°-thalassaemia allele. It seems likely that interaction with a severe β^+-thalassaemia type of allele results in a slightly milder condition but is still a serious disorder, in contrast to the more rare interaction of HbE with a mild β^+-thalassaemia allele, which results in an extremely mild, almost symptomless, disorder.

3 Globin chain synthesis

This technique may be useful in fetal diagnosis when the putative father is not available for tests. Guidelines to the analysis of globin chain biosynthesis in adult blood samples for carrier status determination may be found in the review by Clegg (1983); those relating to the determination of globin chain synthesis in fetal blood samples for fetal diagnosis can be found in the review by Alter (1989).

4 Deoxyribonucleic analysis

Fetal DNA for prenatal diagnostic studies can be isolated from amniotic fluid cells or chorionic villus biopsies (Old, 1993). Sufficient DNA (10–70 µg) is usually obtained from a chorionic villus sample (CVS) for both polymerase chain reaction (PCR) and Southern blot techniques. However, 20 ml of amniotic fluid will yield approximately only 7 µg DNA and sometimes much less than this or occasionally even none at all. Thus it is an unreliable source of DNA and, although usually sufficient DNA is obtained for PCR, the amount will be borderline for Southern blot analysis; therefore the establishment of a back-up cell culture is recommended for amniocyte DNA diagnosis.

4.1 Southern blot analysis

This technique is used for identifying α- and β-globin gene rearrangements caused by the various α^+- and α^o-thalassaemia deletion genes, $\delta\beta^o$-thalassaemia deletions and the hereditary persistence of fetal haemoglobin (HPFH) deletions. Prenatal diagnosis or α^o thalassaemia is achieved by hybridizing Southern blots of BamH I and Bgl II digested DNA to ^{32}P-labelled α-gene and ζ-gene probes. The homozygous state for α^o thalassaemia is diagnosed by the presence of abnormal ζ-gene-containing fragments in combination with the absence of normal α-gene-containing fragments (Old & Ludlam, 1991). The procedure usually takes 10–14 days to get a result. Southern blot analysis gives an overall picture of the α-globin gene arrangement and is still very useful for carrier diagnosis of α thalassaemia and for the confirmation of prenatal diagnosis results obtained by PCR.

4.2 Polymerase chain reaction techniques

Polymerase chain reaction-based techniques are now used for the diagnosis of α thalassaemia, β thalassaemia, some $\delta\beta$ thalassaemias and HPFH deletions, the analysis of β-globin restriction fragment length polymorphisms (RFLPs) and the detection of the genes for HbS, HbC, HbD, HbE and HbO^{Arab}. A fetal diagnosis result is usually obtained in 1–2 days if the mutations requiring analysis are known. If the mutations have not been identified beforehand, the parental DNA samples will have to be analysed first before the fetal DNA, and the fetal diagnosis will take 2–5 days.

4.2.1 Detection of known mutations

There are three PCR-based techniques in general use in fetal diagnosis laboratories: (i) the hybridization of ^{32}P-labelled allele-specific oligonucleotide probes, either to amplified DNA fixed to nylon filters by dot-blotting (Saiki *et al.*, 1986) or by reverse dot-blotting with the probes fixed to the filter (Saiki *et al.*, 1989); (ii) the use of allele-specific primers (Old *et al.*, 1990); and (iii) agarose or polyacrylamide gel electrophoresis. The first two techniques detect point mutations and require a battery of specific probes – one for every mutation likely to be encountered. The task of screening parental DNA samples for β-thalassaemia mutations is greatly simplified by the knowledge of the ethnic origin of each individual. The DNA is then screened first for the common mutations in that particular ethnic group, and then, if the tests prove negative, analysis is made for the rarer mutations. In this manner, it is possible to identify the mutations carried by both partners in more than 95% of couples. The remaining few per cent of individuals with an unidentifiable mutation either have an undescribed one or a rare one from a different ethnic group. In these cases, fetal diagnosis can often be carried out by the indirect methods of RFLP linkage or denaturing gradient gel electrophoresis (DGGE).

The mutations for HbS, HbE, HbD and HbO^{Arab} affect a restriction enzyme site in the β-globin gene and are detected directly by amplification followed by restriction enzyme digestion of the product and agarose gel electrophoresis (Old & Ludlum, 1991). Similarly, 13 β-thalassaemia mutations can be detected in this way (Kazazian, 1989), and this method provides an alternative approach to check prenatal diagnosis results involving these mutations. Gel electrophoresis of amplified product is used for diagnosing the β-thalassaemia deletion mutations (Faa *et al.*, 1992), α$^\circ$ thalassaemia (Bowden *et al.*, 1992), Hb Lepore (Camaschella *et al.*, 1990) and δβ thalassaemia (Ghanem *et al.*, 1933). Primers which are complementary to sequences flanking the deletion are used to generate a specific product only in the presence of the mutation (with the exception of β thalassaemia, normal DNA is not amplified because the primers are too far apart). Normal DNA is amplified using a flanking primer in combination with one complementary to the deleted sequence.

4.2.2 Detection of unknown mutations

There are now several PCR methods for characterizing β-thalassaemia mutations that are undefined by direct detection methods. These are DGGE, chemical mismatch cleavage analysis and single-stranded conformation polymorphism (SSCP) analysis, followed by direct sequencing of amplified single-stranded DNA. The method most widely used is DGGE, a polyacrylamide gel system that separates DNA fragments as a function of the melting temperature and it has been found to be particularly useful for the diagnosis of β thalassaemias in geographical areas where a very heterogeneous spectrum of mutations occurs (Losekoot *et al.*, 1991).

4.2.3 Indirect detection by restriction fragment length polymorphisms

Nearly all the β-globin RFLPs discovered by Southern blotting can now be analysed by PCR and restriction enzyme digestion (Old & Ludlam, 1991). By carrying out a family study with DNA from children and/or grandparents, the linkage phase of informative RFLPs can be established and β-thalassaemia genes can be diagnosed indirectly in fetal DNA without identifying the mutations involved. The technique has a slightly higher risk of error (0.3%) than a direct method because of the chance of recombination between the RFLP and the mutation locus. Restriction fragment length polymorphism linkage analysis provides a useful alternative approach to the diagnosis of β thalassaemia in the 80% of families that are found to be informative and should be used for confirmation of a diagnosis obtained by direct mutation analysis whenever possible.

4.2.4 Polymerase chain reaction errors

Misdiagnosis may occur through a number of technical reasons, i.e. failure to amplify one of the two target DNA segments, maternal DNA contamination, contamination with previously amplified target DNA sequences through aerosol contact, mispaternity, sample exchange, incomplete digestion of amplified product by restriction endonucleases and incorrect phenotype information resulting in a missed allele or incorrect assignment of polymorphic markers. These errors can be countered by careful laboratory practice in setting up PCR reactions and running appropriate controls, duplicate analysis of the fetal sample, the use of the minimum number of amplification cycles, the use of a second different diagnostic approach and the amplification of a suitable polymorphic marker, such as a variable number of tandem repeats (VNTR) sequence, to monitor the presence of maternal contamination (Decorte *et al.*, 1990).

5 Requirements for prenatal diagnosis

When a potentially at-risk couple is detected, they will require counselling and, if fetal diagnosis is requested, it will be necessary to: (i) confirm the parental phenotypes as determined by the first centre; (ii) send family or parental blood samples to a specialist DNA diagnostic laboratory; and (iii) arrange for fetal sampling and for sending correctly the fetal sample for fetal diagnosis. Ideally, confirmation of the parental phenotypes and identification of the DNA mutations involved should be done before arrangements are made for fetal sampling, in order to define the exact nature of risk and to avoid unnecessary invasion of a pregnancy not at risk. To diagnose α in combination with β thalassaemia or β thalassaemia with normal HbA_2 and low mean corpuscular haemoglobin (MCH) may require a combination of careful family studies, globin chain synthesis and DNA analysis.

5.1 Carrier state determination

This requires a blood count, including red cell indices, haemoglobin electrophoresis, a sickle solubility test and an estimation of HbA_2 and HbF (see Chapter 9). These tests should be repeated at the centre which is referring blood and fetal samples for DNA analysis from an at-risk couple. The referral form (see Appendix 10.1) should be completed and accompany the blood samples to the DNA diagnostic laboratory. Details of the ethnic origin (not place of birth) are particularly important for DNA analysis.

5.1.1 Alpha thalassaemia

The typical haematological features for α-thalassaemia carriers are shown in Table 9.1 in Chapter 9. Some important points to note are that carriers for $α^+$ thalassaemia are haematologically normal or have only slightly reduced indices (e.g. MCH 24–30 pg). The indices for $α^°$-thalassaemia trait usually fall below the normal range (MCH 28–32 pg) in the absence of iron deficiency, but are indistinguishable from those found in individuals with homozygous $α^+$ thalassaemia (e.g. MCH 19–24 pg) (Higgs, 1993). Therefore definitive carrier diagnosis can only be done by DNA studies. It is recommended that all pregnant women of Chinese, South-east Asian or eastern Mediterranean origin should be screened for $α^°$-thalassaemia trait and offered prenatal diagnosis when indicated.

5.1.2 Beta thalassaemia

The haematological phenotype of heterozygous β thalassaemia can be modified by interacting genetic or environmental factors. The coinheritance of α thalassaemia (usually the deletion of two α-globin genes) may raise the MCH and MCV sufficiently, in some cases, to values that lie within the normal range. However, α thalassaemia does not affect the HbA_2 level, unlike iron deficiency, which may decrease the HbA_2 value although it normally remains within the β-thalassaemia carrier range. Therefore, in any population in which α and β thalassaemia occur together, the best method of screening for β thalassaemia in pregnancy is to measure the HbA_2 level.

A subgroup of β-thalassaemia alleles exists in which heterozygotes have normal or minimally increased levels of HbA_2. The ones with reduced red cell indices may be confused with heterozygous $α^°$ thalassaemia. Those with normal red cell indices are truly silent (the only abnormality being an imbalance of the β/α-globin chain synthesis) and are not detectable by haematological screening techniques. Fortunately, the latter are both rare and very mild alleles hitherto found only in one or both parents of patients affected by thalassaemia intermedia. These alleles are the Mediterranean −101 mutation and the Indian cap site mutation CAP + 1 mutation. The triple α-globin gene arrangement is another truly silent allele, which, in combination with a β-thalassaemia mutation, can result in the phenotype of β thalassaemia intermedia.

Normal HbA$_2$ β thalassaemia with reduced red cell indices is usually caused by the double heterozygosity for δ and β thalassaemia. The mutation causing defective δ-gene expression may be *cis* or *trans* to the β-thalassaemia allele, which may be a mild allele, such as codon 27 (Hb Knossos) or intervening sequence (IVS)-I-5 (Corfu δβ thalassaemia), or severe, such as IVSI-110, IVSII-745 and the β° codon 39 mutation. However, several β-thalassaemia mutations by themselves have been observed in individuals with borderline to normal HbA$_2$ values, the best-known example being the Mediterranean mutation IVSI-6. Finally, adults heterozygous for the rare condition of (γδβ)° thalassaemia have red cell indices typical of β-thalassaemia trait but with normal levels of HbA$_2$ and HbF.

Adults with normal or low MCV/MCH, normal or reduced HbA$_2$ level and high HbF are heterozygous for δβ thalassaemia or HPFH. Although the distinction between the two conditions is not always clear-cut, in general heterozygotes fo δβ thalassaemia have 5–15% HbF, hypochromic microcytic red cells and a heterogeneous distribution of HbF in peripheral red blood cells; those with HPFH have 15–25% HbF, normal indices and a homogeneous distribution of HbF. A definitive diagnosis can be made by globin chain synthesis (normal in HPFH, unbalanced in δβ thalassaemia) and by DNA analysis.

5.2 Sample requirements

Adult blood samples in heparin or ethylenediamine tetra-acetic acid (EDTA) for carrier determination by globin chain synthesis have to be fresh (i.e. received by the laboratory within a few hours) and are best transported at 4°C. It is essential to contact the referral laboratory about transport arrangements for blood samples for such tests before arranging for the patient to attend. Fetal blood sampling is usually carried out at the prenatal diagnosis centre.

Blood samples in heparin or EDTA for DNA analysis can be sent by overnight delivery or first-class post without refrigeration. The maximum delay before deterioration is about 3 days, so blood taken on a Friday is best stored in a fridge until Monday and then posted to arrive Tuesday. Ten millilitres of anticoagulated blood (EDTA or heparin) is normally sufficient from each parent. If RFLP linkage analysis is to be performed in addition to direct detection of β-thalassaemia mutations, then additional blood samples are required from either: (i) a homozygous normal child or an affected child with β thalassaemia major; (ii) a child with β-thalassaemia trait plus one set of grandparents; or (iii) if no children are available then both sets of future grandparents would be required. The samples should be clearly labelled and be accompanied with a request form (see Appendix 10.1) detailing the following relevant particulars:

1 Haematological details: haemoglobin, red blood cells (RBC), MCV, MCH, sickle test, haemoglobin electrophoresis, HbA_2, HbF, HbH bodies, ferritin, serum iron and total iron-binding capacity (TIBC).

2 Patient particulars: surname, first name, date of birth, address, ethnic origin, referring consultant, gestational age.

3 Details of family history and previous children.

4 Confirmation that the family has been counselled as to the nature of the disease and obstetric risks/error rates.

5 Name and address of contact for arrangement of follow-up studies.

Chorionic villus samples must be dissected free of any contaminating maternal decidua by microscopic dissection before sending to the fetal diagnosis referral centre. The CVS can be sent by overnight delivery, either in tissue culture medium or, preferably, in a special lysis buffer obtainable from the DNA diagnosis laboratory. Amniotic fluid samples (15–20 ml) are best sent to the DNA laboratory as quickly as possible and must be received within 24 hours. If a longer transit time is anticipated, the amniocytes should be sent resuspended in tissue culture medium. In many cases, it is now possible to arrange for the fetal sample to go to a regional molecular genetics laboratory for DNA extraction. The fetal DNA can then be posted to the haemoglobinopathy diagnosis laboratory without risk of deterioration if delayed in transit.

5.3 Risks and misdiagnosis rates

Since both chorionic villus sampling and fetal DNA analysis are still in the stages of development, it is vital that parents are given accurate advice about the current fetal loss rate and also the likely misdiagnosis rate. Current figures suggest that the fetal loss rate following chorionic villus sampling in the first trimester is in the 2–3% range. The error in DNA analysis due to such factors as genetic recombination, technical problems in the laboratory and maternal contamination of CVS specimens has been determined to be 1% for fetal diagnoses carried out by the Southern blot technique. There are not yet sufficient data to give an absolutely accurate assessment of the misdiagnosis rate for the recently introduced PCR-based techniques but experience to date suggests it may be in a similar range of 1–2%.

It is essential that follow-up data are obtained on all cases that have undergone fetal diagnosis by CVS DNA analysis; ideally this should include both haematological and developmental assessment, as well as any fetal abnormalities. These data should be available to both the DNA laboratory and the referral centre:

1 Information on date of birth and birthweight and any information observed in the neonatal period.

2 Neonatal study of cord blood (electrophoresis or globin biosynthesis), or standard carrier test at 6 months or later.

3 Confirmation of genotype by DNA analysis.

5.4 Counselling

No couple should be offered fetal diagnosis without proper counselling, involving properly trained counsellors. Counselling requires an accurate determination of the parental genotypes and a good understanding of clinical outcomes of the haemoglobin disorders and their various interactions. It must include: (i) the nature and prognosis of the disorder involved and the treatment available; (ii) the genetic risks and possible methods of fetal diagnosis; and (iii) the obstetric risks and risk of misdiagnosis.

6 Summary of guidelines for centres sending samples for fetal diagnosis

1 A well-run diagnostic service requires a close liaison between haematologists, their obstetric colleagues and the DNA referral laboratory.

2 Haematological findings determined previously elsewhere should be rechecked for accuracy by the referring hospital.

3 Counselling of families requires the accurate determination of parental genotypes, a good understanding of the interactions producing the different haemoglobin disorders and the clinical picture of each disorder and accurate advice on the current fetal loss rate and the likely fetal DNA analysis error rate.

4 All haematology results and patient details should be sent to the DNA referral laboratory. A referral form to accompany blood samples is provided.

5 It is essential to contact the DNA referral laboratory to discuss transport arrangements for samples.

6 Family or parental blood samples for DNA analysis are required for fetal diagnosis of both thalassaemia and SCD.

Blood samples for DNA analysis ideally should be sent at least 1 week before a fetal sample to allow time for mutation identification. However, current techniques now permit sending parental and fetal samples at the same time, on the understanding that the fetal diagnosis may take a few days longer and there is a small chance of diagnostic failure from not being able to identify one of the β-thalassaemia mutations.

7 It is essential to obtain follow-up data for CVS DNA diagnoses. These should always be returned to the DNA laboratory and the referring centre.

7 Summary of guidelines for those carrying out fetal diagnosis

1 Ensure that adequate haematological data have been provided.

2 Ensure that mother (couple) has been adequately counselled.

3 Ensure that CVS have undergone careful microscopic dissection to remove any contaminating maternal decidua.

4 Always analyse parental DNA samples and appropriate control DNAs alongside the fetal DNA sample.

5 Always repeat the fetal DNA analysis test to double-check the result.

6 Use a second alternative DNA analysis test whenever possible to confirm a result.

7 Use a limited number of amplification cycles to minimize coamplification of maternal DNA.

8 Check for maternal DNA contamination by amplification of polymorphic markers.

9 The fetal diagnosis report should detail the types of DNA analysis used and clearly state the risk of misdiagnosis.

8 Useful addresses

1 Characterization of mutations and fetal diagnosis for thalassaemia and SCD is available as a national service from:

Dr John Old,
National Haemoglobinopathy Reference Service
Institute of Molecular Medicine
John Radcliffe Hospital
Oxford OX3 9DU
UK
Tel: 0865 222449
Fax: 0865 222500

2 Fetal diagnosis for thalassaemia and SCD is also provided by the following regional centres:

Dr M. Petrou, Dr B. Modell
Perinatal Centre
Department of Obstetrics and Gynaecology
88–96 Chenies Mews
London WC1E 6HX
UK
Tel: 071-387 9300 ext. 5230
Fax: 071-380 9864

Dr M. Layton
Department of Haematological Medicine
King's College Hospital
Denmark Hill
London SE5 9RS
UK
Tel: 071-326 3239
Fax: 071-326 3514

For SCD only:

Dr M. Patton
SW Thames Regional Genetics Service
St George's Hospital Medical School
Cranmer Terrace
London SW17 ORE
UK
Tel: 081-672 9944

Appendix 10.1:   Fetal diagnosis for sickle cell and thalassaemia: request for deoxyribonucleic acid analysis

Information for 1–5 should be available before arrangements are made to counsel a couple for fetal diagnosis.

1   *Mother*   *Haematology data*

Family name: ....   Date: ....
First name: ....   Hb: ....
Date of birth: ....   RBC: ....
Hospital number: ....   MCV: ....
Ethnic origin: ....   MCH: ....
Consultant: ....   Sickle test: ....
Last menstrual period: ....   Hb electrophoresis: ....
Address: .... HbA_2: ....
....   HbF: ....
....   Others (H bodies, ferritin, serum iron/
                                                         TIBC): ....

2   *Father*

Family name: ....   Date: ....
First name: ....   Hb: ....
Date of birth: ....   RBC: ....
Hospital number: ....   MCV: ....
Ethnic origin: ....   MCH: ....
Consultant: ....   Sickle test: ....

Address: ....   Hb electrophoresis: ....
....   HbA$_2$: ....
....   HbF: ....
                                           Others (H bodies ferritin, serum iron/
                                           TIBC): ....

3 Previous children and their genotypes: ....

4 Relevant family history: ....

5 Hence fetus at risk of: ....

6 Has the family been:
   (a) Counselled as to the nature of the disease ....

   (b) Told about obstetric risks and error rate ....

7 Follow-up arrangements: name of person who can be contacted:
   .... Tel. no.: ....

   Address: ....

   Postnatal arrangements (if applicable): ....

References

Alter B.P. (1989) Antenatal diagnosis using prenatal blood. In Alter B.P. (ed.) *Methods in Haematology*, pp. 114–133. Churchill Livingstone, Edinburgh.

Bowden D.K., Vickers M.A. & Higgs D.R. (1992) A PCR-based strategy to detect the common severe determinants of α-thalassaemia. *British Journal of Haematology* **81**, 104–108.

Camaschella C., Alfarano A., Gottardi E., Travi M., Primignani P., Cappio F.C. & Saglio G. (1990) Prenatal diagnosis of fetal hemoglobin Lepore–Boston disease on maternal peripheral blood. *Blood* **75**, 2102–2106.

Clegg J.B. (1983) Haemoglobin synthesis. In Weatherall D.J. (ed.) *Methods in Haematology*, pp. 54–73. Churchill Livingstone, Edinburgh.

Decorte R., Cuppens H., Marynen P. & Cassiman J.-J. (1990) Rapid detection of hypervariable regions by the polymerase chain reaction technique. *DNA and Cell Biology* **9**, 461–469.

Faa V., Rosatelli M.C., Sardu R., Meloni A., Toffoli C. & Cao A. (1992) A simple electrophoretic procedure for fetal diagnosis of β-thalassaemia due to short deletions. *Prenatal Diagnosis* **12**, 903–908.

Ghanem N., Vidaud M., Plassa F., Martin J. & Goossens M. (1993) Direct carrier detection and prenatal diagnosis of Sicilian and Spanish (δβ)°-thalassaemias. *Molecular and Cellular Probes* **7**, 167–168.

Gonzalez-Redondo J.M., Stoming T.A., Kutlar A. *et al.* (1989) A C → T substitution at nt-101 in a conserved DNA sequence of the promoter region of the β globin gene in association with 'silent' β thalassemia. *Blood* **73**, 1705–1711.

Higgs D.R. (1990) The molecular genetics of the α globin gene family. *European Journal of Clinical Investigation* **20**, 340–347.

Higgs D.R. (1993) α-Thalassaemia. In Higgs D.R. & Weatherall D.J. (eds) *Baillière's Clinical*

Haematology. International Practice and Research: The Haemoglobinopathies, pp. 117–150. Baillière Tindall, London.

Huisman T.H.J. (1990) Frequencies of common β-thalassaemia alleles among different populations: variability in clinical severity. *British Journal of Haematology* **75**, 454–457.

Kazazian H.H. Jr (1989) Use of PCR in the diagnosis of monogenic disease. In Erlich H. (ed.) *PCR Technology*, pp. 153–169. Stockton Press, New York.

Kazazian H.H. Jr (1990) The thalassemia syndromes: molecular basis and prenatal diagnosis in 1990. *Seminars in Hematology* **27**, 209–228.

Losekoot M., Fodde R., Harteveld C.L., Van Heeren H., Giordano P.C. & Bernini L.F. (1991) Denaturing gradient gel electrophoresis and direct sequencing of PCR amplified genomic DNA: a rapid and reliable diagnostic approach to beta thalassaemia. *British Journal of Haematology* **76**, 269–274.

Old J.M. (1993) Fetal DNA analysis. In Davies K.E. (ed.) *Human Genetic Disease Analysis: a Practical Approach*, pp. 1–20. Oxford University Press, Oxford.

Old J.M. & Ludlam C.A. (1991) Antenatal diagnosis. In Hann I.M. & Gibson B.E.S. (eds) *Baillière's Clinical Haematology – Paediatric Haematology*, pp. 391–428. Baillière Tindall, London.

Old J.M., Varawalla N.Y. & Weatherall D.J. (1990) The rapid detection and prenatal diagnosis of β thalassaemia in the Asian Indian and Cypriot populations in the UK. *Lancet* **ii**, 834–837.

Padmos M.A., Roberts G.T., Sackey K. *et al.* (1991) Two different forms of homozygous sickle cell disease occur in Saudi Arabia. *British Journal of Haematology* **79**, 93–98.

Petrou M., Brugiatelli M., Old J. *et al.* (1992) Alpha thalassaemia hydrops fetalis in the UK: the importance of screening pregnant women of Chinese, other South East Asian and Mediterranean extraction for alpha thalassaemia trait. *British Journal of Obstetrics and Gynaecology* **99**, 985–989.

Powars D.R. (1991) β^s-Gene cluster haplotypes in sickle cell anemia. *Hematology and Oncology Clinics of North America* **5**, 475–493.

Saiki R.K., Bugawan T.L., Horn G.T., Mullis K.B. & Erlich H.A. (1986) Analysis of enzymatically amplified β globin and HLA-DQ α DNA with allele-specific oligonucleotide probes. *Nature* **324**, 163–166.

Saiki R.K., Walsh P.S., Levenson C.H. & Erlich H.A. (1989) Genetic analysis of amplified DNA with immobilized sequence-specific oligonucleotide probes. *Proceedings of the National Academy of Science USA* **86**, 6230–6234.

Thein S.L., Hesketh C., Taylor P. *et al.* (1990) Molecular basis for dominantly inherited inclusion body β-thalassaemia. *Proceedings of the National Academy of Science USA* **87**, 3924–3928.

Wainscoat J.S., Thein S.L. & Weatherall D.J. (1987) Thalassaemia intermedia. *Blood Reviews* **1**, 273–279.

Weatherall D.J. & Clegg J.B. (1981) *The Thalassaemia Syndromes*, 3rd edn. Blackwell Scientific Publications, Oxford.

11 Immunophenotyping in Acute Leukaemia*

Prepared by the
General Haematology Task Force

1 Summary

We have outlined here the value of and the need for the immunophenotypic analysis of leukaemic cells for the precise diagnosis of acute leukaemias (AL), cases of blast transformation of chronic myeloproliferative disorders and myelodysplasia.

The various techniques that can be applied to perform marker studies, their description, advantages and disadvantages, and a number of recommendations to avoid pitfalls are also detailed.

Because of the increasing numbers of monoclonal antibodies (McAb) and the wide range of commercially available reagents, we recommend the use of a restricted panel of McAb which allow the identification with certainty of the cell lineage of the leukaemic cells and thus are useful for the diagnosis of acute leukaemias.

2 Introduction

Immunophenotypic analysis of the reactivity of leukaemic cells with McAb has proved to be useful and nowadays essential in the diagnosis of AL. This was first shown to be relevant in the characterization and classification of acute lymphoblastic leukaemias (ALL) of various cell types (Greaves et al., 1981; Janossy et al., 1989), as there is no specific and reliable cytochemical marker to recognize lymphoblasts. Subsequently, immunological markers have also been demonstrated to be important in the diagnosis of acute myeloblastic leukaemias (AML), particularly when the nature of the blasts cannot be defined by morphology and cytochemistry. Examples of these 'undifferentiated' AL are cases with poorly differentiated myeloblasts (AML-M0) (Chan et al., 1985; Matutes et al., 1987;

---

* Reprinted with permission from *Journal of Clinical Pathology*, 1994, **47**, (in press).

Bennett *et al.*, 1991) or those derived from early erythroid and megakaryocytic precursors (Buccheri *et al.*, 1992).

There is currently a large panel of McAb (>1000) available which detect different molecules (>70) on normal haemopoietic and leukaemic cells of various lineages. The McAb are grouped according to the molecule or antigen that they recognize under a cluster designation (CD) number which extend from 1 to 76. Only a minority of these reagents have been shown to be helpful for the diagnosis of AL; these comprise McAb which recognize antigens in lymphoid/myeloid cells from the earlier stages of differentiation and which, with few exceptions, are cell-lineage-restricted.

An outline will be given of:

1 The panel of McAb which are of practical use in the diagnosis of AL.

2 The advantages and disadvantages of the different techniques which can be applied to detect the cell reactivity with a McAb.

3 A number of considerations or recommendations related to the methodology and interpretation of the findings.

4 Detailed description of the methodologies for immunophenotyping.

5 Selection of reagents.

6 Indications for immunophenotyping.

3 Panel of monoclonal antibodies for the diagnosis of acute leukaemias

The most useful reagents for characterizing and distinguishing B- and T-cell-derived ALL (B-ALL and T-ALL) and AML are illustrated in Fig. 11.1. Thus, a

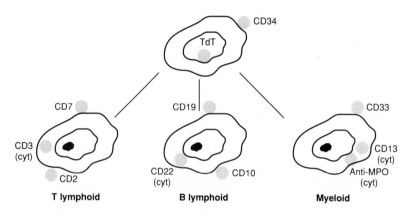

Fig. 11.1 A first-line panel of monoclonal antibodies for characterizing and distinguishing B- and T-cell-derived acute lymphoblastic leukaemias and acute myeloid leukaemias.

first-line panel of McAb will include 10 reagents:
- three B-cell-associated markers: CD19, CD22(cytoplasmic) (CD22(cyt)), CD10;
- three T-cell-associated markers: CD7, CD3(cyt), CD2;
- three myeloid-associated markers: CD33, CD13(cyt), antimyeloperoxidase (anti-MPO);
- the nuclear enzyme terminal deoxynucleotidyltransferase (TdT).

With the use of these 10 reagents, it is possible to detect all types of B-ALL (TdT$^+$, CD19$^+$, CD22(cyt)$^+$, CD10$^{+/-}$), all T-ALL (TdT$^+$, CD7$^+$, CD3(cyt)$^+$, CD2$^{+/-}$) and AML (CD33$^{+/-}$, CD13(cyt)$^{+/-}$, anti-MPO$^{+/-}$).

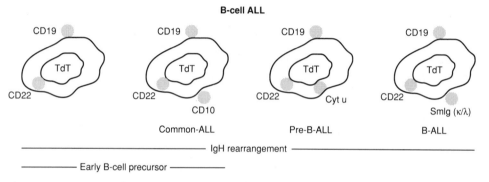

Fig. 11.2 Monoclonal antibodies for subclassifying B-cell-derived acute lymphoblastic leukaemias.

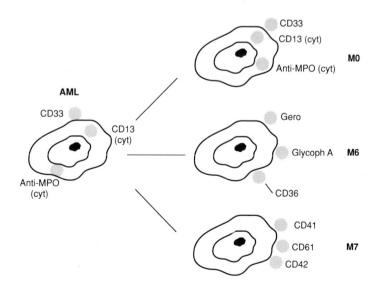

Fig. 11.3 Monoclonal antibodies for detecting acute myeloblastic and megakaryoblastic leukaemias and erythroleukaemias.

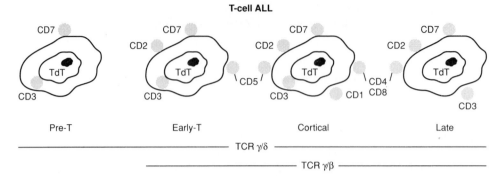

Fig. 11.4 Monoclonal antibodies for further characterization of T-cell derived acute lymphoblastic leukaemias.

A second panel of McAb can be used to dissect further the various ALL and AML subtypes, but these are not essential and are only of value in particular cases:

● Cytoplasmic μ chain (cyt μ) and surface immunoglobulins (SmIg) to subclassify further the various B-ALL into: early-B-ALL (CD19$^+$, CD22(cyt)$^+$), common-ALL (CD10$^+$), pre-B-ALL (cyt μ$^+$) and B-ALL (SmIg$^+$) (Fig. 11.2).

● CD41 (antiplatelet glycoprotein IIb/IIIa) or CD61 (antiplatelet glycoprotein IIIa) to detect megakaryoblastic (M7)-AML and the McAb antiglycophorin A for the diagnosis of erythroleukaemias (Fig. 11.3). These may be of great value for the diagnosis of some acute 'undifferentiated' leukaemias, when all the markers used in the screening panel are negative.

● Other T-associated markers (CD5, CD1, CD4, CD8) are recommended to further characterize T-ALL and to support this diagnosis when the phenotype is TdT$^+$, CD7$^+$, CD3(cyt)$^+$, CD2$^+$ (Fig. 11.4).

4 Methodology

Essentially there are two types of techniques which can be applied for routine immunophenotyping:

1 immunofluorescence on viable, unfixed cells in suspension;

2 immunoenzymatic methods: immunoperoxidase (IP) and immunoalkaline phosphatase–antialkaline phosphatase (APAAP) on fixed cells on slides.

The two techniques are reliable and the use of one or the other or both will depend on the facilities of each laboratory, although the immunoenzymatic methods are recommended for a district general hospital.

The advantages and disadvantages of the two methods are summarized in Table 11.1.

Table 11.1 Advantages and disadvantages of two immunological methods applied on cell suspensions and fixed cells in smears

Immunofluorescence (cell suspension)	Immunoenzymatic (slides – fixed cells)
Advantages	
Preservation of antigens, as cells are unfixed	Performance of retrospective studies
Quantitates antigenic sites	Detection of membrane and cytoplasmic antigen
Analyses a large number of cells (flow cytometry)	Allows identification of the morphology of positive cells
Permits double-labelling on a routine basis	Results can be reviewed as slides are kept
	Requires only ordinary light microscope
Disadvantages	
Requires a fluorescence microscope or flow cytometer	Some antigens may be destroyed by the fixative
No detection of cytoplasmic antigens with standard method	No discrimination between cytoplasm/membrane staining
Retrospective studies are not possible	Quantitative measurement of antigenic sites is not possible
Difficulties in interpretation of data in heterogeneous samples or those with few blasts	

5 Recommendations

A laboratory that is going to set up one or both methodologies for immunophenotyping has to take into account a number of considerations:

1 Before setting up the technique, the laboratory worker should spend at least a week in a unit with experience in immunophenotyping.

2 Normal samples should be tested before analysing leukaemia specimens.

3 Results must be interpreted in the context of the sample analysed, particularly in those with a mixture of leukaemic and normal cells.

4 Results should be interpreted with knowledge of cytological features, and a 'composite' phenotype has always to be considered. For example, reactivity with CD19 and CD22, when no assessment of TdT has been made, may correspond to a B-cell lymphoma as well as to ALL. The specificity of the markers needs also to be considered, e.g. the McAb CD7 on its own does not ascribe as T-ALL a particular blast population, as *c*. 20% of AML are CD7$^+$.

5 Some McAb – CD3, CD22, CD13, anti-MPO – are useful reagents when reactivity is detected in the cytoplasm of the cells, as they are expressed first in the cytoplasm and later in the membrane (Pombo de Oliveira *et al.*, 1988; Van

Dongen *et al.*, 1988; Janossy *et al.*, 1989). Therefore these markers should be assessed on fixed cells.

6 Blood and bone marrow samples must be collected on anticoagulant. Preservative-free heparin is a suitable anticoagulant, as it ensures that samples are also suitable for cytogenetic studies and other laboratory tests. Nevertheless, dipotassium ethylenediamine tetra-acetatic acid (K_2EDTA) and K_3EDTA are also satisfactory for cell marker studies.

7 Samples may be stored for 24 hours at room temperature or at 4°C prior to immunophenotyping. When the specimens are not fresh (over 24 hours), a viability test should be performed to exclude false binding by non-viable cells. Addition of tissue culture medium (e.g. RPMI-1640) is recommended when the samples are stored beyond 24 hours. For the immunoenzymatic techniques, the slides should be dried at room temperature for 24–48 hours and thereafter the test must be carried out or the slides should be wrapped in foil paper and kept at −20°C until the test is performed. The fixative recommended for the immuno-enzymatic methods is acetone for 10 minutes.

8 Dilutions of the McAb and the second-layer reagents should be carefully set up in each laboratory to avoid false positive or negative results. In this context, positive and negative controls should always be used. This is absolutely essential when a new batch of reagents is applied.

6 Methodology for immunophenotyping

Peripheral blood and bone marrow samples are collected in anticoagulant and mononuclear cells are isolated by Ficoll density centrifugation and washed twice in phosphate-buffered saline (PBS) with 1% bovine serum albumin (Sigma), 0.05% sodium azide and 2% human AB serum (pH 7.6) (PBS-bovine serum albumin (BSA)-azide-AB buffer). Cells from pleural fluid, ascites and cerebrospinal fluid (CSF) are also resuspended in the same buffer, which is used in all washes.

6.1 Immunofluorescence

For the detection of cell surface antigens by indirect immunofluorescence, 50 µl of a cell suspension (10^6 cells) is incubated with 50 µl of the optimally titrated McAb for 30 minutes at 4°C. Following two washes with the PBS-BSA-azide-AB buffer, the cells are incubated with the fluorescein-conjugated (FITC) antimouse immunoglobulin (optimally diluted) for 30 minutes at 4°C and washed again twice in the buffer. The cell pellet is resuspended in glycerol/PBS (1/1), mounted on a glass slide, covered with a coverslip and sealed to be evaluated under the fluorescence microscope.

The same procedure is applied for flow cytometry analysis but, following the incubation with the FITC antimouse immunoglobulin and subsequent washes, the cell pellet is resuspended in 500 µl of Isoton and assessed on the flow cytometer. If the sample is analysed after 4 hours from staining, the cell pellet should be fixed in 1% paraformaldehyde in 0.85% saline instead of being resuspended in Isoton.

Whole blood can also be tested by flow cytometry, without the need to isolate the mononuclear fraction. For this purpose, 100–200 µl of blood are spun down and the cell pellet is resuspended in 50 µl of buffer (PBS-azide). The methodology is identical to that described above but the buffer used does not contain human serum and the pellet, following the immunostaining, is treated with 1 ml of lysing solution for 10 minutes at room temperature and washed twice in buffer (PBS-azide). Finally, the cell pellet is resuspended in 250 µl of Isoton and the reading is performed in the flow cytometer.

Negative control preparations will be set up by replacing the relevant McAb with a mouse immunoglobulin of the same isotype and, when possible, positive controls will be performed, using normal or leukaemic blood samples. For practical purposes, a mixture of mouse immunoglobulins of the various isotypes can be used as a negative control.

6.2 Immunoalkaline phosphatase–antialkaline phosphatase

This may be carried out on smears or on a layer of mononuclear cells prepared on a cytocentrifuge. Both will be air-dried for at least 6 hours before proceeding to the test, and the location of the cells will be marked by encircling the area with a glass pencil. Fixation is done in pure acetone for 10 minutes at room temperature. A water repellent (Sigmacote) is applied around the circle and the slides are placed in a humid chamber and incubated with 50 µl of optimally titrated McAb for 30 minutes. From now on, do not let the cells dry. Following a wash with 0.05 M tris(hydroxymethyl)aminomethane (TRIS)-buffered saline (TBS) (pH 7.6), the slides are incubated with 50 µl of a rabbit antimouse immunoglobulin, diluted 1/20 in TBS, and 2% human serum for 30 minutes, washed again in TBS and incubated for 45 minutes in the APAAP complexes, diluted 1/60 in TBS. Following a wash in TBS, the spread cells are incubated for 20 minutes in a previously filtered developing solution, which contains napthol AS-Mx phosphate, levamisole, *N,N*-dimethylformamide and FAST red TR salt, rinsed in distilled water and counterstained with Harris haematoxylin for 10–20 seconds. The slides are mounted with Glycergel (Dako) without letting them dry, and assessed under an ordinary light microscope. To assess the nuclear enzyme TdT, an extra incubation step is required following the fixation and initial incubation with the rabbit anti-TdT antibody; this requires incubating the cells for 30 minutes with a mouse antirabbit immunoglobulin, followed by the incubations with the rabbit antimouse immunoglobulin and the APAAP complexes, as outlined above.

Negative controls are set up by replacing the McAb with a mouse immunoglobulin of the same isotype, and smears from normal blood and bone marrow are used as positive controls when required.

7 Selection of reagents

Different antibodies with the same CD number are not always equally satisfactory as diagnostic reagents. Reagents will be selected on the basis of their well-established specificity, stability and potential for use in detecting membrane and cytoplasmic antigens and also their cost, which is generally high. Polyclonal antibodies are preferable for the detection of immunoglobulin light chains (κ and λ).

8 Indications for immunophenotyping

Immunophenotypic analysis should be systematically performed in all AL, blast transformation of chronic myeloid leukaemia or other myeloproliferative disorders (e.g. myelofibrosis) and myelodysplasia.

This analysis is mandatory when the leukaemic blasts are morphologically undifferentiated and negative for the cytochemical reactions characteristic of myeloid cells: Sudan black B and myeloperoxidase for the granulocytic line and non-specific esterases for the monocytic line. In these cases, immunophenotypic analysis will clarify whether they correspond to one of the subtypes of ALL or are AML-M0, early erythroleukaemias or megakaryoblastic leukaemias.

In the remaining AL cases, in which the blasts are shown to be myeloid by standard light-microscopy morphology and cytochemistry (e.g. presence of Auer rods or MPO activity), the immunological markers are not essential, as in the group outlined above. Still, it is recommended that the immunological profile of these blasts be investigated in order to rule out cases of biphenotypic/mixed-lineage AL, in which the blasts have myeloid and lymphoid features, despite presenting as AML (Greaves *et al.*, 1986; Catovsky *et al.*, 1991).

Immunological markers are not useful and should not be performed in those cases of chronic myeloproliferative disorders and myelodysplasia with no evidence of blast transformation.

References

Bennett J.M., Catovsky D., Daniel M.T., Flandrin G., Galton D.A.G., Gralnick H.R. & Sultan C. (1991) Proposal for the recognition of minimally differentiated acute myeloid leukaemia. *British Journal of Haematology* **78**, 325–329.

Buccheri V., Shetty V., Yoshida N., Morilla R., Matutes E. & Catovsky D. (1992) The role of an anti-myeloperoxidase antibody in the diagnosis and classification of acute leukaemia: a comparison with light and electron microscopy cytochemistry. *British Journal of Haematology* **80**, 62–68.

Catovsky D., Matutes E., Buccheri V., Shetty V., Hanslip J., Yoshida N. & Morilla R. (1991) A classification of acute leukaemia for the 1990s. *Annals of Haematology* **62**, 16–21.

Chan L.C., Pegram S.M. & Greaves M.F. (1985) The contribution of immunophenotype to the classification and differential diagnosis of acute leukaemia. *Lancet* **i**, 475–479.

Greaves M.F., Janossy J., Peto J. & Kay H. (1981) Immunologically defined subclasses of acute lymphoblastic leukaemia in children: their relationship to presentation features and prognosis. *British Journal of Haematology* **48**, 179–197.

Greaves M.F., Chan L.C., Furley A.J.W., Watt S.M. & Molgaard H.V. (1986) Lineage promiscuity in hemopoietic differentiation and leukemia. *Blood* **67**, 1–11.

Janossy G., Coustan-Smith E. & Campana D. (1989) The reliability of cytoplasmic CD3 and CD22 antigen expression in the immunodiagnosis of acute leukemia – a study of 500 cases. *Leukemia* **3**, 170–181.

Matutes E., Pombo de Oliveira M., Foroni L., Morilla R. & Catovsky D. (1987) The role of ultrastructural cytochemistry and monoclonal antibodies in clarifying the nature of undifferentiated cells in acute leukaemia. *British Journal of Haemotology* **69**, 205–211.

Pombo de Oliveira M., Matutes E., Rani S., Morilla R. & Catovsky D. (1988) Early expression of MCS2 (CD13) in the cytoplasm of blast cells from acute myeloid leukaemia. *Acta Haematologica* **80**, 61–64.

Van Dongen J.J.M., Krissansen G.W., Wolvers-Tettero I.L.M., Comans-Bitter W.M., Adriaansen H.J., Hooijkas H., Van Wering E.R. & Terhorst C. (1988) Cytoplasmic expression of the CD3 antigen as a diagnostic marker for immature T cell malignancies. *Blood* **71**, 603–612.

12 Immunophenotyping in the Diagnosis of Chronic Lymphoproliferative Disorders*
Prepared by the General Haematology Task Force

1 Summary

The chronic lymphoproliferative disorders include a variety of diseases which result from the clonal proliferation of B and T lymphocytes at different stages of cell maturation and/or activation. The availability of a number of immunological markers that recognize B and T lymphoid subpopulations, together with more careful attention to the cell morphology and histopathology, has resulted in a more exact characterization and classification of the chronic lymphoproliferative disorders. The role of immunophenotyping in the diagnosis and characterization of the various lymphoid neoplasms is described. Guidelines will be defined for methodology, the panel of markers useful for diagnostic purposes and the demonstration of clonality in B-cell conditions, interpretation of results and finally indications for immunophenotyping.

2 Introduction

As in the acute leukaemias, immunophenotyping has been shown to be useful in the characterization and classification of the chronic lymphoproliferative disorders (Bennett *et al.*, 1989; Matutes & Catovsky, 1991a). This term refers to a group of diseases which result from the clonal proliferation of B and T lymphocytes. Recognition of the various disease entities is essential because of major implications for prognosis and patient management. The diagnosis of lymphoproliferative disorders requires use of multiple technologies, including immunological markers, cell morphology and, in some cases, histopathology of the involved tissues and molecular and cytogenetic investigations (Matutes & Catovsky, 1991a). Immunophenotyping is a key laboratory procedure in the exact diagnosis of these conditions.

This chapter discusses the role of immunological markers in the diagnosis and

---

* Reprinted with permission from *Journal of Clinical Pathology*, 1994, **47**, (in press).

characterization of the lymphoproliferative disorders and provides guidance on:
- methodological aspects;
- panels of markers useful for diagnostic purposes;
- interpretation of results;
- indications for immunophenotyping.

3 Role of immunological markers in the characterization of lymphoproliferative disorders

The value of immunological marker studies as a diagnostic tool in chronic lymphoproliferative disorders can be summarized as follows:

1 Markers are essential to distinguish:

(a) immature/acute lymphoblastic leukaemias (ALL), which, with the exception of Burkitt's or L3-ALL, are, as a rule, terminal deoxynucleotidyltransferase (TdT)$^+$, from mature/chronic lymphoproliferative disorders, which are TdT$^-$. This is important when the clinical and cytological features of a chronic lymphoproliferative disorder resemble those of acute leukaemia, as may be the case with large-cell lymphomas in leukaemic phase (Bain *et al.*, 1991).

(b) B-cell from T-cell lymphoid neoplasms.

2 Immunophenotyping permits the establishment of clonality in B-cell malignancies and the distinction from non-neoplastic reactive lymphocytosis. This is possible by demonstrating the expression of only one of the two types of immunoglobulin (Ig) light chain (κ or λ) on the surface or in the cytoplasm of lymphocytes. In contrast, in reactive conditions, both κ$^+$ and λ$^+$ B cells will be present.

There is no immunological marker to demonstrate clonality in T cells; however, aberrant phenotypes which are not present or are very uncommon among normal T cells are suggestive of a clonal T-cell proliferation (Matutes & Catovsky, 1991b).

3 Markers are useful to confirm or establish the diagnosis of a particular disease entity. Despite the lack of specificity of markers for the different lymphoid disorders, there are some well-defined phenotypes, such as that of B-cell chronic lymphocytic leukaemia (B-CLL) and hairy cell leukaemia, which are of great value for the recognition of these diseases, particularly when other clinical and laboratory features are atypical.

4 Recommendations

4.1 Specimens

Peripheral blood specimens are often more suitable than bone marrow for immunophenotyping of chronic lymphoproliferative disorders. Immunophenotyping of bone marrow cells is indicated only when the bone marrow is infiltrated and there are few or no abnormal cells in the peripheral blood.

4.2 Immunophenotyping techniques

Immunophenotyping in mature lymphoproliferative disorders can be carried out either by immunofluorescence on unfixed cells in suspension or by immunoenzymatic methods on fixed cells spread on slides. The use of techniques applied to cell suspensions is recommended as routine for the following reasons:

1 Information is provided on the density of expression of an antigen on the cells. This is very important when investigating the expression of Ig or of antigens recognized by certain monoclonal antibodies (McAb), e.g. cluster designation CD22, which discriminate phenotypes typical of B-CLL from those seen in other B-cell disorders.

2 Some antigens, such as that recognized by the McAb FMC7, are usually destroyed by fixatives and therefore findings will be reliable only when they relate to unfixed cells in suspension.

On the other hand, immunoenzymatic techniques may be helpful and are recommended in two situations:

1 In cases of plasma-cell leukaemia, which, as a rule, are negative with the majority of immunological markers when tested in suspension, whereas the testing of fixed cells permits the demonstration of cytoplasmic Ig.

2 When B-cell clonality is not shown by membrane staining with anti-κ or anti-λ reagents, as a consequence of strong membrane expression of IgG receptors – Fc$_\gamma$ receptors – which non-specifically bind the anti-Ig reagents. These are usually blocked by the fixative used in the immunoenzymatic methods.

5 Methodology for immunophenotyping

Recommendations for immunofluorescence and immunoenzymatic techniques in the study of chronic lymphoproliferative disorders are described below and are identical to those given in the study of acute leukaemias (see Chapter 11), except for the detection of surface Ig (SmIg) – heavy and light chains.

Peripheral blood or bone marrow is collected in anticoagulant (e.g. heparin, ethylene diamine tetra-acetic acid (EDTA)) and mononuclear cells are obtained by Ficoll density centrifugation. The cells are washed twice in phosphate-buffered saline (PBS) and resuspended in PBS containing 1% bovine serum albumin (BSA) (Sigma), 0.05% sodium azide and 2% human AB serum (pH 7.6) (PBS-BSA-azide-AB buffer), except for the staining of SmIg.

5.1 Immunofluorescence on cell suspensions

For the detection of cell membrane antigens by indirect immunofluorescence,

50 µl of a cell suspension (10^6 cells) is incubated with an appropriate volume (ranging from 5 to 50 µl) of optimally diluted McAb for 30 minutes at 4°C. Following two washes in PBS-BSA-azide-AB buffer, the cells are incubated with the fluorescein-conjugated (FITC) antimouse IgF(ab)$_2$ fragment (optimally diluted) for 30 minutes at 4°C and washed twice in the buffer. The cell pellet is resuspended with two drops of PBS/glycerol (1/1), mounted on a glass slide, covered with a coverslip and sealed to be evaluated by fluorescence microscopy. An antifade reagent, e.g. 1,4-diazabicyclo-2,2,2-octane, may be added to the mounting medium to facilitate reading under the microscope. A phase-contrast microscope with adequate filters is recommended and at least 200 cells should be analysed for the fluorescence stain. A reaction is considered positive when the cell has multiple fluorescent dots on the membrane.

The same procedure is applied for flow cytometry, but the cell pellet, instead of being resuspended in glycerol/PBS, is resuspended in 500 µl of Isoton and assessed on the flow cytometer. If analysis of the sample is performed more than 4 hours after staining, the cell pellet should be fixed in 1% paraformaldehyde in 0.85% saline, instead of being resuspended in Isoton.

Whole blood can also be tested by flow cytometry, except for the detection of SmIg. The manufacturer's instructions for the lysing procedure should be followed. Usually, 100–200 µl of blood are incubated with the McAb and subsequently with the FITC antimouse Ig. The methodology is similar to that described above, but the buffer does not contain human AB serum and the pellet, following the immunostaining, is treated with 1 ml lysing solution for 10 minutes at room temperature. This is followed by two washes in PBS-BSA-azide buffer. Reading is performed in the flow cytometer after resuspending the pellet in 250 µl of Isoton.

As in the biphenotypic acute leukaemias, it may be useful in some circumstances to apply a double-immunolabelling technique to determine if a single cell population coexpresses two different antigens in the membrane. For example, it may be informative to investigate the coexpression of a B-cell marker, CD19, and CD5 in cases of B-CLL or that of CD4 and CD8 in T-cell proliferations. Usually this is performed by a direct immunofluorescence technique, using two McAb directly conjugated to two fluorochromes (e.g. fluorescein and phycoerythrin). The McAb should be independently titrated and the methodology is similar to that for indirect immunofluorescence, omitting the second incubation step.

In general terms, use of the indirect immunofluorescence as the routine method is recommended for the following reasons: (i) the direct technique is less sensitive for the detection of an antigen when expression on the membrane is weak; (ii) some McAb are not commercially available as reagents directly conjugated to fluorochromes; and (iii) the indirect method is less expensive. The direct immunofluorescence method is recommended when double-immunolabelling is performed.

Negative control preparations are always set up, by replacing the McAb with a mouse Ig of the same isotype, and, when possible, positive controls are carried out on normal or leukaemic samples. For practical purposes, a mixture of mouse Ig of the various isotypes can be used as negative control.

5.2 Surface immunoglobulin staining

The methodology for detection of Ig (heavy and light chains) on the cell membrane is similar to that described above, with slight modifications. Prior to the immunological reaction, the isolated cells are resuspended in tissue culture medium and incubated at 37°C for 30–60 minutes to remove extrinsic Ig bound by the Fc_γ receptors present on B cells. Following this, the cells are washed once in PBS with 0.2% BSA and are subsequently stained with the anti-Ig reagents, following standard techniques except that the buffer used for all washes does not contain 2% human AB serum.

5.3 Immunoalkaline phosphatase–antialkaline phosphatase on fixed cells (Cordell *et al.*, 1984)

This may be carried out on smears or on a layer of mononuclear cells on a cytocentrifuge slide for all McAb, except for the detection of Ig expression, which should always be carried out on isolated mononuclear cells. The location of the cells is marked by encircling the area with a glass pencil. Smears and cytocentrifuge slides should be air-dried for at least 6 hours and up to 48 hours prior to the test. Fixation is done in pure cold acetone for 10 minutes at room temperature. A water repellent (Sigmacote) is applied around the circle; the slides are placed in a humid chamber and incubated with 50 µl of optimally diluted McAb for 30 minutes. From now on, the cells must not be permitted to dry and all the steps are carried out at room temperature. After a wash with 0.05 M tris(hydroxymethyl) aminomethane (TRIS)-buffered saline (TBS) (pH 7.6), the slides are incubated with 50 µl of a rabbit antimouse Ig diluted 1/20 in TBS and 2% human serum for 30 minutes, washed again in TBS and incubated in the immunoalkaline phosphatase–antialkaline phosphatase (APAAP) complexes diluted 1/60 in TBS for 45 minutes. Following a wash in TBS, the cells are incubated for 20 minutes in a previously filtered developing solution which contains naphthol AS-Mx phosphate, levamisole, *N,N*-dimethylformamide and FAST red TR salt, rinsed in distilled water and counterstained with Harris haematoxylin for 10–20 seconds. The slides, still wet, are mounted with Glycergel (Dako) and assessed under the ordinary microscope. Cells positive with a McAb will be seen with red stain in the cytoplasm or on the cell surface.

Negative controls are set up by replacing the McAb with a mouse Ig of the same isotype, and normal blood and bone marrow smears are used as positive control when required.

6 Interpretation of results

Results have to be considered in the context of the cell morphology, and the proportion of leukaemic cells has to be estimated in the samples analysed. Therefore, the cut-off point to consider a marker positive will vary. For instance, for samples from primary leukaemias, such as B-CLL or prolymphocytic leukaemia (PLL), which usually contain over 80% leukaemic cells, a cut-off point of 30% of cells stained with a marker can be considered to be positive. In contrast, in diseases such as non-Hodgkin's lymphomas in leukaemic phase or hairy-cell leukaemia, the proportion of malignant cells ranges from small to large. Therefore, results must be interpreted in each case and for each particular marker, according to whether such marker is or is not expressed in normal blood lymphocytes. For instance, 10% of positive cells with the McAb B-ly-7, which is consistently negative in normal lymphocytes, can be considered a positive finding, whereas the interpretation will be different with the marker CD2, which is positive in most normal blood T lymphocytes.

The lack of specificity of most of the markers also needs to be considered and results must be interpreted taking into consideration findings with the whole panel of markers investigated and not a marker in isolation. For example, CD5 is a T-cell marker but is also positive in B-CLL cells and in a proportion of B-cell non-Hodgkin's lymphoma cells; CD38 is positive in activated T cells but also in lymphoplasmacytic cells and plasma cells.

7 Recommended panel of monoclonal antibodies for the characterization of chronic lymphoproliferative disorders

The first panel (Fig. 12.1) of markers to be tested is aimed at:
- distinguishing B- from T-cell disorders;
- assessing clonality in B-cell proliferations;
- distinguishing a phenotype typical of B-CLL from those seen in other B lymphoproliferative disorders.

The first panel should include the following reagents:
- A pan-T marker: CD2.
- A pan-B maker: CD20, CD19 or CD37 (the latter McAb is also weakly positive in a subset of T cells).
- A marker expressed on T cells and a subset of B cells (most B-CLL and a few lymphomas): CD5.
- Two markers to assess clonality: anti-immunoglobulin light chains – anti-κ and anti-λ.
- Three markers which will help to discriminate between B-CLL and other B-cell conditions: CD23, FMC7 and CD22.

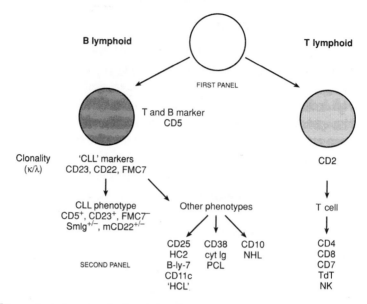

Fig. 12.1 Immunological markers in chronic lymphoid disorders. CLL, chronic lymphocytic leukaemia; HCL, hairy-cell leukaemia; PCL, plasma-cell leukaemia; NHL, non-Hodgkin's lymphoma; NK, natural killer.

With the use of these eight reagents in the first screen, it is possible to distinguish:

- T-cell disorders: $CD2^+$, $CD5^{+/-}$, pan-B$^-$, anti-κ/λ^-;
- B-cell disorders: $CD2^-$, pan-B$^+$, anti-κ or anti-λ^+, $CD5^{+/-}$;
- a typical B-CLL phenotype ($CD2^-$, $CD5^+$, anti-κ or anti-λ weakly positive, pan-B$^+$, $CD23^+$, FMC7$^-$, mCD22$^-$ or weakly positive) from phenotypes seen in other B-cell malignancies ($CD2^-$, $CD5^{+/-}$, anti-κ or anti-λ strongly positive, pan-B$^+$, $CD23^{+/-}$, FMC7$^+$, membrane expression of CD22 (mCD22$^+$)) (Catovsky *et al.*, 1981; Matutes & Catovsky, 1991a).

8 Second panel of reagents

The cell reactivity with a second panel (Fig. 12.1) of reagents should be investigated when the first panel indicates a phenotype consistent with a T-cell disorder or with a clonal B-cell disorder with a marker profile atypical for B-CLL. In contrast, if the first panel shows an immunological profile characteristic of B-CLL, no further immunophenotyping is needed.

In the cases with a T-cell phenotype ($CD2^+$, $CD5^{+/-}$), use of the following McAb is recommended (Matutes & Catovsky, 1991b; Matutes *et al.*, 1991):

- CD3, CD7, CD4 and CD8 to confirm the T-cell nature of the lymphocytes and to see whether a particular subset (e.g. CD4 or CD8) is expanded and whether leukaemic cells have a phenotype atypical among normal T lymphocytes.

● TdT and CD1a to distinguish thymic/immature (TdT$^+$, CD1a$^{+/-}$) lymphoid neoplasms (i.e. T-cell ALL) from post-thymic/mature (TdT$^-$, CD1a$^-$) T-cell proliferations.

● Optional markers which are sometimes of relevance are: (i) McAb that recognize antigens of natural killer and killer cells (CD11b, CD16, CD56 and CD57), which may provide some information in the study of proliferations of large granular lymphocytes; and (ii) McAb that recognize antigens in activated T cells (CD25, CD38 and class II human leucocyte antigen DR (HLA-DR) determinants) in the analysis of suspected adult T-cell leukaemia/lymphoma and large-cell T-lineage non-Hodgkin's lymphomas.

In the cases in which the first panel shows a clonal B-cell disorder with a phenotype atypical for B-CLL, the second panel of markers to be used needs to be tailored according to the diagnosis suspected from clinical features and cell morphology. For instance, if a diagnosis of hairy-cell leukaemia is entertained, the McAb panel − B-ly-7, CD25, CD11c and HC2 − will be useful to confirm the diagnosis and distinguish hairy-cell leukaemia from other B-cell conditions, such as the hairy-cell leukaemia variant (Mulligan *et al.*, 1990; Sainati *et al.*, 1990) or splenic lymphoma with villous lymphocytes, with which it may be confused.

Optional markers which sometimes give relevant information are CD10 when a diagnosis of follicular lymphoma in leukaemic phase is suspected (Melo *et al.*,

Table 12.1 Immunological markers in mature B-cell disorders

Marker	Leukaemias					Lymphomas		
	CLL	B-PLL	HCL	HCL-V	PCL*	SLVL	FL	McL
SmIg	Weak	Strong	Strong	Strong	−	Strong	Strong	Strong
CD5	++	−/+	−	−	−	−/+	−/+	++
Pan-B	++	++	++	++	−	++	++	++
CD23	++	−	−	−	−	−/+	−/+	−/+
FMC7	−/+	++	++	++	−	++	++	+
mCD22	Weak or −	++	++	++	−	++	++	+
CD25†/HC2	−	−	++	−	−	−/+	−	−
B-ly-7	−	−	++	+	−	−/+	−	−

*Expression of cytoplasmic Ig (light-chain-restricted) and CD38.
†CD25 may be identified in other conditions when using sensitive techniques.
CLL, chronic lymphocytic leukaemia; B-PLL, B-cell prolymphocytic leukaemia; HCL, hairy-cell leukaemia; HCL-V, hairy-cell leukaemia variant; PCL, plasma-cell leukaemia; SLVL, splenic lymphoma with villous lymphocytes; FL, follicular lymphoma; McL, mantle-cell lymphoma; SmIg, surface (membrane) immunoglobulin; −, negative or positive in less than 10% of cases; −/+, positive in 10–25% of cases; +, positive in 25–75% of cases; ++, positive in more than 75% of cases.

Table 12.2 Immunological markers in mature T-cell disorders

Marker	T-PLL	ATLL	SS	LGL-L	T-NHL
CD2/CD5	++	++	++	++	+
mCD3*	+	+	++	++	+
CD7	++	−/+	+	+	+
CD4	++	++	++	−/+†	+
CD8	+‡	−	−	++	+‡
CD25	−/+	++	−/+	−	+

All cases have a mature (TdT⁻, CD1a⁻) phenotype.
* mCD3: membrane expression. All cases express CD3 in the cytoplasm.
† Coexpressed with natural killer markers.
‡ Coexpressed with CD4 or with negative CD4.
T-PLL, T-cell prolymphocytic leukaemia; ATLL, adult T-cell leukaemia lymphoma; SS, Sézary syndrome; LGL-L, large granular lymphocyte leukaemia; T-NHL, post-thymic T-cell non-Hodgkin's lymphoma; −, negative or positive in less than 10% of cases; −/+, positive in 10–25% of cases; +, positive in 25–75% of cases; ++, positive in more than 75% of cases.

1988) and CD38 in cases in which lymphoplasmacytic differentiation or plasma-cell leukaemia is suspected from morphological examination.

A situation that may arise is that in which all the markers tested in the first panel are negative. The diagnosis of plasma-cell leukaemia should then be suspected and tests on fixed cells to detect cytoplasmic Ig light chains and tests with the McAb CD38 should be carried out (Parreira *et al.*, 1985).

The most characteristic immunophenotypic profiles on the various chronic B and T lymphoproliferative disorders are shown in Tables 12.1 and 12.2.

9 Indications for immunophenotyping

Immunophenotypic analysis is indicated on blood and/or bone marrow samples from all chronic lymphoproliferative disorders, including:
1 primary lymphoid leukaemias;
2 leukaemia/lymphoma syndromes or non-Hodgkin's lymphoma in leukaemic phase, when there are at least 10% circulating abnormal cells;
3 non-Hodgkin's lymphoma with bone marrow infiltration.

References

Bain B., Matutes E., Robinson D., Lampert I.A., Brito-Babapulle V., Morilla R. & Catovsky D. (1991) Leukaemia as a manifestation of large cell lymphoma. *British Journal of Haematology* **77**, 301–310.

Bennett J.M., Catovsky D., Daniel M.-T., Flandrin G., Galton D.A.G., Gralnick H.R. & Sultan C. (1989) Proposals for the classification of chronic (mature) B and T lymphoid leukaemias. *Journal of Clinical Pathology* **42**, 567–584.

Catovsky D., Cherchi M., Brooks D., Bradley J. & Zola H. (1981) Heterogeneity of B-cell leukemias demonstrated by the monoclonal antibody FMC7. *Blood* **58**, 406–408.

Cordell J.L., Falini B., Erber W.N., Ghosh A.K., Abdulaziz Z., MacDonald S., Pulford K.A.F., Stein H. & Mason D.Y. (1984) Immunoenzymatic labelling of monoclonal antibodies using immuno complexes of alkaline phosphatase and monoclonal anti-alkaline phosphatase (APAAP complexes). *Journal of Histochemistry and Cytochemistry* **14**, 291–302.

Matutes E. & Catovsky D. (1991a) The classification of lymphoid leukaemias. *Leukaemia and Lymphoma Supplement* **5**, 153–155.

Matutes E. & Catovsky D. (1991b) Mature T-cell leukaemias and leukaemia/lymphoma syndromes: review of our experience in 175 cases. *Leukaemia and Lymphoma* **4**, 81–91.

Matutes E., Brito-Babapulle V., Swansbury J., Ellis J., Morilla R., Dearden C., Sempere A. & Catovsky D. (1991) Clinical and laboratory features of 78 cases of T-prolymphocytic leukemia. *Blood* **78**, 3269–3274.

Melo J.V., Robinson D.S.F., de Oliveira M.P., Thompson I.W., Lampert I.A., Ng J.P., Galton D.A.G. & Catovsky D. (1988) Morphology and immunology of circulating cells in leukaemic phase of follicular lymphoma. *Journal of Clinical Pathology* **41**, 951–959.

Mulligan S.P., Travade P., Matutes E., Dearden C., Visser L., Poppema S. & Catovsky D. (1990) B-ly-7, a monoclonal antibody reactive with hairy cell leukemia, also defines an activation antigen on normal CD8$^+$ T cells. *Blood* **76**, 959–964.

Parreira A., Robinson D.S.F., Melo J.V., Ayliffe M., Ball S., Hedge U., Baugham A., Fairhead S., Talavera J.G., Katzmann J.A. & Catovsky D. (1985) Primary plasma cell leukaemia: immunological and ultrastructural studies in 6 cases. *Scandinavian Journal of Haematology* **35**, 433–441.

Sainati L., Matutes E., Mulligan S.P., de Oliveira M.P., Rani S., Lampert I.A. & Catovsky D. (1990) A variant form of hairy cell leukemia resistant to alpha-interferon: clinical and phenotypic characteristics of 17 patients. *Blood* **76**, 157–162.

13 Testing for the Lupus Anticoagulant*
Prepared by the
Haemostasis and Thrombosis Task Force

In 1988 the results of a questionnaire from the Lupus Anticoagulation Working Party for the Haemostasis and Thrombosis Task Force showed that there was considerable preanalytical and analytical variability among UK laboratories which perform tests for the lupus anticoagulant. In a subsequent quality control exercise, these variables influenced the success of the various tests in identifying the presence of such inhibitors. One hundred British laboratories participated in a further exercise, using standardized methodology for two tests – namely, the dilute Russell's viper venom time (DRVVT) and the kaolin clotting time (KCT). This improved the rate of correct detection of lupus anticoagulant compared with the earlier study. As a result of these observations, methodological guidelines for laboratories wishing to test for the presence of lupus anticoagulant were formulated.

The detection and positive identification of the lupus-like anticoagulant has become an important procedure for routine coagulation laboratories. Lupus anticoagulant is associated with arterial and venous thromboembolism and neurological disease. It has also been implicated in recurrent spontaneous abortion (Hughes, 1983, 1988). These inhibitors usually prolong the activated partial thromboplastin time (APTT) (Mannucci et al., 1979), and investigation for lupus anticoagulant is often prompted by an unexplained prolonged APTT result.

The activity of the inhibitor seems to be directed towards coagulation-active phospholipid complexes in the coagulation cascade. Several phospholipid-dependent coagulation tests have been advocated as being more sensitive and specific than the APTT, but there is no consensus on the most appropriate laboratory method. Anticardiolipin antibodies (ACA) have also been shown to be associated with lupus anticoagulant (Hughes, 1983, 1988).

The unrelated behaviour of lupus anticoagulant and ACA in the course of disease and in individual patients indicates that both assays are required when the antiphospholipid syndrome is suspected. Standardization of methods for ACA

* Reprinted with permission from *Journal of Clinical Pathology*, 1991, **44**, 885–889.

138

Table 13.1 Criteria for lupus anticoagulants

1 Prolongation of a phospholipid-dependent clotting test
2 Clotting time of a mixture of test and normal plasma should be longer than the clotting time of normal plasma
3 There should be a relative correction of the defect by the addition of lysed platelets or phospholipids

assays has been recommended and has recently been reviewed (Harris, 1990). A Working Party of the International Society on Thrombosis and Haemostasis (ISTH) on acquired inhibitors of coagulation made recommendations regarding definition and test procedures in 1983 (Green *et al.*, 1983), but recent evidence suggests that a significant number of patients will be misdiagnosed using these criteria. Any definition of the lupus anticoagulant must include the phospholipid dependency of the inhibitory activity in clotting testing and the relative correction by lysed platelets or increased phospholipid concentration (Table 13.1). The definition has recently been reviewed by the Lupus Anticoagulant Subcommittee of the Scientific and Standardization Committee of the ISTH (Exner *et al.*, 1991).

In view of the undoubted clinical importance of lupus anticoagulants and the lack of standardization in their detection (Exner *et al.*, 1990), a detailed national UK survey and quality control exercises in lupus anticoagulant testing have been undertaken (Lupus Anticoagulant Working Party, 1990).

Factors which influence the performance of these tests have been identified, and standardized methodology evaluated. As a result of these studies, recommendations for standardized procedures for testing for lupus anticoagulants have been formulated and these are set out below.

1 Background

Lupus anticoagulant is frequently requested in routine coagulation laboratories. The methods of sample collection and handling before testing strongly influence lupus anticoagulant results. Inadequate removal of platelets in the test plasma adversely affects test results (Exner, 1985; McGlassin *et al.*, 1989; Taberner *et al.*, 1989; Lupus Anticoagulant Working Party, 1990) and, furthermore, tests are frequently performed on frozen samples, which inevitably leads to the presence of platelet fragments and lupus anticoagulant-bypassing activity if the original plasma is not platelet-free. Filtering or double-centrifugation seems desirable (Exner, 1985; Taberner *et al.*, 1989; Lupus Anticoagulant Working Party, 1990).

Various methods have been proposed, but the APTT is the most frequently used screening test for lupus anticoagulant (Lupus Anticoagulant Working Party, 1990). Studies have shown that sensitivity to the lupus anticoagulant defect varies considerably with different APTT reagents (Mannucci *et al.*, 1979; Taberner & Poller, 1985). Reagents with low phospholipid content are the most sensitive (Mannucci *et al.*, 1979; Taberner & Poller, 1985; Stevenson *et al.*, 1986). Control and patient mixtures are often performed but a weak lupus anticoagulant defect may be corrected by a 50/50 mixture. These findings were confirmed in the recent UK survey (Lupus Anticoagulant Working Party, 1990). The Austen and Rhymes (1975) modification of the APTT, using aluminium hydroxide absorption and heat stability, has not proved a reliable test (Lupus Anticoagulant Working Party, 1990). The dilute thromboplastin time test (Schleider *et al.*, 1976) (tissue thromboplastin inhibition test) is prolonged by factor deficiencies as well as the lupus anticoagulation defect (Triplett *et al.*, 1983), and sensitivity depends on thromboplastin dilution (Lupus Anticoagulant Working Party, 1990). Some immunoglobulin M (IgM) lupus anticoagulants do not prolong this test, although they do prolong others (Thiagarajan *et al.*, 1986). In a recent review (Triplett & Brandt, 1989), the lack of specificity of the dilute thromboplastin time test was noted. The KCT (Exner *et al.*, 1978) and DRVVT (Thiagarajan *et al.*, 1986) are particularly sensitive to lupus anticoagulants (Lesperance *et al.*, 1988; Lo *et al.*, 1989). The mixture of normal and test plasma in the KCT offers some degree of specificity. The platelet correction procedure (PCP) with the DRVVT, using freeze–thawed or lyophilized platelets, offers a good degree of specificity. This PCP can also be used with the APTT (Howard & Firkin, 1983; Triplett *et al.*, 1983), but experience with this test is limited.

Table 13.2 Situations in which lupus anticoagulant screening may be indicated

---

Venous thromboembolic disease, especially:
Spontaneous venous thrombosis at age younger than 40 years
Recurrent venous thrombosis
Unusual venous thrombosis, such as Budd–Chiari syndrome
Thromboembolic pulmonary hypertension

Arterial thrombotic disease, particularly:
Unexplained arterial occlusion at younger than 30 years
Unusual cerebrovascular events

Other conditions:
Recurrent unexplained fetal loss and early severe pre-eclampsia
Systemic lupus erythematosus and some other collagen vascular disorders
Immune thrombocytopenic purpura
Livedo reticularis

And
False positive serological tests for syphilis
Unexplained prolonged APTT; undue sensitivity of APTT to heparin

---

2 Recommended methods

Conditions where testing for the lupus anticoagulant may be required to assist in diagnosis and management are listed in Table 13.2.

2.1 Sample collection and handling

Careful blood collection, using a 19-gauge needle and minimal stasis, is advised to avoid platelet activation. Blood should be processed as soon as possible and ideally within 1 hour of collection. It is important to obtain plasma with a platelet count of less than $10 \times 10^9/l$ and to achieve this it is suggested that either double-centrifugation or filtration is used.

2.1.1 Double-centrifugation

1 Platelet-poor plasma (PPP) is prepared by centrifuging citrated blood at 2000 $\times$ g for 10 minutes, then removing the plasma, avoiding the plasma–buffy-coat interface, and transferring to a plastic tube.

2 The plasma is then recentrifuged at 2000 $\times$ g for 10 minutes (or ideally in a microcentrifuge at 10 000 $\times$ g for 5 minutes) and the plasma again removed avoiding the interface.

2.1.2 Filtration

Slow filtration of PPP through a 0.22-μm cellulose acetate syringe filter is adequate (Minisart R, Sartorius Ltd, GB-Belmont, Surrey, or Anotec, Banbury, Oxford). Where possible, tests should be performed on fresh plasma. When frozen plasma is used, rigorous care in preparation of the fresh platelet-free plasma is advised.

Normal control plasma must be carefully prepared in a similar way to the test plasma. Commercial normal plasmas might not be free of platelet fragments and may therefore be unsuitable. Advice and specifications should be obtained from the manufacturer.

2.2 Test procedures

These inhibitors are heterogeneous in their behaviour in phospholipid-dependent coagulation tests and no single test for their identification is sufficient. At least two tests are advisable, one of which could be the screening test, the APTT. A flow diagram for the laboratory investigation for lupus anticoagulant is given in Fig. 13.1.

A coagulation screen, including prothrombin time, APTT, with thrombin time or fibrinogen estimation, is required before proceeding to lupus anticoagulant testing, in order to exclude abnormalities unrelated to lupus anticoagulant.

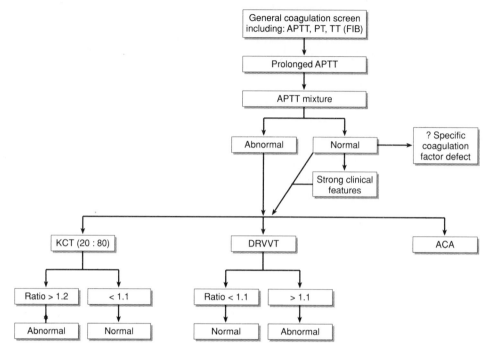

Fig. 13.1 Flow diagram for laboratory investigation when lupus anticoagulant is suspected. To confirm the presence of lupus anticoagulant two positive tests are advisable, one of which could be the screening APTT test. PT, prothrombin time; TT, thrombin time; FIB, fibrinogen estimation.

2.3 Screening with activated partial thromboplastin time

The APTT should be performed on freshly prepared patient PPP, on pooled normal PPP, and on a mixture of four parts patient PPP to one part normal PPP (80%:20% mixture). Even the most sensitive APTT method will not detect all inhibitors and so an additional specific test should be performed in suspected cases of lupus anticoagulant, even if the APTT is normal.

2.4 Confirmatory tests

These must confirm that the inhibitor activity is due to lupus anticoagulant, directed against procoagulant phospholipids, and not to an inhibitor to a single clotting factor. Although some degree of specificity can be achieved using mixtures of patient and control plasmas, better specificity is provided by use of a PCP.

For two tests, the KCT and the DRVVT, standardized methodology has been shown to improve performance (Table 13.3) and is therefore recommended (see below). For other tests, firm data evaluating their performance as regards speci-

Table 13.3 Interpretations in UK lupus anticoagulant surveys

	Plasma					
	01	02	03	04	05	06
Dilute Russell's viper venom time						
Defect	Weak	Strong	Absent	Absent	Moderate	Moderate
Methodology	Non-standardized			Standardized		
Proportion correct	42%	61%	55%	93%	87%	66%
Kaolin clotting time						
Defect	Weak	Strong	Absent	Absent	Moderate	Moderate
Methodology	Non-standardized			Standardized		
Proportion correct	43%	83%	67%	98%	81%	85%

Plasmas 01, 02 and 03 were included in the first UK lupus quality control survey (Exner *et al.*, 1990). The KCT and DRVVT results from this survey are tabulated.

In a second exercise, three further lyophilized plasmas, 04, 05 and 06, were included, which were, respectively, normal and two moderate-intensity lupus-positive samples. Participants were requested to test by KCT or DRVVT with standardized methodology, using method sheets included in the survey. These results are tabulated for comparison with the results of the first survey. The standardized methods form the basis for the recommendations in these guidelines for KCT and DRVVT.

ficity are still awaited and so these tests have not been included in the present recommendations.

3 Kaolin clotting time (Exner *et al.*, 1978)

3.1 Reagents and materials

- Plastic or glass coagulation tubes – for example, 75 × 10 mm polystyrene.
- Calcium chloride ($CaCl_2$) (0.025 M).
- Owren's buffer:
  5.825 g sodium diethylbarbiturate;
  7.335 g sodium chloride (NaCl);
  dissolve in 750 ml distilled water;
  add 0.1 M hydrochloric acid (HCl) to give pH 7.35;
  adjust volume to 1000 ml with distilled water.
- Kaolin (20 mg/ml in Owren's buffer, pH 7.35).
- Normal control plasma.

3.2 Test procedure

Perform tests in duplicate on normal plasma, on test plasma and on a 1:4 mixture of test and normal plasma. A full curve is not essential, but the ratios of test to normal and of the 1:4 mixture to normal are calculated, as shown below:

$$\text{Test ratio} = \frac{\text{test (seconds)}}{\text{normal (seconds)}}$$

$$\text{Mixture ratio} = \frac{1:4 \text{ mixture (seconds)}}{\text{normal (seconds)}}$$

1 Place 0.2 ml plasma in the plastic tube at 37°C.
2 Add 0.1 ml kaolin and tilt three times.
3 Incubate for 3 minutes at 37°C.
4 Add 0.2 ml $CaCl_2$, start stop-watch and tilt three times.
5 At 60 seconds, slowly tilt and record time of end point.

3.3 Interpretation

A test ratio of >1.2 indicates an abnormal result; a mixture ratio of >1.2 should be considered a positive result for lupus anticoagulant and a ratio between 1.1 and 1.2 equivocal.

Note: A control time of less than 60 seconds suggests contamination of the normal control plasma with platelet fragments and invalidates the results.

4 Dilute Russell's viper venom test and platelet correction procedure (Thiagarajan & Shapiro, 1983)

4.1 Reagents and materials

- Glass tubes (75 × 10 mm rimless).
- $CaCl_2$ (0.025 M).
- Imidazole buffer (0.05 M, pH 7.3):
  3.4 g imidazole (glyoxaline);
  5.85 g NaCl;
  dissolve in 900 ml distilled water;
  adjust pH with HCl;
  make volume to 1000 ml with distilled water.
- 100 mM ethylenediamine tetra-acetatic acid (EDTA) in buffer.
- 3.74 g disodium (Na_2) EDTA diluted in 100 ml of buffer to achieve this concentration.
- Imidazole buffer with albumin:
  dissolve 0.1 g bovine serum albumin (fraction V, 99% pure – for example, Sigma Chemical Co. Ltd, Dorset, Poole) in 10 ml imidazole buffer (pH 7.3); store at −20°C and then thaw for use, or use during the working day.
- Calcium-free Tyrode's buffer (pH 6.5):
  8.0 g NaCl;
  0.2 g potassium chloride (KCl);
  0.065 g sodium acid phosphate ($NaH_2PO_4.2H_2O$);

0.415 g magnesium chloride (MgCl$_2$.6H$_2$O);

1.0 g sodium bicarbonate (NaHCO$_3$);

dissolve in 900 ml distilled water, adjust pH to bring to 1 l.

- 1 μg Iloprost (Schering, UK) or Epoprostenol (Wellcome, Dartford, Essex) diluted 1:100 in buffer (that is, 10 ng/ml).

- Tris(hydroxymethyl)aminomethane (TRIS)-buffered saline (TBS):

  stock solution;

  60.5 g TRIS per litre water with HCl to pH 7.6;

  working buffer;

  dilute stock solution 1:10 in 0.15 M saline;

  10 mM EDTA in buffer;

  0.37 g Na$_2$EDTA in 100 ml buffer.

- Russell's viper venom (Diagnostic Reagents, Thame, Oxford, Wellcome Diagnostics, or Sigma Chemical Co. Ltd: all are suitable): reconstitute to give a stock solution containing 1 mg/ml and store in 20-μl aliquots at −20°C or below.

- Phospholipid – use cephalin, such as Diagen 'Bell and Alton' phospholipid reagent (Diagnostic Reagents Ltd, UK), which does not contain activator, from a sensitive APTT method; reconstitute according to the manufacturer's instructions for use in the APTT.

4.2 Reagent preparation

4.2.1 Dilute Russell's viper venom

The stock solution is thawed and 10 μl is added to 5 ml imidazole buffer with albumin. The venom concentration is further adjusted to give a Russell's viper venom (RVV) clotting time of between 30 and 35 seconds in a mixture of 0.1 ml of RVV, 0.1 ml normal control PPP, 0.1 ml of undiluted phospholipid and 0.1 ml CaCl$_2$ at 37°C. Store the RVV solution on ice and use within 4 hours.

4.2.2 Dilute phospholipid

The RVV test is repeated, using normal control PPP, dilute RVV and phospholipid diluted in imidazole buffer 1:2, 1:4, 1:8 and 1:16. From these results, a dilution of phospholipid is selected which gives a DRVVT of between 35 and 40 seconds (2−5 seconds greater than the time with undiluted phospholipid). This is subsequently used in testing normal control and patients' plasmas.

4.2.3 Freeze–thawed washed platelets

Platelet-rich plasma (PRP) is prepared by centrifuging citrated whole blood at 170 × *g* for 10 minutes. The supernatant PRP is carefully removed and placed in a plastic tube. The platelets are washed three times in either: (i) calcium-free Tyrode's buffer plus 10 ng/ml Iloprost, or Epoprostenol, and 10 mM EDTA; (ii) imidazole buffer (pH 7.3) plus 10 mM EDTA; or (iii) TBS (pH 7.6) plus 10 mM

EDTA, by repeated suspension in buffer, followed by recentrifugation at 2000 × g for 10 minutes. Finally, they are resuspended at a concentration of 200–500 × 10^9 in the selected buffer, without Iloprost, Epoprostenol or EDTA, and stored in plastic phials at −20°C or below. It is advisable to dilute the PRP 1:2 with buffer (and inhibitors where appropriate) before the first centrifugation step. The platelets are rapidly thawed for use, mixed well and used in place of the dilute phospholipid in the DRVVT as part of the DRVVT PCP. Some commercial platelet preparations – for example, Biodata platelet extract reagent (Lep Scientific, Milton Keynes) – are available, which are designed for use in lupus anticoagulant tests.

4.3 Dilute Russell's viper venom time and platelet correction procedure method

1 Into clean glass tubes at 37°C, pipette:
   (a) 0.1 ml diluted phospholipid;
   (b) 0.1 ml normal control plasma.
2 Mix and incubate for 30 seconds.
3 0.1 ml dilute RVV reagent.
4 Incubate for exactly 30 seconds and then add 0.1 ml $CaCl_2$ and time clot formation.
5 Repeat steps **1–4** with patient plasma.
6 If the result with patient plasma is longer than that with normal control plasma, repeat steps **1–4** for normal and patient plasmas, substituting washed freeze–thawed platelets for the dilute phospholipid reagent.
7 Calculate the ratio of patient clotting times to normal clotting times for both DRVVT and PCP.

4.4 Interpretation

1 Normal ratio 0.9–1.09.
2 Ratios of >1.1 in DRVVT should be retested using the PCP, and a significant shortening (10%) of the DRVVT is suggestive of the presence of lupus anticoagulant.
3 A normal control plasma must be tested with each batch of patient plasmas, and should be repeated at regular intervals (at least every hour) to check for loss of activity of the RVV reagent.

5 Lupus anticoagulant testing in the presence of anticoagulation treatment

There are no reliable methods for testing for the presence of the lupus anticoagulant when the patient is receiving heparin or oral anticoagulants. If the patient is receiving heparin, testing should be delayed until treatment with heparin has stopped. Mixtures of patient and normal plasma may correct the coumarin defect, without neutralizing the lupus anticoagulant inhibitory activity. Consequently, a 50% normal to 50% test mixture giving a ratio of more than 1.1 with the DRVVT is suggestive of the presence of lupus anticoagulant. Similarly, an 80% normal to 20% test mixture giving a ratio of more than 1.2 with KCT suggests the presence of the lupus anticoagulant inhibitor. Firm conclusions cannot be made, however, unless testing is repeated after discontinuing oral anticoagulation.

6 Discussion

The clinical diversity of the primary antiphospholipid syndrome has recently become widely recognized (Asherson *et al.*, 1989) and the identification of the lupus anticoagulant is important in the diagnosis and management of this condition. Consequently, lupus anticoagulant testing has become an essential routine procedure for haemostasis laboratories. Nevertheless, there is considerable controversy about the most appropriate methods for detecting lupus anticoagulant (Triplett & Brandt, 1989). Further problems were highlighted in the first UK national survey by the Lupus Anticoagulant Working Party (1990), when three freeze-dried samples were distributed to 183 laboratories. These problems included preanalytical and analytical factors, as well as choice of test type. Based on these results, the methodology for two of the most widely used confirmatory tests was specified as described above.

The benefits of this approach for improving the identification and interpretation of the lupus anticoagulant test were shown when a second group of three freeze-dried samples were distributed to routine laboratories. Standardization of the two confirmatory tests led to considerable improvement in the correct identification of negative and moderately positive lupus anticoagulant samples. The relative ease with which this methodology can be introduced into a laboratory was shown by a successful wet workshop, when over 60 participants performed the standardized assays satisfactorily.

The main aim of these guidelines and the Lupus Anticoagulant Working Party is to encourage standardized methodology for laboratories wishing to test for lupus anticoagulant. The current recommendations suggest that laboratories should perform at least one standardized confirmatory test in addition to the APPT screening test.

Correct reporting of a positive lupus anticoagulant test will generate increased confidence in the diagnosis of the antiphospholipid syndrome. This will allow multicentre clinical trials to determine the incidence and treatment response of the thrombotic episodes and recurrent fetal loss which are associated with this condition.

References

Asherson R.A., Khamashta M.A., Ordi-Ros J. *et al.* (1989) The primary antiphospholipid syndrome: major clinical and serological features. *Medicine* **68**, 366–374.

Austen D.E. & Rhymes I.L. (1975) DLE inhibitor test. *Laboratory Manual of Blood Coagulation*, pp. 650–651. Blackwell Scientific Publications, Oxford.

Exner T. (1985) Comparison of two simple tests for the lupus anticoagulant. *American Journal of Clinical Pathology* **83**, 215–218.

Exner T., Rickard A. & Kronberg H. (1978) A sensitive test demonstrating lupus anticoagulant and its behavioural patterns. *British Journal of Haematology* **40**, 143–151.

Exner T., Triplett D.A., Taberner D.A., Howard M.A. & Harris E.N. (1990) Comparison of test methods for the lupus anticoagulant: international survey on lupus anticoagulants – 1 (ISLA-1). *Thrombosis and Haemostasis* **64**, 478–480.

Exner T., Triplett D.A., Taberner D. & Machin S.J. (1991) Guidelines for testing and revised criteria for lupus anticoagulants. *Thrombosis and Haemostasis* **65**, 320–322.

Green D., Hougie C., Kazmier F.J., Lechner K., Mannucci P.M., Rizza C. & Sultan Y. (1983) Report of the Working Party on Acquired Inhibitors: studies of the 'lupus' anticoagulant. *Thrombosis and Haemostasis* **49**, 144–146.

Harris E.N. (1990) Anticardiolipin antibodies. *British Journal of Haematology* **74**, 1–9.

Howard M.A. & Firkin B.G. (1983) Investigation of the lupus-like inhibitor by-passing activity of platelets. *Thrombosis and Haemostasis* **50**, 775–779.

Hughes G.R.V. (1983) Thrombosis, abortion, cerebral disease and the lupus anticoagulant. *British Medical Journal* **287**, 1088–1089.

Hughes G.R.V. (1988) An immune mechanism in thrombosis. *Quarterly Journal of Medicine* **258**, 753–754.

Lesperance B., David M., Rauch J., Infante-Rivard C. & Rivard G.E. (1988) Relative sensitivity of different tests in the detection of low titre lupus anticoagulants. *Thrombosis and Haemostasis* **60**, 217–219.

Lo S.C.L., Oldmeadow M.J., Howard M.A. & Firkin B.G. (1989) Comparison of laboratory tests used in identification of the lupus anticoagulant. *American Journal of Hematology* **30**, 213–220.

Lupus Anticoagulant Working Party (1990) Detection of the lupus-like anticoagulant: current laboratory practice in the United Kingdom. *Journal of Clinical Pathology* **43**, 73–75.

McGlassin D.L., Brey R.L., Strickland D.M. & Patterson W.R. (1989) Differences in kaolin clotting times and platelet counts resulting from variations in specimen processing. *Clinical and Laboratory Science* **2**, 109–110.

Mannucci P.M., Canciani M.T., Mari D. & Meuycci P. (1979) The varied sensitivity of partial thromboplastin and prothrombin reagents in the demonstration of lupus-like anticoagulants. *Scandinavian Journal of Haematology* **22**, 423–432.

Schleider M.A., Nachman R.L., Jaffe E.A. & Coleman M. (1976) A clinical study of the lupus anticoagulant. *Blood* **48**, 499–509.

Stevenson K.J., Easton A.C., Curry A., Thomson J.M. & Poller L. (1986) The reliability of activated partial thromboplastin time methods and the relationship to lipid composition and ultrastructure. *Thrombosis and Haemostasis* **55**, 250–258.

Taberner D.A. & Poller L. (1985) Detection of inhibitors using the activated partial thromboplastin time test. *British Journal of Haematology* **61**, 565–569.

Taberner D., Machin S., Mackie I., Giddings J., Malia R. & Greaves M. (1989) Quality control of the lupus anticoagulant test in the UK. *Postgraduate Medical Journal* **65**, 698–699.

Thiagarajan P. & Shapiro S.S. (1983) Lupus anticoagulants. In Coleman M.A. (ed.) *Methods in Haematology: Disorders of Thrombin Formulation other than Haemophilia*, pp. 223–247. Churchill Livingstone, Edinburgh.

Thiagarajan P., Pengo V. & Shapiro S.S. (1986) The use of the dilute Russell viper venom time for the diagnosis of lupus anticoagulants. *Blood* **68**, 869–872.

Triplett D.A. & Brandt J.T. (1989) Laboratory identification of the lupus anticoagulant. *British Journal of Haematology* **73**, 139–142.

Triplett D.A., Brandt J.T., Kaczar D. & Schaeffer J. (1983) Laboratory diagnosis of lupus inhibitors: a comparison of the tissue thromboplastin inhibition procedure with a new platelet neutralisation procedure. *American Journal of Clinical Pathology* **79**, 678–682.

14 The Use and Monitoring
of Heparin*

Prepared by the
Haemostasis and Thrombosis Task Force

1 Properties of unfractionated and low-molecular-weight heparin

1.1 Chemistry of heparin

Unfractionated heparin is a naturally occurring glycosaminoglycan produced by the mast cells of most species. It is extracted from porcine or bovine mucosa, all the products currently used in the UK being of porcine origin. It consists of alternating chains of uronic acid and glucosamine, sulphated to varying degrees, and has a molecular weight range of 5000–35 000, with a mean of about 12 000–14 000.

Low-molecular-weight heparin is manufactured from unfractionated heparin by controlled depolymerization, using chemical (nitrous acid or alkaline hydrolysis) or enzymatic (heparinase) methods. Although these processes yield different end groups, there is no evidence that these differences in chemical structure affect biological function. The biological properties of any low-molecular-weight heparin are primarily determined by its molecular weight distribution. The products currently available have an average molecular weight between 4000 and 6000, and 60–80% of the total polysaccharides lie between 2000 and 8000.

1.2 Anticoagulant activities

All anticoagulant activities of unfractionated heparin and low-molecular-weight heparin depend on the presence of a specific pentasaccharide sequence which binds with high affinity to antithrombin III (ATIII) and potentiates its activity (Lindahl et al., 1979); this sequence is present in about one-third of the chains in unfractionated heparin but in lower proportions in low-molecular-weight heparin because some of these sequences are destroyed by the depolymerization process. Acceleration of inhibition of factor Xa (anti-Xa activity) requires only the pentasaccharide sequence (approximate molecular weight 1700), but potentiation

---

* Reprinted with permission from *Journal of Clinical Pathology*, 1993, **46**, 97–103.

of thrombin inhibition (anti-IIa activity; also prolongation of activated partial thromboplastin time (APTT)) requires a minimum total chain length of 18 saccharides (molecular weight approximately 5400) (Lane *et al.*, 1984). Therefore, in all low-molecular-weight heparin preparations the anti-Xa activity is greater than the anti-IIa or APTT activity. In the low-molecular-weight heparins currently available, the ratio of anti-Xa to anti-IIa activity ranges from 1.8 to 3.5.

1.3 Standardization

When initially developed, low-molecular-weight heparins were assayed against the unfractionated heparin standard by a variety of different methods, and the units for the different products could not readily be compared. An international standard for low-molecular-weight heparin was established in 1986 (Barrowcliffe *et al.*, 1988) and all manufacturers now use it to calibrate their products for both anti-Xa and anti-IIa activities. In some published and conference presentations, however, other units are still quoted. In particular, the Sanofi product, Fraxiparine, is often described in 'Institut Choay units' (ICU) – these being a measure of anti-Xa activity – but they should be divided by about 2.5 to obtain the equivalent in international units (IU) of anti-Xa activity. When this is done, the dose requirement for prophylaxis of deep-vein thrombosis in general surgery falls within a fairly narrow range for all products: from 2000 to 3500 IU of anti-Xa activity, once a day subcutaneously.

1.4 Pharmacology

Unfractionated heparin is available as sodium or calcium salt. After subcutaneous injection of equal amounts, the overall anticoagulant activity is lower with calcium than with sodium salt, but this does not affect clinical efficacy. There may be a lower incidence of ecchymoses after subcutaneous injection of the calcium than of the sodium salt, but there is no clear evidence for any major differences in the incidence of haemorrhagic effects. All low-molecular-weight heparins are in the sodium form except Fraxiparine, which is a calcium salt.

Both unfractionated heparin and low-molecular-weight heparin are given parenterally, by either intravenous or subcutaneous injection. Metabolism is by a saturable mechanism, involving binding to endothelial cells and clearance by the reticuloendothelial system, and a non-saturable mechanism, involving mainly renal clearance. Both mechanisms are important for unfractionated heparin, but renal clearance predominates for low-molecular-weight heparin. There is no evidence that either unfractionated heparin or low-molecular-weight heparin crosses the placenta.

1.5 Differences between unfractionated heparin and low-molecular-weight heparin

The principal aspects in which low-molecular-weight heparin differs from unfractionated heparin are as follows.

1.5.1 Pharmacokinetics

Low-molecular-weight heparin has a longer half-life than unfractionated heparin, by both intravenous and subcutaneous injection (Albada *et al.*, 1989; Boneu *et al.*, 1990). The intravenous half-life is about 2 hours, measured as anti-Xa activity, although it is somewhat shorter (about 80 minutes) when measured by anti-IIa assay. The half-life of unfractionated heparin is dose-dependent but at normal intravenous doses is 45–60 minutes by both assay methods. The subcutaneous half-life of low-molecular-weight heparin is about 4 hours, measured as anti-Xa activity. Unlike unfractionated heparin, which has a bioavailability of less than 50%, all low-molecular-weight heparins have a bioavailability after subcutaneous injection of 100%. These differences in pharmacokinetics and bioavailability are responsible for the successful use of once-daily subcutaneous injections of low-molecular-weight heparin for prophylaxis of deep-vein thrombosis. There is no evidence for differences in pharmacokinetics between the different low-molecular-weight heparins.

1.5.2 Interaction with proteins

Several proteins interact strongly with heparin to antagonize its anticoagulant activity, the most important being platelet factor 4 (PF4) and protamine. Binding affinity to these proteins is reduced with decreasing molecular weight, so that low-molecular-weight heparin preparations require higher concentrations of PF4 or protamine to neutralize their activity than does unfractionated heparin. Below 18-saccharide heparin chains become increasingly resistant to neutralization by either of these agents, so that all low-molecular-weight heparin preparations have a portion of their anti-Xa activity which is non-neutralizable (Lane *et al.*, 1984; Harenberg *et al.*, 1986). Animal studies indicate, however, that this does not affect the ability of protamine to neutralize the haemorrhagic action of low-molecular-weight heparins (Van Ryn-McKenna *et al.*, 1990).

1.5.3 Interaction with cells

Low-molecular-weight heparin binds less strongly than unfractionated heparin to endothelial cells, and this is partly responsible for the difference in pharmacokinetics, because endothelial binding and processing is an important mechanism of clearance for unfractionated heparin. Low-molecular-weight heparin also interacts with platelets less readily than unfractionated heparin, whether measured as potentiation of spontaneous aggregation or as inhibition of agonist-induced aggregation (Salzman *et al.*, 1980).

1.5.4 *Release of lipase*
Low-molecular-weight heparin, when given in similar doses to unfractionated heparin, releases lower concentrations of the enzymes lipoprotein lipase and hepatic lipase from the vascular endothelium.

2 Clinical use of heparin

Heparin is used in the treatment of established thromboembolic disease (therapeutic administration) and to prevent thrombosis and embolism (prophylactic administration). It is also valuable in the maintenance of extracorporeal circuits in cardiopulmonary bypass and haemodialysis.

3 Therapeutic administration

3.1 Indications
Therapeutic heparin is given to treat conditions in which thrombosis or embolism has occurred. More heparin is required for this purpose than for prophylaxis.

Currently accepted indications are: deep-vein thrombosis; pulmonary embolism; myocardial infarction; unstable angina pectoris; and acute peripheral arterial occlusion.

At present, only unfractionated heparin can be recommended for therapeutic use in normal circumstances, although clinical trials of low-molecular-weight heparin are being conducted and already indicate a potential role in the out-patient management of deep-vein thrombosis (Hirsh & Levine, 1992; Hull *et al.*, 1992).

Where possible, a coagulation screen and platelet count should be performed before beginning treatment.

3.2 Route
Heparin can be given either intravenously by continuous infusion, using an infusion pump, or by intermittent subcutaneous injection into the anterior or antero-lateral wall of the abdomen near the iliac crest or thigh, using small-volume syringes with small-bore needles so that a precise dose can be delivered (Bentley *et al.*, 1980). The recommended concentration for subcutaneous administration is 25 000 IU/ml.

3.3 Dosage
3.3.1 *Deep-vein thrombosis and pulmonary embolism*
In adults, an intravenous loading dose of 5000 IU is given, save in severe pulmonary embolism, when 10 000 IU may be advisable. Anticoagulation is maintained by intravenous infusion of 1000–2000 IU/hour or subcutaneous injection of 15 000 IU 12-hourly, adjusted in each case by laboratory monitoring, 4–6 hours after the treatment has started.

Children or small adults should receive a lower loading dose, and maintenance therapy can be calculated on the basis of 15–25 IU/kg/hour intravenously or 250 IU/kg 12-hourly subcutaneously.

3.3.2 Myocardial infarction
Heparin is used to prevent the following.

Coronary reocclusion after thrombolysis
Current regimens include: (i) 2000 IU intravenously, followed by 12 500 IU subcutaneously 12-hourly after streptokinase (SCATI Group, 1989; International Study Group, 1990); and (ii) 5000 IU followed by 1000 IU/hour intravenously after tissue plasminogen activator (Hsia *et al.*, 1990).

Mural thrombosis
Subcutaneous injection of 12 500 IU 12-hourly for at least 10 days is effective (SCATI Group, 1989; Turpie *et al.*, 1989).

3.3.3 Unstable angina pectoris
An intravenous regimen is used. The same doses as for deep-venous thrombosis and pulmonary embolism given above apply (Theroux *et al.*, 1988).

3.3.4 Acute peripheral arterial occlusion
Surgical treatment is often used in this condition, and thrombolytic treatment or full therapeutic heparin treatment or both are frequently used.

3.3.5 Disseminated intravascular coagulation
The use of heparin in disseminated intravascular coagulation (DIC) is not established, but its use is logical where the manifestations are predominantly vaso-occlusive. Because of the risk of bleeding, it is unusual to administer more than 1000 IU/hour.

3.4 Laboratory monitoring
Daily laboratory monitoring is essential when therapeutic heparin is prescribed. The APTT technique is the most widely used for this purpose, and a value of 1.5–2.5 times the midpoint of the normal range is common practice. Depending on the APTT reagents used, this roughly corresponds to a heparin concentration of 0.2–0.4 IU/ml (Hirsh, 1991). The calcium thrombin time is an alternative test. The APTT and calcium thrombin time are not sensitive to low-molecular-weight heparin and are inappropriate for monitoring treatment with this drug.

3.5 Adjustment of dose

Routine APTT tests should be performed at the same time each day and in the same relationship to subcutaneous doses. An interval of 4–6 hours between injection and testing is appropriate. An increased dose may require a small bolus injection of 3000–5000 IU if an immediate effect is desired. If a reduction of dose is necessary, it is advisable to stop the intravenous infusion for 30–60 minutes before reducing the dosage.

Where necessary, protamine can be given intravenously to neutralize the effect of heparin. The effect is instantaneous and 1 mg of protamine is roughly equivalent to 100 IU of heparin. If heparin neutralization is required 60 minutes after heparin injection, only 50% of the theoretical calculated dose of protamine should be given, while after 2 hours from heparin injection only 25% of the calculated dose is appropriate. Dose can also be calculated by a protamine neutralization test. Protamine should be given slowly over 10 minutes because it can cause hypotension and bradycardia, and not more than 40 mg of protamine should be given in any one injection, except in the context of cardiopulmonary bypass. Treatment may have to be repeated, because protamine is cleared from the circulation more rapidly than heparin. Allergic and even anaphylactic reactions may occur, particularly in diabetics who have received protamine zinc insulin.

3.6 Duration of treatment

Parenteral treatment should continue until it is no longer required or until oral anticoagulants have achieved a therapeutic effect. This generally takes at least 3 days, even if the International Normalized Ratio (INR) falls within the appropriate therapeutic range earlier, because of the different half-lives of the vitamin-K-dependent factors. Four to 5 days of heparin treatment is usually sufficient, but longer courses of 9–10 days may be advisable for patients with massive iliofemoral thrombosis or major pulmonary embolism (Gallus *et al.*, 1986; Hull *et al.*, 1990).

3.7 Contraindications

There are no absolute contraindications to heparin, but the main risk is abnormal bleeding.

Full treatment is more hazardous after major trauma or recent surgery (especially to the eye or nervous system).

It is not desirable to treat patients who are severely thrombocytopenic with heparin, because the drug itself can reduce the platelet count (see complications) and because of the additional haemostatic defect. If it is necessary to give heparin to patients with thrombocytopenia, a reduced loading and maintenance dose should be given.

Other relative contraindications include: congenital or acquired haemorrhagic diatheses; recent cerebral haemorrhage; uncontrolled hypertension; hepatic dysfunction, including oesophageal varices; renal failure; peptic ulceration; and known hypersensitivity to heparin.

4 Prophylactic administration

4.1 Indications

Prophylactic heparin is given to prevent deep-venous thrombosis and pulmonary embolism, particularly in patients at risk when undergoing a surgical procedure under general anaesthesia which lasts for over 30 minutes and requires a stay in hospital after surgery.

In the context of general surgery, high-risk patients include those aged over 40, those who are obese, those who have a malignancy, those who have had prior deep-vein thrombosis or pulmonary embolism, those with an established thrombophilic disorder and those undergoing large or complicated surgical procedures. Any patient undergoing major orthopaedic surgery has a higher risk of thromboembolism, and special techniques have been developed to address this problem. The prevention of deep-vein thrombosis and pulmonary embolism in these and other situations was the subject of a consensus conference held by the US National Institutes of Health in 1986 (Consensus conference, 1986). This remains a useful source of information and advice, although low-molecular-weight heparin was not available at that time. It also contains a valuable review of the indications for other methods of prophylaxis, such as low-dose warfarin, dextran, external pneumatic compression and graduated-compression elastic stockings. A more recent account of the prophylaxis of deep-vein thrombosis has been published (Turpie, 1991).

4.1.1 General surgery

The recommended regimen for general surgery using unfractionated heparin is (International Multicentre Trial, 1975):
- Preoperative 2 hours – 5000 IU subcutaneously.
- Postoperative – 5000 IU subcutaneously every 8–12 hours for 7 days or until the patient is mobile.

Low-molecular-weight heparins have not been shown to be more effective than unfractionated heparin in this group. There is no consistent evidence of a clinically important alteration in postoperative bleeding (Samama & Desnoyers, 1991).

Dose requirements for each product have been established following extensive clinical trials, and manufacturers' dose recommendations should be strictly followed. It should be noted that overdosage with low-molecular-weight heparins may cause bleeding without a significant prolongation of the APTT.

No laboratory monitoring is necessary for standard prophylactic doses of unfractionated heparin or low-molecular-weight heparins. If it is decided that monitoring of prophylactic heparin is desirable, then anti-Xa assays should be used. These assays may be performed by coagulation methods but are simpler by chromogenic substrate techniques, and commercial assay kits are available. Both methods should be controlled by the appropriate international heparin standard. In the event of overdose, it may be more difficult to neutralize the effect of low-molecular-weight heparin because of its longer half-life and lesser sensitivity to protamine.

4.1.2 Orthopaedic surgery
Standard heparin prophylaxis can reduce the risk of thromboembolism in patients undergoing major orthopaedic procedures, but, despite its use, 25% of patients will still develop deep-vein thrombosis (Collins *et al.*, 1988). Several solutions have been proposed.

Adjusted-dose heparin
A dose-adjusted regimen, using APTT monitoring to maintain minimal prolongation of the test, has been shown to reduce further the incidence of thrombosis in hip surgery (Leyvraz *et al.*, 1983; Taberner *et al.*, 1989). This approach requires close cooperation between surgical and laboratory staff.

Low-molecular-weight heparin
Several studies have shown that low-molecular-weight heparin in a fixed dose can reduce the incidence of venous thrombosis to about 15% (Samama & Desnoyers, 1991).

Turpie and colleagues (1986) conducted a randomized trial of enoxaparin compared with placebo in patients undergoing total hip replacement, using a fixed-dose regimen, and showed a fourfold reduction in thrombosis. The overall incidence of venous thrombosis in the treated group was 12%, with a 4% incidence of proximal thrombosis. There was no evidence of an increase in bleeding. Leyvraz and colleagues (1991) compared their adjusted-dose unfractionated heparin regimen with a fixed dose of Fraxiparine and showed that the low-molecular-weight heparin was more effective in preventing proximal venous thrombosis after hip replacement, with comparable bleeding complications.

Thus low-molecular-weight heparin seems to be the treatment of choice in major orthopaedic surgery to the lower limb, because of its effectiveness and because the once-daily regimen requires no laboratory monitoring.

Warfarin prophylaxis
Although this is effective, some surgeons are reluctant to operate on patients taking warfarin.

Heparin plus dihydroergotamine
Dihydroergotamine 0.5 mg subcutaneously is given with each standard heparin dose (Kakkar *et al.*, 1979). The disadvantage of this approach is the risk of peripheral ischaemia.

4.2 Other preparations

Several other preparations are being developed which may have a role in the prevention of venous thromboembolism. Of these, dermatan sulphate, heparan sulphate and the low-molecular-weight heparinoids are related to heparin and have been considered by Samama and Desnoyers (1991).

5 Pregnancy

Heparin is the drug of choice for women who require anticoagulation during pregnancy, because it does not cross the placenta. It does carry the risk of causing maternal osteoporosis, however, particularly if the dose exceeds 20 000 IU/24 hours for more than 5 months (Hirsh, 1991). There are no conclusive scientific data on this subject and information is often contradictory. Dahlman and colleagues (1990) found no correlation between osteoporosis and heparin dose or duration of treatment in pregnancy, and in their study the changes were reversible in most cases, findings which contrast with those of the earlier study by de Swiet and colleagues (1983). It should be remembered that oral anticoagulation can be reintroduced immediately after delivery where necessary and that women taking warfarin may safely breastfeed.

5.1 Prophylaxis of thromboembolism

To prevent thromboembolism in mothers with a history of deep-vein thrombosis or pulmonary embolism, an initial dose of 5000 IU 12-hourly by self-administered subcutaneous injection has been recommended. An increase in dose may be needed in the last trimester to prolong the APTT to 1.5 times an average control value at the midinterval (Turpie, 1991), although this can be difficult to achieve. Letsky (1985) recommends 10 000 IU 12-hourly subcutaneously throughout the antenatal period, only changing the dose by reducing it if levels of more than 0.3 IU/ml are found by anti-Xa assay. Titrated heparin has been used successfully in the management of ATIII deficiency, ATIII concentrate being used to cover delivery (Hellgren *et al.*, 1982). Some authorities caution against the prescription of warfarin at any stage of pregnancy, because of the risk of embryopathy in the first trimester and fetal haemorrhage later, but others approve its use from 16 to 36 weeks, maintaining the INR between 2.0 and 3.0. The exact time at which any prophylaxis is started will depend on the nature of the risk, the previous obstetric history and the mother's own wishes, but it may be possible to delay drug treatment until late in pregnancy, when the greatest risk of thromboembolism develops.

Patients receiving full therapeutic doses of heparin must reduce their heparin dose on the day of delivery to a dose of 10 000–15 000 IU/24 hours intravenously (or 5000–7500 12-hourly subcutaneously). Patients receiving prophylactic doses of heparin should generally continue their treatment unchanged during labour and delivery. In any event, the APTT must be checked to ensure that anticoagulation is not excessive.

Epidural analgesia for those women who have been receiving heparin during pregnancy remains a difficult and controversial problem, but, providing the coagulation screen is within normal limits, it is probably safe to introduce an epidural catheter (Letsky, 1991).

5.2 Antiphospholipid syndromes

Patients with lupus anticoagulant or anticardiolipin antibodies, or both, who have experienced previous thrombotic episodes should also receive heparin prophylaxis. Where patients have suffered recurrent miscarriages despite low-dose aspirin treatment, heparin prophylaxis should be considered in subsequent pregnancies. If heparin monitoring is performed, the APTT test may be unreliable, and an anti-Xa assay is better.

5.3 Prosthetic heart valves

The management of pregnant women with prosthetic heart valves is difficult and controversial. The problems have been highlighted by Iturbe-Alessio and colleagues (1986). They found that low-dose heparin 5000 IU 12-hourly sub-cutaneously was ineffective in preventing valve thrombosis, while the incidence of embryopathy in patients receiving coumarin derivatives from the 6th to the 12th week of gestation was between 25 and 30%. A higher dose of heparin (15 000 IU 12-hourly subcutaneously) has been recommended by Hirsh (1991). Women with artificial heart valves who wish to become pregnant therefore require careful counselling. It is important to emphasize that there is no perfect solution to the problem and that the choices of management will lie between the following:

1 Continuing warfarin throughout pregnancy and accepting the risk of embryopathy.

2 Using heparin throughout pregnancy and accepting the risk of osteoporosis, as well as a possible increased risk of thrombosis.

3 Using heparin until 12–16 weeks, followed by warfarin up to 36 weeks, and then reverting to heparin until delivery.

When using the higher-dose heparin prophylaxis, it would be wise to monitor APTT, aiming to achieve values about 1.5 times an average control value at the midinterval.

5.4 Low-molecular-weight heparin

It is still too early to give any specific recommendations on these preparations in pregnancy. They have the advantage of once-daily administration, but there is no reason to believe that osteoporosis will be less likely to occur with prolonged use.

In circumstances where higher doses are required, anti-Xa assays are necessary for laboratory monitoring.

6 Extracorporeal circulation and haemodialysis

6.1 Cardiopulmonary bypass

Heparin is universally used as the anticoagulant during cardiopulmonary bypass procedures.

The bypass machine is primed with a crystalloid solution, to which 1000 IU of heparin are added to each 500 ml. If stored blood is also used for priming, 3000 IU are added to each unit of blood.

Before the cannulation of the heart and major blood vessels, which is required before bypass surgery can begin, heparin is given intravenously through a cannula placed in a large central vein. The dose is determined on the basis of the surface area or weight of the patient. Usually the initial dose is 300 IU/kg.

The administration of heparin is controlled both before, during and after bypass, by monitoring the activated clotting time (ACT) in an automated system in the operating theatre. Estimations are made every 30 minutes. In patients not receiving heparin, the normal ACT in one system is 100–140 seconds. During cardiopulmonary bypass, the safe range is between 400 and 500 seconds, and further increments of 5000 IU are given to maintain this level, as necessary (Kamath & Fozard, 1980).

When bypass is discontinued, heparin can be reversed readily with protamine. A standard dose is usually given, but it is more sophisticated, though more time-consuming, to titrate the dose of protamine with ACT measurements, using ACT tubes to which known amounts of protamine have been added (Keeler *et al.*, 1991).

Protamine, unlike heparin, may have toxic effects on the cardiopulmonary circulation, and it is usual to administer protamine cautiously after bypass.

6.2 Haemodialysis and haemofiltration

None of the membranes used in haemodialysis and haemofiltration is sufficiently biocompatible to enable the dialysis process to be carried out without anticoagulation of the circuit. In modern haemodialysis machines, a heparin pump is incorporated and heparin is infused directly into the exit line of the extracorporeal circuit. Current clinical practice is to administer a loading dose of heparin at the start of the session, and to give a continuous infusion, which is usually discontinued about 1 hour before dialysis is due to stop, to allow adequate haemostasis to take place when the dialysis needles are removed.

The dose requirements of the patients receiving dialysis vary widely according to the individual. The anticoagulant effect is usually monitored by whole-blood clotting time and, in patients without potential bleeding complications, the clotting time is usually maintained in excess of 40 minutes. In practice, to achieve this will require a loading dose which varies from 1000 to 5000 IU and a maintenance dose of 1000–2000 IU/hour, which gives a heparin concentration of >0.5 IU/ml (Ireland *et al.*, 1988). The dose variability depends on the weight of the patient, the volume of the extracorporeal circuit, the pump speed, which can vary from 150 to 450 ml/minute, and the biocompatibility of the dialysis membrane. In patients who are actively bleeding or who have a known bleeding tendency, it is possible to dialyse for short periods without heparin, using high pump speeds and short dialysis circuits. Usually, however, lines will begin to clot between 60 and 120 minutes after starting dialysis. Alternatively, regional heparin treatment can be given; heparin is infused into the circuit as the blood leaves the patient and a neutralizing dose of protamine is infused into the circuit as the blood is returned to the patient.

6.2.1 Low-molecular-weight heparins

A potential advance in this area has been the introduction of low-molecular-weight heparins, which have a much prolonged half-life in renal failure and therefore may have the advantage of avoiding maintenance infusion. Lipolytic effects tend to be less. Interestingly, patients receiving maintenance haemodialysis will be anticoagulated with heparin for about 900 hours a year, and the question of whether heparin induces osteoporosis has been much discussed. This bony lesion has been very difficult to extrapolate from the complex picture of renal osteodystrophy, however, and there is no hard evidence that it is a major clinical problem or that low-molecular-weight heparins will be less likely to contribute to it.

Monitoring of low-molecular-weight heparins in haemodialysis by anti-Xa assays is still not fully established (although the low-molecular-weight international standard will be useful), and the new technique has not yet achieved wide acceptance.

7 Complications

7.1 Haemorrhage

Haemorrhage usually results from excess dose or idiosyncratic response to conventional dose. Serious concurrent illness, chronic heavy consumption of alcohol and concomitant use of aspirin have also been implicated (Hirsh, 1991).

The management of heparin overdose has already been considered in the section on adjustment of dosage.

7.2 Thrombocytopenia

This is a rare complication of heparin treatment in the UK and may be commoner with the bovine than the porcine preparation. It can occur at any dose and whether heparin is given by the intravenous or subcutaneous route. Both unfractionated heparin and low-molecular-weight heparin are associated with thrombocytopenia, and regular monitoring of the platelet count is advisable.

Clinically important thrombocytopenia is usually delayed, occurring 6–10 days after the start of treatment, and is immune-mediated. Paradoxical thrombosis is common and the heparin should be stopped immediately (Hirsh, 1991).

Heparin from a different source or low-molecular-weight heparin may be tried, but cross-reactivity has been described and it is difficult to judge the appropriate dose of low-molecular-weight heparin for therapeutic use. The heparinoid Danaparoid has minimal cross-reactivity with heparin. Hirudin and ancrod are other potential alternative drugs.

An immediate decline in the platelet count after starting therapy is also occasionally observed; it is thought to be a direct effect due to platelet aggregation and probably does not occur with low-molecular-weight heparin. It is of little clinical importance.

7.3 Osteoporosis

This complication of heparin treatment has only been described with prolonged use and is probably independent of molecular size. It is discussed in the section on pregnancy.

7.4 Abnormal liver function tests

An increase in serum aminotransferase activity has been reported in patients who are being treated with heparin. This does not seem to be of any clinical importance (Salomon & Schmid, 1991).

7.5 Other side-effects

Localized skin necrosis and anaphylaxis caused by hypersensitivity have been described. Alopecia is very rare.

8 Medical audit

The use and monitoring of heparin treatment are suitable topics for medical audit, which might include local reviews of indications, therapeutic and prophylactic doses and control.

Protocols might be drawn up for the use of heparin in pregnancy and agreement reached on the indications for the various heparin preparations available.

9 Note on guidelines

These guidelines should be read in conjunction with BCSH (1990) and Guidelines on the prevention, investigation and management of thromboembolism in pregnancy (see Chapter 16), which have also been prepared by the Haemostasis and Thrombosis Task Force.

References

Albada H., Nieuwenhuis H.K. & Sixma J.J. (1989) Pharmacokinetics of standard and low molecular weight heparin. In Lane D.A. & Lindahl U. (eds) *Heparin – Chemical and Biological Properties – Clinical Applications*, pp. 417–432. Edward Arnold, London.

Barrowcliffe T.W., Curtis A.D., Johnson E.A. & Thomas D.P. (1988) An international standard for low molecular weight heparin. *Thrombosis and Haemostasis* **60**, 1–7.

BCSH Haemostasis and Thrombosis Task Force (1990) Guidelines on oral anticoagulation: second edn. *Journal of Clinical Pathology* **43**, 177–183.

Bentley P.G., Kakkar V.V., Scully M.F., MacGregor I.R., Webb P., Chan P. & Jones N. (1980) An objective study of alternative methods of heparin administration. *Thrombosis Research* **18**, 177–187.

Boneu B., Caranobe C. & Sie P. (1990) Pharmacokinetics of heparin and low molecular weight heparin. In Hirsh J. (ed.) *Antithrombotic Therapy. Baillière's Clinical Haematology*, pp. 531–544. Baillière Tindall, London.

Collins R., Scrimgeour A., Yusuf S. & Peto R. (1988) Reduction in fatal pulmonary embolism and venous thrombosis by perioperative administration of subcutaneous heparin. *New England Journal of Medicine* **318**, 1162–1173.

Consensus conference (1986) Prevention of venous thrombosis and pulmonary embolism. *Journal of the American Medical Association* **256**, 744–749.

Dahlman T., Lindvall N. & Hellgren M. (1990) Osteopenia in pregnancy during long-term heparin treatment: a radiological study post partum. *British Journal of Obstetrics and Gynaecology* **97**, 221–228.

de Swiet M., Dorrington Ward P., Fidler J. *et al.* (1983) Prolonged heparin therapy in pregnancy causes bone demineralization. *British Journal of Obstetrics and Gynaecology* **90**, 1129–1134.

Gallus A., Jackaman J., Tillett J., Mills W. & Wycherley A. (1986) Safety and efficacy of warfarin started early after submassive venous thrombosis or pulmonary embolism. *Lancet* **ii**, 1293–1296.

Harenberg J., Wurzner B., Zimmermann R. & Schettler G. (1986) Bioavailability and antagonization of the low molecular weight heparin CY 216 in man. *Thrombosis Research* **44**, 549–554.

Hellgren M., Tengborn L. & Abildgaard U. (1982) Pregnancy in women with congenital antithrombin III deficiency: experience of treatment with heparin and antithrombin. *Gynecological and Obstetric Investigations* **14**, 127–141.

Hirsh J. (1991) Heparin. *New England Journal of Medicine* **324**, 1565–1574.

Hirsh J. & Levine M.N. (1992) Low molecular weight heparin. *Blood* **79**, 1–17.

Hsia J., Hamilton W.P., Kleiman N., Roberts R., Chaitman B.R. & Ross A.M. (1990) A comparison between heparin and low-dose aspirin as adjunctive therapy with tissue plasminogen activator for acute myocardial infarction. *New England Journal of Medicine* **323**, 1433–1437.

Hull R.D., Raskob G.E., Rosenbloom D. *et al.* (1990) Heparin for 5 days as compared with 10 days in the initial treatment of proximal venous thrombosis. *New England Journal of Medicine* **322**, 1260–1264.

Hull R.D., Raskob G.E., Pineo G.F. *et al.* (1992) Subcutaneous low molecular weight heparin compared with continuous intravenous heparin in the treatment of proximal-vein thrombosis. *New England Journal of Medicine* **326**, 975–982.

International Multicentre Trial (1975) Prevention of fatal post operative pulmonary embolism by low doses of heparin. *Lancet* **ii**, 45–51.

International Study Group (1990) In hospital mortality and clinical course of 20 891 patients with suspected acute myocardial infarction randomised between alteplase and streptokinase with or without heparin. *Lancet* **336**, 71–75.

Ireland H., Lane D.A. & Curtis J.R. (1988) Objective assessment of heparin requirements for haemodialysis in humans. *Journal of Laboratory and Clinical Medicine* **103**, 643–652.

Iturbe-Alessio I., del Carmen Fonseca M., Mutchinik O., Santos M.A., Zajarias A. & Salazar E. (1986) Risks of anticoagulant therapy in pregnant women with artificial heart valves. *New England Journal of Medicine* **315**, 1390–1393.

Kakkar V.V., Stamatakis J.D., Bentley P.D., Lawrence D., de Haas H.A. & Ward V.P. (1979) Prophylaxis for post operative deep venous thrombosis: synergistic effect of heparin and dihydroergotamine. *Journal of the American Medical Association* **241**, 39–42.

Kamath B.S.K. & Fozard J.R. (1980) Control of heparinisation during cardiopulmonary bypass. *Anaesthesia* **35**, 250–256.

Keeler J.F., Shah M.V. & Hansbro S.D. (1991) Protamine – the need to determine the dose. *Anaesthesia* **46**, 925–928.

Lane D.A., Denton J., Flynn A.M., Thunberg L. & Lindahl U. (1984) Anticoagulant activities of heparin oligosaccharides and their neutralization by platelet factor 4. *Biochemistry Journal* **218**, 725–732.

Letsky E.A. (1985) *Coagulation Problems During Pregnancy*. Churchill Livingstone, Edinburgh.

Letsky E.A. (1991) Haemostasis and epidural anaesthesia. *International Journal of Obstetric Anesthesia* **1**, 51–54.

Leyvraz P.F., Richard J., Bachmann F., Van Melle G., Treyvaud J.-M., Livio J.-J. & Candardjis G. (1983) Adjusted versus fixed-dose subcutaneous heparin in the prevention of deep vein thrombosis after total hip replacement. *New England Journal of Medicine* **309**, 954–958.

Leyvraz P.F., Bachmann F., Hoek J., Büller H.R., Postel M., Samama M. & Vandenbroek M.D. (1991) Prevention of deep vein thrombosis after hip replacement: randomised comparison between unfractionated heparin and low molecular weight heparin. *British Medical Journal* **303**, 543–548.

Lindahl U., Backstrom G., Hook M., Thunberg L., Fransson L. & Linker A. (1979) Structure of the antithrombin-binding site in heparin. *Proceedings of the National Academy of Sciences USA* **76**, 3198–3202.

Salomon F. & Schmid M. (1991) Heparin. *New England Journal of Medicine* **325**, 1585.

Salzman E.W., Rosenberg R.D., Smith M.H., Lindon J.N. & Favreau L. (1980) Effect of heparin and heparin fractions on platelet aggregation. *Journal of Clinical Investigation* **65**, 64–73.

Samama M. & Desnoyers P. (1991) Low-molecular weight heparins and related glycosaminoglycans in the prophylaxis and treatment of venous thromboembolism. In Poller L. (ed.) *Recent Advances in Blood Coagulation*, Vol. 5, pp. 177–222. Churchill Livingstone, Edinburgh.

SCATI Group (1989) Randomised controlled trial of subcutaneous calcium–heparin in acute myocardial infarction. *Lancet* **ii**, 182–186.

Taberner D.A., Poller L., Thomson J.M., Lemon G. & Weighill F.J. (1989) Randomised study of adjusted versus fixed low dose heparin prophylaxis of deep vein thrombosis in hip surgery. *British Journal of Surgery* **76**, 933–935.

Theroux P., Ouimet H., McCans J. *et al.* (1988) Aspirin, heparin or both to treat acute unstable angina? *New England Journal of Medicine* **319**, 1105–1111.

Turpie A.G.G. (1991) Prophylaxis of deep vein thrombosis. In Poller L. (ed.) *Recent Advances in Blood Coagulation*, Vol. 5, pp. 161–176. Churchill Livingstone, Edinburgh.

Turpie A.G.G., Levine M.N., Hirsh J. *et al.* (1986) A randomized controlled trial of a low molecular weight heparin (enoxaparin) to prevent deep-vein thrombosis in patients undergoing elective hip surgery. *New England Journal of Medicine* **315**, 925–929.

Turpie A.G.G., Robinson J.G., Doyle D.J. *et al.* (1989) Comparison of high-dose with low-dose subcutaneous heparin to prevent left ventricular mural thrombosis in patients with acute transmural anterior myocardial infarction. *New England Journal of Medicine* **320**, 352–357.

Van Ryn-McKenna J., Cai L., Ofosu F.A., Hirsh J. & Buchanan M.R. (1990) Neutralization of Enoxaparine-induced bleeding by protamine sulfate. *Thrombosis and Haemostasis* **63**, 271–274.

15 Investigation and Management of Haemorrhagic Disorders in Pregnancy*
Prepared by the
Haemostasis and Thrombosis Task Force

1 Introduction

Bleeding and blood loss associated with pregnancy and delivery remain important causes of morbidity. Although catastrophic bleeding is nowadays fairly uncommon, haemorrhage, particularly postpartum, is still one of the leading causes of maternal mortality (Department of Health *et al.*, 1991).

Obstetric haemorrhage may be associated with specific complications of pregnancy or labour or may be due to an inherited or acquired bleeding diathesis. Obstetricians confronted with a patient who is bleeding or who gives a past history or family history of bleeding or excessive bruising should be alert to the possibility of an underlying inherited or acquired haemostatic defect. Each hospital should have a set of management guidelines for severe haemorrhage and must have 24-hour ready access to diagnostic laboratory facilities and advice from a designated haematologist. Although modern alternatives to blood exist, rapid access to blood and blood products is an absolute requirement for acceptable obstetric practice. Therefore, laboratory facilities for blood grouping and compatibility testing should be on site close to the maternity unit.

2 Haemostatic changes in normal pregnancy

Normal pregnancy is associated with major changes in the coagulation and fibrinolytic systems, the concentration of many coagulation factors increasing and plasma fibrinolytic activity decreasing as the levels of plasminogen activator inhibitors progressively rise. Fibrinogen increases from early pregnancy onwards to almost double its prepregnancy value by term. Both factor VIII (FVIII) and von Willebrand factor (vWf) rise steadily throughout pregnancy. Factor VII and FX also increase very significantly during pregnancy, but the other vitamin-K-dependent clotting factors, FII and FIX, and FXII

* Reprinted with permission from *Journal of Clinical Pathology*, 1994, **47**, 100–108.

show a less significant or no rise and FXI and FXIII may fall slightly.

The platelet count does not normally change significantly during pregnancy, although some authors have reported a slight drop in the count in the third trimester. The bleeding time remains normal throughout pregnancy.

Screening tests used for the investigation of bleeding – the activated partial thromboplastin time (APTT) and the prothrombin time (PT) – are within the normal adult ranges during pregnancy, but in the third trimester the PT and the APTT are at the lower (shorter) limits of normal or slightly shortened, and this must be taken into account when assessing coagulation screen results from pregnant women.

3 Inherited bleeding disorders

In general, pregnant patients with inherited bleeding disorders and the female partners of men with these defects should be managed by an obstetric unit allied with a haemophilia centre and a neonatal intensive care unit.

The most common inherited bleeding defects involve FVIII deficiency (haemophilia A), FIX deficiency (haemophilia B) and vWf deficiency (von Willebrand's disease (vWD)). These will be discussed at length and the more uncommon inherited bleeding disorders mentioned briefly thereafter.

3.1 Haemophilia A and haemophilia B

The prevalences of haemophilia A and haemophilia B in the UK population are 90 in 1 000 000 and 20 in 1 000 000 respectively. The majority of female carriers of these X-linked recessive disorders do not have significant bleeding problems, but in 10–20% of carriers extreme Lyonization results in marked reduction of FVIII or FIX levels respectively (to <40 international units (IU)/dl) and, at the lowermost levels, a significantly increased risk of bleeding. Statistically, 50% of the male children of carrier females will have haemophilia and be at risk of serious bleeding.

Very rarely, homozygous haemophilia A or B may occur when a female is the offspring of a haemophiliac father and a carrier mother. These women have the same risk of major haemorrhage as do affected males.

3.2 Von Willebrand's disease

Von Willebrand's disease is the most common clinically significant inherited abnormality of coagulation affecting women. Because of the very wide spectrum of clinical presentation, it is difficult to ascertain precisely the prevalence of all forms of vWD, but it is more common than generally realized and may be as high as 1% (Rodeghiero *et al.*, 1987).

Broadly, vWD falls into three classes (Table 15.1). Type I vWD – the com-

Table 15.1 Simplified classification of von Willebrand's disease

Type	Bleeding time	FVIIIC	vWf antigen	vWf activity	Multimers
I	N or P	R	R	R	All present
IIA	P	N or R	N or R	R	Large and intermediate absent
IIB	P	N or R	N or R	R	Large absent
III	P	R or ND	R	ND	ND

N, normal; ND, not detectable; P, prolonged; R, reduced.

monest type (approximately 75% of patients) – is characterized by a reduction in all forms of vWf, with the highest-molecular-weight forms remaining detectable. Its inheritance can be autosomal dominant or recessive and its expression very variable. In non-pregnant patients with type I vWD, the vWf levels (by antigen and by activity assay) are between 10 and 40 IU/dl, as is the FVIII clotting activity (FVIIIC). The bleeding time may be slightly to moderately prolonged but is often normal and the bleeding tendency is generally mild.

The feature common to all subvariants of type II vWD is the loss of the highest-molecular-weight vWf multimers. Inheritance is usually autosomal dominant. In type II vWD, the vWf is functionally impaired, the bleeding time is usually prolonged and bleeding episodes tend to be more severe and more common, especially in type IIA (the commonest type II subvariant – 10% of all vWD patients), than in type I. In subtype IIB (7% of all vWD patients) the abnormal vWf has enhanced interaction with platelet glycoprotein 1b (Gp1b). These patients often have mild to moderate thrombocytopenia. Infusion of desmopressin (1-desamino-8-D-arginine vasopressin (DDAVP)) may cause a further fall in the platelet count in these patients and should therefore be avoided in type IIB vWD.

Type III vWD is clinically the most severe. The prevalence in the UK of type III vWD is approximately 1 in 10^6. Type III vWD patients have no detectable or only trace amounts of vWf in their circulation. Probably many type III vWD patients are homozygous, but some may be compound heterozygotes. The condition is more prevalent in cultures where consanguinity is common. In general, the parents are clinically unaffected or only mildly affected, although their vWf levels may be at or just below the lower limits of normal. Type III vWD patients have only 1–2 IU/dl FVIIIC and therefore have a bleeding tendency which mimics moderately severe haemophilia A, with the added mucosal and subcutaneous bleeding characteristic of vWD. Parents who have had a child with type III vWD require follow-up and careful counselling with respect to the management of future pregnancies and the availability of prenatal diagnosis.

Most women with vWD show an increase in their FVIII and vWf concentrations during pregnancy, and the majority do not suffer excessive bleeding. When bleeding does occur, it happens more frequently postpartum than during pregnancy and is usually associated with surgical delivery and perineal damage. This tendency is accentuated by the rapid fall in the levels of FVIII and vWf after delivery (Krishnamurthy & Miotti, 1977). Some patients show variable responses of their FVIII and vWf during pregnancy (Adashi, 1980; Hill *et al.*, 1982) and measurement of bleeding time, FVIIIC activity, vWf antigen and vWf activity are not always predictive of patients who will bleed (Lipton *et al.*, 1982; Greer *et al.*, 1991).

In general, patients with type I vWD increase FVIII and vWf levels during pregnancy and do not bleed excessively. On the other hand, type II and type III patients do have an increased tendency to bleed. In patients with type IIA vWD, it has been shown that the large multimers of vWf antigen do not rise in all patients during pregnancy (Takahashi, 1983). This may explain the greater risk of haemorrhage in women with type IIA vWD than in those with type I vWD. Type IIB patients may develop worsening thrombocytopenia during pregnancy and type III vWD patients show little or no increase in their FVIII and vWf levels.

4 Preconception counselling

As far as possible, it is essential that families with heritable bleeding disorders understand the genetic implications of their particular disorder and that young family members are presented for investigation. Haematologists responsible for providing haemophilia services must see these family studies and counselling as an important aspect of their remit and they may want to involve an interested obstetrician at this time. Female carriers of haemophilia A or B and women with vWD or other inherited bleeding disorders should be reviewed at intervals during their reproductive life, even if they remain asymptomatic.

Pregnancy planning should be encouraged and patients with inherited bleeding disorders and carriers or potential carriers should seek specialist medical advice from their haematologist and, if possible, also an obstetrician prior to conception. This is most evident where the affected patient is female, but couples in which the potential father has a heritable bleeding defect must also be offered prepregnancy counselling to discuss the possibility of antenatal diagnosis and other aspects of the management of the planned pregnancy. Women who may require blood product therapy and who are not immune should be immunized against hepatitis B. This should be carried out before their first pregnancy, but immunization during pregnancy is safe, although not ideal, and may be necessary for women not previously immunized. Because of recent reports of outbreaks of hepatitis A in some haemophiliacs, immunization against hepatitis A is now being offered to non-immune haemophiliacs and to patients with vWD who may require blood products.

It is important that, as far as possible, carriers of haemophilia are identified prior to pregnancy so that appropriate genetic counselling may be offered and women at increased risk of bleeding recognized. Considerable overlap exists between clotting factor values in normal women and in obligatory carriers of haemophilia A or B; thus not all carriers are identifiable by phenotype analysis. Details of carrier identification are beyond the scope of this chapter and readers are referred to published papers (Peake *et al.*, 1993). Genetic analysis is becoming more widely available and greatly improves the correct assignment of carrier status. Where there is any doubt about a woman's carrier status, genetic testing should be offered. The possibility of antenatal diagnosis (Old & Ludlam, 1991) should be discussed with carriers and facilities made available, when appropriate, for those who wish it.

Women who first present with a history suggestive of an inherited bleeding disorder when they are already pregnant may need to be managed empirically and full investigation delayed until 3–6 months after delivery – although, with increasing identification of genetic defects, it may be possible, in some instances, to make a diagnosis in pregnancy despite a normal phenotype. A previously undiagnosed congenital bleeding disorder should be considered in a patient who is otherwise well but bleeds and bruises excessively, either spontaneously or following venepuncture or at delivery.

5 Management of pregnancy

Women with vWD and carriers of haemophilia A or B require regular review (at least every 8–12 weeks) at a haemophilia centre throughout pregnancy for

Table 15.2 Obstetric management of women with inherited bleeding disorders – general principles

Prepregnancy diagnosis, counselling, hepatitis B immunization
Regular clinical and haemostasis monitoring during pregnancy
Ultrasound 'sexing' of fetus
Avoid unnecessary invasive procedures
On admission for delivery:
FBC and platelets
Coagulation investigations
Blood group and retain serum
Minimize maternal and fetal trauma at delivery
Access to blood product replacement may be necessary
Avoid intramuscular injections
Collect cord blood sample for investigation
Give neonate vitamin K_1 orally
Immunizations to infant by intradermal route
Consider hepatitis B immunization for infant

FBC, full blood count.

monitoring, including coagulation factor activity and, if appropriate, the levels of vWf antigen, vWf activity, platelet count and bleeding time (Table 15.2). Monitoring during the third trimester (around 34–36 weeks) is particularly important, as it allows final planning and discussion of the management of the forthcoming delivery.

The uptake of prenatal diagnosis in most centres is surprisingly low, with between 20 and 30% of known carriers opting for chorion villous sampling (CVS). Modern ultrasound scanning equipment allows visualization of fetal external genitalia and offers non-invasive techniques for identifying most male fetuses by 18–20 weeks. Information about the sex of the fetus is invaluable in managing pregnancy and delivery in carriers of haemophilia A or B where prenatal diagnosis has not been performed. It should be noted that, although the diagnosis of a male fetus is almost always correct, the diagnosis of a female fetus is less accurate.

5.1 Invasive procedures during pregnancy

The potential benefits and risks of invasive procedures during pregnancy, which may result in accidental maternal, fetal or placental bleeding, must be carefully considered on an individual patient basis. Rational decisions about these procedures require input from experts experienced in the management of pregnant women with bleeding disorders. Because of the risk of haemorrhage, even CVS for prenatal diagnosis may be hazardous and should be performed only after careful consideration and full discussion of risks and benefits with the parents.

Maternal coagulation factor activity and levels of vWf do not rise significantly until the second trimester. Chorion villous sampling and other invasive procedures, such as pregnancy termination, spontaneous abortion or general surgery, during the first trimester may therefore be complicated by serious maternal haemorrhage unless coagulation factor activity is raised to 50 IU/dl.

6 Management of delivery

If there is any concern over the coagulation factor activity level in the mother, a planned delivery date is advised. On admission, a maternal blood sample should be sent for full blood count and platelet count, coagulation screen and appropriate coagulation factor or vWf assays and for blood grouping and antibody screening, with a request to the blood bank to retain serum for compatibility testing if that should become necessary (Table 15.2).

In the absence of obstetric contraindication, vaginal delivery is usual, but caesarean section should be considered if labour fails to progress steadily. An early recourse to caesarean section is recommended for carriers of haemophilia A or B with a known male fetus if any problem develops and the chance of an easy vaginal delivery is less likely. Operative or instrumental delivery (if necessary) should be performed by the most experienced member of staff available. Ventouse extraction should be avoided in a suspected affected fetus. Scalp electrodes or scalp vein blood sampling can cause massive haematomata and should be avoided if possible if the fetus may have vWD and in haemophilia A or B carriers when the fetus is known to be male or its sex is unknown. Every effort must be made to minimize maternal genital tract or perineal trauma, as this greatly increases the risk of postpartum bleeding. After a difficult delivery, particularly if instruments have been required, the neonate may need blood product replacement therapy and this should be readily available.

6.1 Blood product therapy

Factor VIII levels usually rise during pregnancy and, in general, also in haemophilia A carriers. In type I vWD, providing the FVIIIC activity exceeds 40 IU/dl, no blood product replacement therapy is required to cover uncomplicated vaginal delivery. Coagulation factor activity levels should be rechecked between 34 and 36 weeks' gestation in case emergency admission or caesarean section is required. If caesarean section is planned or becomes necessary, FVIIIC activity should be in excess of 50 IU/dl and infusion of FVIII concentrate may occasionally be necessary to raise a type I vWD or a haemophilia A carrier's level of FVIIIC.

Normally FIX activity does not rise as much as FVIII during pregnancy, and female carriers of haemophilia B with low FIX activity more frequently require specific replacement therapy to raise their FIX activity to safe levels for vaginal delivery (40 IU/dl) or caesarean section (50 IU/dl). High-purity FIX concentrate should be used as FIX concentrates containing FII, FVII and FX are potentially thrombogenic.

In carriers of haemophilia A or B, following delivery FVIIIC and FIX levels should be maintained above 40 IU/dl for at least 3–4 days or for 4–5 days if post caesarean section. In the presence of bleeding or wound infection, a longer duration of therapy may be necessary.

Frequently type III and type IIA vWD and occasionally type IIB vWD patients require blood product therapy to raise their FVIII and vWf complex levels to cover delivery – even if vaginal delivery is anticipated (Table 15.3). Prophylactic infusion of factor concentrates should commence at the onset of labour, aiming to raise FVIIIC and vWf activity to above 40 IU/dl. Factor VIII concentrates which contain significant amounts of the larger vWf multimers should be used, e.g. 8Y (Blood Products Laboratory) or Haemate P (Hoechst) (UK Regional Haemophilia Centre Directors Organisation, 1992). Caesarean section is major surgery and vWD patients with reduced FVIII and vWf levels must be given appropriate FVIII and vWf replacement (as above) to raise their FVIIIC and vWf activity to above 50 IU/dl prior to surgery. Factor VIIIC activity levels are used to monitor the response to infusion in patients with type I vWD and vWf

Table 15.3 Management of delivery and puerperium in von Willebrand's disease

vWD type	Delivery	Postpartum
I	Occasionally require blood product therapy Regard CS as major surgery	Treat bleeds with blood products or desmopressin
IIA IIB	May require blood products Regard CS as major surgery	Treat bleeds with blood products Do not use desmopressin in type IIB
III	Treat as major surgery and offer blood products	Prophylactic blood products for 3–5 days

CS, caesarean section.

activity in type II patients. Levels must be maintained at above 40 IU/dl for 3–4 days after vaginal delivery and for 4–5 days after caesarean section.

Carriers of haemophilia A and a proportion of patients with type I or type IIA vWD may respond to infusion of desmopressin (DDAVP) with a rise in their FVIII and vWf complex levels. Some haematologists and obstetricians recommend, however, that desmopressin is avoided during pregnancy and intrapartum because of its oxytocic effect. Desmopressin infusion may be used after delivery or following abortion or termination, when a moderate rise in FVIII activity is required for a few days only. Desmopressin infusions after surgery may cause water retention and hyponatraemia (Lowe *et al.*, 1977); hence blood urea and electrolytes should be monitored and excessive fluid input (e.g. dextrose infusions) avoided. Type IIB vWD patients should not be given desmopressin because of the risk of causing platelet aggregation and thrombocytopenia, due to binding of abnormal intermediate-sized multimers of vWf antigen to platelets and subsequent platelet aggregation (Rick *et al.*, 1987).

6.2 Analgesia

Intramuscular analgesia should be avoided and intravenous or subcutaneous analgesia used, if necessary. Providing the coagulation screen is normal, the Simplate bleeding time less than 10 minutes and the platelet count greater than $100 \times 10^9/l$, it has been stated that there should be no contraindication to inserting an epidural catheter (Letsky, 1991). Care must be exercised before removing the catheter and, in those patients with an inherited bleeding tendency, it is suggested that a further coagulation screen and platelet count are performed prior to withdrawal of the epidural catheter. In cases of elective surgery, spinal anaesthesia may be the safer option.

7 Less common inherited bleeding defects

7.1 Fibrinogen abnormalities

Women with hereditary hypofibrinogenaemia may suffer recurrent pregnancy loss or excessive bleeding, but successful pregnancy outcome has been described with regular replacement therapy throughout pregnancy (Grech *et al.*, 1991).

7.2 Other coagulation factor deficiencies

There is very limited recorded experience of pregnancy management in women with other coagulation factor deficiencies (for review, see Bern, 1990). As far as possible, females with these defects should be identified and counselled before pregnancy and should be managed in obstetric units allied to a haemophilia centre.

7.3 Congenital platelet disorders

Congenital platelet function disorders are uncommon without being rare and are usually associated with a mild bleeding diathesis. Families with disorders such as familial thrombocytopenia, Glanzmann's thrombasthenia, Bernard–Soulier syndrome, storage pool defects and disorders of platelet secretion should attend a haemophilia centre and be offered counselling and care similar to those offered to families with inherited coagulopathies.

Pregnancy and delivery are documented in only a few patients with severe platelet function disorders (Sundqvist *et al.*, 1981; Michalas *et al.*, 1984), but, in general, management involves the strict avoidance of unnecessary platelet transfusions, the search for platelet antibodies in patients who have previously received donor platelets and, in some patients, the use of single-donor platelets or platelet type-specific donor platelets. In patients with storage pool defects and a history of bleeding, DDAVP may be helpful at the time of delivery.

8 Postpartum follow-up

A cord sample should be collected for investigation. Because some haemostatic factors are physiologically relatively reduced in neonates, it may be difficult to exclude a mild to moderate inherited defect at birth (e.g. in haemophilia B, vWD or FXI deficiency). In these children, repeat investigation at 3–6 months is necessary.

Intramuscular injections must be avoided in children of either sex with proved or possible vWD and in male children of carriers of haemophilia A or B (unless they have been proved to be unaffected). In these neonates, therefore, prophylactic vitamin K_1 must be given orally and their general practitioner informed and asked to ensure that routine immunizations are given carefully intradermally or subcutaneously. Immunization against hepatitis B should be offered. Arrangements to review mother and baby at the haemophilia centre must be made before they are discharged from the maternity unit.

9 Acquired bleeding disorders

Acquired bleeding disorders developing during pregnancy, at delivery or following delivery present a different set of problems from those faced in women with an inherited bleeding tendency. Women with inherited bleeding problems are most frequently known and otherwise well. With careful counselling, planning and, if necessary, prophylaxis, they generally progress through pregnancy and delivery in a reasonably predictable fashion. Women who develop an acquired bleeding disorder during pregnancy or delivery do so acutely, are usually unwell and are sometimes very ill. Their bleeding disorder further complicates their progress and management and may in some instances dominate their clinical presentation.

9.1 Thrombocytopenia

The causes of thrombocytopenia in pregnancy are so numerous and varied that these will be the subject of a separate guidelines document (in preparation).

9.2 Disseminated intravascular coagulation

Disseminated intravascular coagulation (DIC) is associated with a wide variety of clinical situations which complicate pregnancy. It is never a primary event but is always a secondary phenomenon triggered by the release of procoagulant material into the circulation or by damage to the vascular endothelium. Depending on the triggering event, the manifestations of DIC range from a chronic, compensated state through to acute life-threatening haemorrhage. The chronic DIC which occurs in pre-eclampsia or with hydatidiform mole is associated with laboratory evidence of increased platelet turnover and mildly reduced fibrinogen levels but not usually with excessive bleeding. Many obstetric complications – for example, placental abruption, amniotic fluid embolism or septic abortion – are, however, associated with a more acute release of tissue thromboplastin into the circulation, with resultant marked depletion of coagulation factors, increased fibrinolytic activity and consumption of platelets and subsequent clinical bleeding.

10 Management of acute life-threatening haemorrhage in obstetric patients

The immediate management of haemorrhage in obstetric patients is essentially the same, whether or not the bleeding is caused or augmented by DIC. There should be a routine planned procedure, agreed by obstetricians, midwives, anaesthetists and haematologists, to deal with acute haemorrhage whenever it arises. Agreed protocols should be produced and given to all staff concerned and be available in the labour ward. Early and continuing reliable communication with laboratory staff is mandatory, although the urgency of the clinical situation often demands intervention before full test results are available.

Acute obstetric bleeding is usually obvious, as blood escapes from the genital tract. It may, however, be very difficult to estimate the volume of blood loss from the circulation, as much of the loss may be concealed behind the placenta and in the myometrium, within the uterine cavity or the broad ligament. Total blood loss is often dangerously underestimated. In some cases of abruption, there is no visible vaginal bleeding, with all the haemorrhage concealed. Rate of blood loss is probably more important than volume of blood loss, at least initially.

10.1 Source of blood loss

Obstetric bleeding occurs most commonly from the placental bed. Antepartum, this may be the result of a placenta implanted in the lower uterine segment (placenta praevia) or the result of abruption of a normally sited placenta. After delivery, poor myometrial contraction, due to hypotonia or to retained products of conception (placenta or membranes) or blood clot, may allow continuing blood loss from the placental site. Intrapartum and postpartum, bleeding may also be the result of trauma – rupture of the uterine wall, tearing of the cervix or vagina or damage to the perineum or vulval varicosities.

It is imperative that the source of bleeding is identified and dealt with as soon as possible. Shock may trigger DIC, which will further complicate the bleeding tendency. Active steps to restore blood volume and oxygen-carrying capacity must be instituted as a matter of urgency (Table 15.4).

10.2 Laboratory investigation

A sample of venous blood should be sent for full blood count, coagulation screening and cross-matching. Emergency packs, with all necessary sample tubes and forms, should be kept available in a labour ward refrigerator. Results of

---

Table 15.4 Management of acute obstetric haemorrhage

Secure venous access and insert central venous pressure monitor
Summon additional help
Collect blood samples for cross-matching and coagulation screen
Contact haematologist and blood bank
Maintain blood volume – with unmatched blood if necessary (same ABO and Rh D group as patient)
Seek and deal with source of bleeding
Blood product replacement therapy if necessary

---

coagulation screening tests must always be interpreted bearing in mind that normally in the third trimester the APTT and PT are at the lower limits of normal. Measurement of products of plasmin digestion of fibrinogen or fibrin provides an indirect test for fibrinolysis, along with a platelet count, and a fibrinogen assay (Clauss method) or thrombin time will quickly distinguish coagulation screen abnormalities due to DIC from those due to other causes.

10.3 Maintenance of blood volume

Severe bleeding is an obstetric emergency. The aim of management should be to maintain the circulation and stop the bleeding. Help from the most senior obstetricians, anaesthetists and midwives available should be sought. The laboratory should be notified immediately of the problem. Venous access should be achieved at two sites, using large-bore cannulae. As the cannulae are sited, blood should be drawn for a full blood count, including platelet count, a coagulation screen and cross-matching of at least six units of blood. Enough serum should be sent to allow further units to be made available. Blood-pressure and pulse should be monitored and a central venous line should be inserted.

Blood is the best fluid to replace blood loss. Wherever possible, this should have been shown to be compatible with the patient's blood before issue; however, in an emergency it may be necessary to issue unmatched blood. Pregnant women who have been attending for antenatal care will have their blood group and antibody status already known. Providing this blood group has been confirmed, unmatched blood of the patient's own ABO and Rh D group is preferable to unmatched group O Rh D negative blood. Immediately on receipt in the laboratory, the patient's blood sample should be ABO and Rh D grouped by rapid techniques and ABO incompatibility with issued units excluded by a rapid-spin cross-match (i.e. a spin agglutination test after 2–5 minutes' incubation at room temperature). It should usually be possible to recheck the patient's blood group and exclude major incompatibility before a significant amount of blood is transfused. Unmatched group O Rh D negative, Kell negative, Duffy negative blood should only be issued in the very rare event of life-threatening haemorrhage in a woman whose blood group is unknown.

Whilst awaiting blood, the blood volume must be expanded with crystalloids, such as Hartmann's solution (up to 2l). However, these leave the circulation rapidly and must be considered as a first-aid measure only. If available, a 4.5% solution of human albumin may be used; otherwise, other colloids, such as Haemaccel (Hoechst) or Gelofusine (Vifor) – up to 1.5l – are preferable to dextrans, which interfere with compatibility testing and with platelet function. Two lines are usually necessary, to allow blood and other products to be infused simultaneously. After the initial transfusion, fluid replacement should be monitored, with central venous pressure monitoring.

10.4 Stopping the bleeding

Although the circulation can be maintained in the short term, survival of the patient is dependent on cessation of the bleeding. How this is done depends on whether the bleeding is antepartum or postpartum.

11 Antepartum haemorrhage

If the bleeding is severe, delivery and the emptying of the uterus is the only way to stop it. If blood loss is not adequately replaced, acute renal tubular necrosis may occur.

11.1 Placenta praevia

In the case of placenta praevia, most of the bleeding will be apparent. Coagulation defects are rare and the main problem is blood replacement. Delivery must be by caesarean section. If the placenta is anterior, further severe haemorrhage may occur during delivery. After the placenta is delivered, the lower uterine segment does not contract as well as the upper segment and bleeding can continue. If bleeding is not controlled at delivery, the management is similar to that required for postpartum haemorrhage.

11.2 Placental abruption

With placental abruption, the blood loss is always underestimated and replacement should take account of this. Since bleeding may largely be retroplacental and several litres of blood may be concealed behind the placenta, the amount of blood issuing from the vagina prior to delivery is no indicator of the extent of placental detachment or of the subsequent blood loss. There is usually a concomitant coagulation defect and it is the most common cause of acute pregnancy-related DIC. The degree of haemostatic disturbance is related to the degree of placental separation.

   The mere suspicion that a patient may have placental abruption should prompt an urgent coagulation screen, full blood count and platelet count and a blood sample for immediate blood group and antibody screen, with compatibility testing if and when appropriate.

   In placental abruption, prevention or correction of hypovolaemia is the primary concern, with expeditious vaginal delivery whenever possible. The bleeding and coagulation defects will not be controlled until after delivery. There should be prompt replacement of blood volume to maintain renal perfusion. Although depleted coagulation factors should be replaced, the consumption will continue until the uterus is emptied. Fresh-frozen plasma (11) is often sufficient to correct the coagulation defect, but severe depletion of fibrinogen (to less than 0.8 g/l) requires the infusion of 10–15 units of cryoprecipitate. Thrombocytopenia (platelet count less than $50 \times 10^9/l$) may require correction by transfusion of platelet concentrates. Further coagulation investigation and platelet counts are required to monitor response to replacement therapy and the ongoing clinical condition, in order to judge the requirement for further replacement.

Having initiated management of hypovolaemia and taken samples for coagulation screening and for blood group, measures to expedite delivery must be addressed. Vaginal examination should be carried out to assess the state of the cervix. In parous women, amniotomy may be enough to stimulate labour and lead to prompt delivery, but others may, in addition, require oxytocin infusion. If the mother is relatively stable, the fetus can tolerate the delay and, providing damage to the birth canal and perineum can be avoided, vaginal delivery is preferable. If there is any sign of fetal distress or if vaginal delivery is not imminent or seems likely to be difficult, caesarean section may be necessary. In this case, blood volume and coagulation factor replacement prior to surgery is essential as far as it is possible. However, delivery should not be delayed to achieve this, as emptying the uterus will stop the consumption and help in the correction of the factor deficiency. Fresh-frozen plasma and platelet infusion can be commenced as the operation is started. If the fetus is already dead, caesarean section is seldom indicated, except where, despite adequate oxytocic stimulation, cervical dilation does not occur.

Once the fetus and placenta are delivered, myometrial retraction will usually dramatically reduce or stop placental site bleeding, but measures to stimulate myometrial function may be essential, and care must be taken to ensure that the uterus remains well contracted. Abdominal or perineal wound healing may be difficult or slow.

Epidural analgesia is potentially hazardous in patients with DIC and should be avoided. Although heparin has been used in DIC (Thiagarajah *et al.*, 1981), in general its use is not recommended in DIC associated with pregnancy where the circulation is not intact because of the placental bed.

12 Postpartum bleeding

Excessive bleeding after delivery can result from one of the above pre-existing antenatal problems or be due to retained products of conception or trauma to the genital tract. Immediate intravenous access should be obtained, as outlined above, and blood drawn for a full blood count, platelet count, a coagulation screen and cross-matching of at least six units of blood. The blood loss should be replaced and coagulation defects, where identified, should be corrected with appropriate blood product replacement therapy, as outlined above.

The placenta and membranes should be re-examined to check for any evidence of retained products. The fundus should be examined to make sure that the uterus is contracted. If the uterus is atonic, an intravenous injection of 10 IU of oxytocin or 0.5 mg of ergometrine should be given. After this, an infusion of oxytocin should be commenced to keep the uterus contracted. If the haemorrhage continues, Hemabate (Upjohn), a prostaglandin F analogue, should be given either intramuscularly or, in extreme circumstances, directly into the myometrium. These actions should be accompanied by bimanual compression of the uterus.

If there is continuing bleeding from the genital tract, the patient should be examined under the appropriate anaesthesia. If the bleeding is coming through the cervix, the cavity should be explored and any retained products removed, followed by the use of oxytocics. If the bleeding is coming from lower in the genital tract, the cervix and vagina should be examined for tears and promptly repaired.

If there are persistent problems, senior help should be summoned promptly. If bleeding continues from the uterus, laparotomy should be carried out to exclude the possibility of uterine rupture. If there is persistent bleeding from the placental site, oversewing of the bleeding points should be considered. Early recourse to hysterectomy may be life-saving, with tying of the internal iliac arteries a further option. Although the urinary tract is at risk in this situation, most damage can be repaired at a later date and haemostasis is the primary aim. In the acute situation, aortic compression, either at laparotomy or by abdominal compression, may control bleeding enough to visualize the bleeding points or for senior support to arrive.

In the presence of persisting severe haemorrhage, coagulation factors may need to be replaced rapidly. A litre of fresh-frozen plasma and 10 units of cryoprecipitate may be thawed and issued empirically before coagulation screening tests are completed. Fresh-frozen plasma contains all of the coagulation factors normally present in plasma. Cryoprecipitate has the advantage of a higher concentration of fibrinogen per volume. If the platelet count has fallen below 50 $\times$ 10^9/l, platelet concentrates may be suggested, but often haemostasis and control of bleeding can be achieved without platelet transfusion.

The risks and disadvantages of fibrinolytic inhibitors (tranexamic acid, aprotinin) outweigh their potential benefits in most obstetric haemorrhages. In a very few cases, where persisting postpartum bleeding can clearly be shown to be associated with excessive fibrinolytic activity (i.e. a shortened euglobulin clot lysis time) and there is no trauma, antifibrinolytic agents may be tried, with caution.

12.1 Management of less severe obstetric bleeding

In patients who are bleeding less severely, management can be tailored on an individual basis, but the broad principles remain the same as for life-threatening haemorrhage. Extra help, including laboratory staff and anaesthetic staff, must be alerted early on, blood samples for full blood count, coagulation screening and compatibility testing should be dispatched urgently, infusion lines should be in place and a careful search to identify and deal with the source of bleeding should be made. If transfusion is necessary, cross-matched blood is always preferable to unmatched blood.

If time permits, the results of the coagulation screening tests may provide a scientific basis on which to prescribe blood product replacement therapy. In practice, though, this will usually be fresh-frozen plasma in patients without evidence of severe fibrinogen depletion or a combination of fresh-frozen plasma and cryoprecipitate in patients with fibrinogen levels of less than 0.8 g/l.

13 Other causes of acquired obstetric bleeding

13.1 Amniotic fluid embolism

Amniotic fluid embolism is an uncommon, generally fatal, complication of pregnancy. It may occur during or shortly after labour or at caesarean section. If the patient survives the initial event, rapid and virtually total consumption of clotting factors and platelets ensues, leading to catastrophic exsanguinating uterine haemorrhage. Typically, the patient is in or has just completed a strenuous labour with an intact amniotic sac when she suddenly collapses, profoundly shocked, cyanosed with respiratory distress and bleeding from venepuncture sites and from the genital tract.

Cardiopulmonary resuscitation may be necessary and preparation must be made for immediate delivery if this has not occurred. Blood products, including fresh-frozen plasma, cryoprecipitate and platelets, are urgently required and must be used empirically. If occurring postdelivery, 10 000 IU heparin given intravenously (IV) may help to arrest this cycle of coagulation and haemolysis.

13.2 Retained dead fetus

This is now a rare occurrence. To cause detectable consumption of coagulation factors, the fetus has to be retained *in utero* for 3–4 weeks after its demise. Spontaneous labour usually supervenes within 2 weeks of fetal death and current obstetric practice would be to induce labour if it did not occur spontaneously shortly after fetal death. Although significant consumptive coagulopathy is an infrequent complication of a retained dead fetus, it is recommended that a coagulation screen and platelet count is performed on all mothers with a dead fetus *in utero* before inducing labour or as early as possible in a spontaneous labour. Replacement therapy is rarely necessary. If a coagulation defect is found, the presence of antiphospholipid antibodies should be sought, as they could have been contributory to the fetal death rather than caused by it. In the unusual circumstances of a dead twin or selective fetocide, where the dead fetus may remain *in utero* for a number of weeks, a coagulation defect may occur. In this situation, low-dose heparin may be of benefit, but it is not without risk to the mother and her surviving fetus. These pregnancies require close management and advice from centres with previous experience.

13.3 Acquired inhibitors of coagulation

Rarely, a bleeding tendency similar to that observed in haemophilia A may occur secondary to the development of an inhibitor to FVIII. Most cases present 2–3 months after delivery, but the inhibitor may develop during pregnancy (Voke & Letsky, 1977) or cause severe bleeding in the early puerperium (Reece *et al.*, 1984). The inhibitor is usually an immunoglobulin G (IgG) antibody. It may disappear spontaneously or after immunosuppressive therapy with steroids. In at least 50% of women, the inhibitor will be undetectable a year after initial detection (Green & Lechner, 1981) and it rarely recurs with subsequent pregnancies (Vincente *et al.*, 1987). Frequent monitoring of the inhibitor activity is essential to aid planning of therapy if bleeding should occur. A trial of prednisolone or intravenous immunoglobulin may be considered.

Management of bleeding in these patients is very difficult, involving the use of human and/or porcine FVIII or activated prothrombin complex concentrates (Autoplex, Feiba). It is very much the province of haematologists with experience in managing patients with pathological coagulation inhibitors.

13.4 Acute hepatic failure

Acute fatty liver of pregnancy is acute liver failure occurring during pregnancy unrelated to infection, hepatotoxic drugs or chemicals or haemolytic uraemic syndrome (Kaplan, 1985). It can also occur in association with pre-eclampsia. Characteristically, the patient rapidly develops clinical and biochemical evidence of liver failure, in association with a severe coagulopathy, reduced platelet count, elevated fibrin and fibrinogen degradation products, reduced fibrinogen and extremely low antithrombin (AT). The biochemical findings are those of liver function impairment, with low plasma albumin and vitamin K-dependent coagulation factors. The liver enzymes are often not markedly elevated.

It is important to realize the seriousness of this situation. The perinatal mortality is approaching 50%, with a maternal mortality of 30%. If delivery is not expedited, the fetus will die *in utero*, followed by the death of the mother. After delivery, the mother will hopefully recover with supportive management. Some benefits from correction of the coagulopathy after administration of AT have been suggested (Liebman *et al.*, 1983). Infusion of AT-containing material may be worth considering in this dire clinical condition.

14 Acknowledgements

The authors wish to acknowledge the advice and help received from a number of others, including Professor G.D.O. Lowe and Professor I. Peake, who generously gave us their time and expertise during the preparation of this chapter.

References

Adashi E.Y. (1980) Lack of improvement in von Willebrand's disease during pregnancy. *New England Journal of Medicine* **303**, 1178 (abstract).

Bern M.M. (1990) Acquired and congenital coagulation defects encountered during pregnancy and in the fetus. In Bern M.M. & Frigoletto F.D. (eds) *Haematologic Disorders in Maternal–Fetal Medicine*, pp. 395–448. Wiley-Liss, New York.

Department of Health, Welsh Office, Scottish Home & Health Department, Department of Health & Social Services, Northern Ireland (1991) *Report on Confidential Enquiries into Maternal Deaths in the United Kingdom 1985–1987*. HMSO, London.

Grech H., Majumdar G., Lawrie A.S. & Savidge G.F. (1991) Pregnancy in congenital afibrinogenaemia: report of a successful case and review of the literature. *British Journal of Haematology* **78**, 571–572.

Green D. & Lechner K. (1981) A survey on 215 non-hemophilic patients with inhibitors to factor VIII. *Thrombosis and Haemostasis* **45**, 200–203.

Greer I.A., Lowe G.D.O., Walker J.J. & Forbes C.D. (1991) Haemorrhagic problems in obstetrics and gynaecology in patients with congenital coagulopathies. *British Journal of Obstetrics and Gynaecology* **98**, 909–918.

Hill F.G.H., George J. & Enayat M.S. (1982) Changes in VIII:C, VIIIR:AG, VIIIR:WF and ristocetin-induced platelet aggregation during pregnancy in women with von Willebrand's disease. *British Journal of Haematology* **50**, 691 (abstract).

Kaplan M.M. (1985) Acute fatty liver of pregnancy. *New England Journal of Medicine* **313**, 367–370.

Krishnamurthy M. & Miotti A.B. (1977) von Willebrand's disease and pregnancy. *Obstetrics and Gynecology* **49**, 244–247.

Letsky E.A. (1991) Haemostasis and epidural anaesthesia. *International Journal of Obstetric Anaesthesia* **1**, 51–54.

Liebman H.A., McGehee W.G., Patch M.J. & Feinstein D.I. (1983) Severe depression of antithrombin III associated with disseminated intravascular coagulation in women with fatty liver of pregnancy. *Annals of Internal Medicine* **98**, 330–333.

Lipton R.A., Ayromlooi J. & Coller B.S. (1982) Severe von Willebrand's disease during labor and delivery. *Journal of the American Medical Association* **248**, 1355–1357.

Lowe G.D.O., Pettigrew A., Middleton S., Forbes C.D. & Prentice C.R.M. (1977) DDAVP in haemophilia. *Lancet* **ii**, 614 (letter).

Michalas S., Malamitsi-Puchner A. & Tsevrenis H. (1984) Pregnancy and delivery in Bernard–Soulier syndrome. *Acta Obstetrica Gynecologica Scandinavica* **63**, 185–186.

Old J.M. & Ludlam C.A. (1991) Antenatal diagnosis in paediatric haematology. In Hann I.M. & Gibson B.E.S. (eds) *Clinical Haematology: International Practice and Research*, Vol. 4, Part 2, pp. 429–458. Baillière Tindall, London.

Peake I.R., Lillicrap D.P., Boulyjenkov V. *et al.* (1993) Report on joint WHO/WFH meeting on the control of haemophilia: carrier detection and prenatal diagnosis. *Blood Coagulation and Fibrinolysis* **4**, 313–344.

Reece E.A., Romero R. & Hobbins J. (1984) Coagulopathy associated with factor VIII inhibitor: a literature review. *Journal of Reproductive Medicine* **29**, 53–58.

Rick M.E., Williams S.B. & McKeown L.P. (1987) Thrombocytopenia associated with pregnancy in a patient with type IIB von Willebrand's disease. *Blood* **11**, 786–789.

Rodeghiero F., Castaman G. & Dini E. (1987) Epidemiological investigation of the prevalence of von Willebrand's disease. *Blood* **69**, 454–459.

Sundqvist S.B., Nilsson I.M., Svanberg L. & Cronberg S. (1981) Pregnancy and parturition in a patient with severe Glanzmann's thrombasthenia. *Scandinavian Journal of Haematology* **27**, 159–164.

Takahashi N. (1983) Studies on the pathophysiology and treatment of von Willebrand's disease VI. Variant von Willebrand's disease complicating placenta previa. *Thrombosis Research* **31**, 285–296.

Thiagarajah S., Wheby M.S., Jain R., May H.V., Bourgeois J. & Kitchin J.D. (1981) Disseminated intravascular coagulation in pregnancy: the role of heparin therapy. *Journal of Reproductive Medicine* **26**, 17–20.

UK Regional Haemophilia Centre Directors Organisation (1992) Recommendations on the choice of therapeutic products for the treatment of patients with haemophilia A, haemophilia B and von Willebrand's disease. *Blood Coagulation and Fibrinolysis* **3**, 205–214.

Vincente V., Alberca I., Gonzales R. & Alegre A. (1987) Normal pregnancy in a patient with a postpartum factor VIII inhibitor. *American Journal of Hematology* **24**, 107–109.

Voke J. & Letsky E. (1977) Pregnancy and antibody to factor VIII. *Journal of Clinical Pathology* **30**, 928–932.

16 Prevention, Investigation and Management of Pregnancy-Related Thrombosis*

Prepared by the Haemostasis and Thrombosis Task Force

1 Introduction

Although the overall rate of fatal pulmonary thromboembolism (PTE) has fallen over the last 30 years, it remains one of the most common causes of maternal death associated with pregnancy in the UK. The incidence of thromboembolic complications, PTE and deep-vein thrombosis (DVT) presenting during pregnancy is around 1 in 1000, with a further 2 in 1000 women presenting in the puerperium (Letsky, 1985). This means that an average obstetric unit will see between six and 12 cases a year. Deep-vein thrombosis and PTE are not just associated with the risk of mortality, as there is an increased morbidity in those that survive. There is an increased risk of both recurrent DVT and deep-vein insufficiency. This risk is greater than with similar events outside pregnancy. The prompt and accurate diagnosis of these conditions is important. The diagnosis and management of venous thrombotic disease in pregnancy are fraught with problems, because of the fear, on the one hand, of damaging the fetus with irradiation or drugs and, on the other, of failing to prevent, or even causing, serious maternal morbidity with inadequate or inappropriate investigation or with the treatment chosen. Because of these problems, all aspects of thrombosis diagnosis, prevention and management must be fully discussed with affected women, and these patients should be encouraged to involve themselves in decision-making.

2 Investigation of maternal venous thromboembolic disease

Because both treatment and the lack of treatment may carry significant risk, accurate diagnosis is imperative. Since the clinical diagnosis of DVT and pulmonary embolism is difficult and frequently inaccurate (Barnes *et al.*, 1975), there is a positive requirement for 'objective' testing in pregnant women with suspected

* Reprinted with permission from *Journal of Clinical Pathology*, 1993, **46**, 489–496.

DVT or PTE to minimize the exposure of mothers and their unborn children to the hazards of anticoagulant therapy. An uncorroborated positive clinical diagnosis may lead needlessly to long-term complications for women with respect to contraception and the management of future pregnancies.

In the non-pregnant patient, there is a multitude of tests available to investigate for and accurately diagnose DVT and PTE. Contrast venography and impedance plethysmography (IPG) are widely used and validated for the diagnosis of DVT (Barnes *et al.*, 1975; Hull *et al.*, 1978). Other objective tests for DVT diagnosis include radioisotope venography and fibrinogen leg scanning. More recently, duplex ultrasound scanning and Doppler ultrasonography have been shown to be of value and they are of particular interest for use in the obstetric patient.

At least two major problems require consideration with respect to the safety and suitability of these objective tests for use during pregnancy: (i) the risks to the fetus of radiological procedures; and (ii) the potential unreliability of non-invasive tests during the latter stages of pregnancy.

2.1 Risks of *in utero* radiation exposure

Most studies fail to show any increase in teratogenicity following *in utero* exposure to low doses of radiation (Ginsberg *et al.*, 1989a). There may be a slight increase in the relative risk of childhood cancer, but the absolute risk remains small.

It does, however, seem reasonable to assume that, whatever the risks of *in utero* irradiation, they are likely to be dose-related and the fetus will be more susceptible in early pregnancy. Every effort should therefore be made to minimize fetal exposure to radiation – particularly before 12 weeks' gestation. Limited venography with abdominal shielding exposes the fetus to much less radiation than contrast venography without abdominal shielding. The diagnosis of suspected pulmonary embolism during pregnancy presents fewer problems, since pulmonary angiography by the brachial route and ventilation/perfusion lung scanning each expose the fetus to very little radiation.

Screening by measuring the uptake of ^{131}I-labelled fibrinogen is contraindicated throughout pregnancy and the puerperium, because of the hazard to the fetus and neonate. In the antenatal period, the free label is trapped by the fetal thyroid and can cause hypothyroidism and carcinoma. It is secreted in high concentration in breast milk and the same risks therefore apply to breastfed infants.

2.2 Reliability of objective tests during pregnancy

All of the non-invasive approaches to the diagnosis of thrombosis in pregnancy may give false positive results during the later stages of pregnancy. They are unable to differentiate extrinsic compression of the iliac veins or inferior vena cava by the gravid uterus from venous obstruction due to the presence of a thrombus within the vessel. At present, contrast venography remains the most reliable method for differentiating between intraluminal obstruction and extrinsic compression.

Furthermore, although a negative result from a non-invasive test is likely to exclude a proximal-vein thrombosis, none of the non-invasive tests is as reliable as venography for excluding thrombosis in distal (calf) veins.

Equally, a negative result in a limited venogram (with abdominal screening) does not exclude iliac-vein thrombosis.

2.3 Outline of investigation

2.3.1 Clinical history and examination

A diagnosis of DVT or PTE should be considered in all patients presenting with increasing or persisting pain, swelling or discoloration of a limb or sudden onset of chest pain or breathlessness, particularly in those patients in whom the risk of venous thromboembolism may be considered to be increased (older or obese women, multiple pregnancy, varicose veins, past history or strong family history of thrombosis).

2.3.2 Objective tests

In many maternity units, there is access to duplex ultrasound scanning with (sometimes colour) Doppler flow facilities. Real-time ultrasound scanning can be used to visualize the deep vein system directly. In non-pregnant patients, it has been shown to be sensitive and specific (Dauzat *et al.*, 1986; Rosner & Doris, 1988). More recently, Greer and colleagues (1990) have shown similar accuracy in pregnant patients. Compression ultrasonography, where the vein is compressed under ultrasound vision, can detect venous thrombosis in the proximal veins with a sensitivity of 94% and a selectivity of 97%. It has limitations, as it is unable to diagnose distal calf-vein or an isolated iliac-vein thrombosis. Doppler flow analysis consists of listening for the normal venous signal and the responses to respiratory movement. It is also accurate in diagnosing proximal-vein thrombosis, but is less sensitive to calf-vein DVT. It is therefore recommended that, in any case where there is doubt, limited venography should still be performed.

In centres where IPG is routinely available, IPG may be performed initially. If the IPG is positive during the first two trimesters, then it is reasonable to accept a diagnosis of DVT and treat accordingly. During the third trimester, a positive IPG requires further investigation, using limited venography. As with ultrasound, a negative IPG excludes proximal-vein thrombosis but not calf-vein thrombi.

Although the safety of not treating calf-vein thrombosis in non-pregnant patients in whom the IPG remains negative has been established (Hull *et al.*, 1985a), the implications of adopting a policy of non-treatment of calf-vein thrombosis in pregnancy are not known. In theory, at least, venous stasis resulting from compression of the pelvic veins by the uterus may increase the risk of significant extension of calf-vein thrombi during pregnancy. It is therefore suggested that, if the IPG is negative, or in any other case of doubt, limited venography to exclude calf-vein thrombosis should be performed before finally deciding not to treat.

Venography is the only technique that gives information in all parts of the vascular tree. After limited venography, a positive result implies that treatment should be instituted. If the limited venogram is negative, then full venography is indicated to confirm or exclude iliac-vein thrombosis, since the radiation risk to the fetus is outweighed by the risks of not treating a mother with venous thrombosis or unnecessarily treating one who has no venous thrombotic disease.

The diagnosis of PTE during pregnancy may be easier, because the radiation risk to the fetus is less. Initially, chest X-ray is required to exclude conditions which may clinically mimic PTE (pleurisy, pneumothorax, fractured rib). If the chest X-ray is non-diagnostic, ventilation and perfusion lung scans should be performed. If the perfusion scan is negative, PTE can be ruled out (Hull *et al.*, 1985b). If there is a segmental perfusion defect with normal ventilation, then it is reasonable to accept a high probability of PTE and treat accordingly. If there is a subsegmental perfusion defect with normal ventilation or matched perfusion and ventilation defects, then the probability of PTE is only between 10 and 40% (Hull *et al.*, 1985b) and in these cases pulmonary angiography (preferably by the brachial route) is necessary to avoid treating unnecessarily a large percentage of patients. This procedure carries increased risk to the fetus and should be used only if essential.

2.3.3 Laboratory investigation

It must be borne in mind that pregnancy itself alters the levels of haemostatic factors, the procoagulants factor VII (FVII), FVIII and fibrinogen and the natural anticoagulant protein C (PC) increasing particularly in the third trimester and both total and free protein S (PS) decreasing from the first trimester onwards. An acute thrombotic event may be associated with very significant reductions in the levels of natural anticoagulants.

Pregnancy itself may be considered to be a 'thrombotic risk' condition, but all patients with DVT and/or PTE require laboratory investigation to identify or exclude an underlying haemostatic defect. The investigations should include, in the first place, full blood count and platelet count, blood film, coagulation screen (activated partial thromboplastin time (APTT), prothrombin time and thrombin time), functional assays of natural anticoagulants (antithrombin (AT), PC, PS) and tests for lupus inhibitors and other antiphospholipid antibodies.

It is difficult and sometimes impossible to confirm or exclude an underlying thrombophilic condition in a pregnant patient who has recently had a DVT; therefore, follow-up investigation of these patients when they are not pregnant, not anticoagulated and not suffering an acute thrombotic event is recommended. A carefully taken family history and, in some instances (e.g. AT, PC or PS deficiency), testing family members may assist early diagnosis and are essential to confirm the inherited nature of the defect.

3 Treatment of thromboembolism in pregnancy

Careful consideration must be given to whether a particular pregnant patient with thromboembolism should be managed in an obstetric unit or in a medical ward. The final decision will depend on the extent and severity of the thromboembolism and on the assessed needs of the pregnancy and the likelihood of requiring immediate or urgent obstetric or neonatal care. Because of the severity of their thrombotic event, some patients may require transfer to a unit with specialist diagnostic and back-up facilities. Institution of treatment must not be delayed if the clinical suspicion of thromboembolism is high, but objective verification of the diagnosis must be sought as soon as possible. If investigations prove negative, therapy can be stopped.

3.1 Surgery
Life-threatening pulmonary embolism may require surgical intervention. Patients who have massive ileofemoral thrombosis should be managed in centres where expert surgical help is available if urgently needed. In these cases, the transfer of the patient to a unit with the necessary facilities may be required. If the thrombus is free-floating, the risk of embolism is high. The use of caval filters can be life-saving.

3.2 Thrombolysis
Because of the risk of major haemorrhage from the placental site, the use of fibrinolytic agents is not recommended during pregnancy and should be avoided if delivery is imminent or during the first few days after delivery, unless surgical intervention is not possible and fatal pulmonary embolism appears likely.

4 Therapeutic anticoagulation in pregnancy

Anticoagulant therapy during pregnancy is indicated for the treatment or prevention of venous thromboembolic disease and in patients with valvular heart disease and/or prosthetic heart valves to prevent systemic embolism. The use of anticoagulants during pregnancy is problematic and their introduction or continuation must be carefully considered in each individual patient.

The oral anticoagulants, vitamin K antagonists, cross the placenta and potentially cause adverse effects in the fetus. Heparins appear not to cross the placenta and therefore would not be expected to cause adverse fetal effects. However, heparins have the potential to cause adverse effects in the mother.

4.1 Warfarin

Exposure to warfarin during organogenesis may be associated with embryopathy. The incidence of embryopathic changes is very difficult to estimate. Much of the literature on this topic comprises case reports and is therefore subject to bias. In a small prospective study, Iturbe-Alessio and colleagues (1986) reported embryopathy in 10 out of 35 full-term pregnancies (29%; 95% confidence limits 15%– 46%) after exposure to warfarin during the first trimester. Avoiding warfarin during the period from 6 to 12 weeks' gestation appears to reduce the risk of embryopathy very markedly but should not be considered to abolish the risk completely.

Patients on long-term oral anticoagulants should seek medical advice prior to pregnancy so that the desirability and feasibility of substituting heparin for the first trimester of pregnancy may be considered. Patients who conceive whilst on warfarin should seek further medical advice as soon as a pregnancy is suspected.

It has also been suggested that central nervous system (CNS) abnormalities – due to intracranial haemorrhages and to malformations – occur with increased frequency in babies of mothers taking warfarin at any stage of their pregnancy. On examining the evidence in the literature, Ginsberg and colleagues (1989b) conclude that CNS abnormalities are an uncommon complication of warfarin therapy during pregnancy. However, they reaffirm that the use of oral anticoagulants in pregnancy is associated with an increased rate of fetal wastage and congenital malformations.

Letsky (1992) states that the risk of fetal malformation may be overstated, since abnormalities would appear to be uncommon in the UK, and the risk is probably dose-related. The risk of fetal damage must be weighed against the problems and risk of converting the mother to heparin.

Because of the risk of fetal intracranial haemorrhage occurring during delivery, oral anticoagulants should be discontinued no later than 36 weeks' gestation or 2–3 weeks prior to expected delivery and anticoagulation maintained with heparin.

4.2 Heparin

There is no evidence that either unfractionated or low-molecular-weight heparins cross the placenta. They would therefore not be expected to cause direct adverse effects to the fetus. Previous reports (Hall *et al.*, 1980) that the use of heparin in pregnancy may be associated with a high rate of fetal loss are not supported on review. The fetal loss could be explained on the basis of maternal comorbid conditions which were themselves responsible for adverse effects (Ginsberg *et al.*, 1989b).

Osteoporosis is a rare but much feared complication of long-term heparin therapy (Hellgren & Nygard, 1982; Howell *et al.*, 1983). The available evidence would suggest that heparin-associated bone demineralization is dose- and duration-dependent (Levine & Hirsh, 1986), but conclusive evidence about the risks of developing clinically important osteoporosis is difficult to obtain. Women taking 20 000 international units (IU) heparin daily for more than 5 months may be at increased risk (Hirsh, 1991), but the possibility that only a subgroup of patients is susceptible to the effects of heparin on bone density must also be considered (Ginsberg *et al.*, 1990). Originally it was postulated that heparin-induced bone changes were irreversible, but a more recent report (Dahlman *et al.*, 1990) suggests that bone density changes may be reversible. There is no correlation between bone loss and the symptoms relating to it (de Swiet *et al.*, 1983). Ginsberg and colleagues (1990) concluded that heparin therapy used for over 1 month is associated with a very small risk of symptomatic osteoporosis but causes a reduction in bone density in the axial skeleton and long bones.

Because of the degree of susceptibility to these bone density changes, their reversibility in individual patients and the possibility that affected women may be at increased risk of the complications of osteoporosis following the menopause, it is recommended that wherever possible the dose and duration of heparin therapy are minimized.

Thrombocytopenia is a rare complication of heparin therapy in the UK. Two distinct groups are described: a mild symptomless thrombocytopenia of early onset, probably due to a direct action of heparin on platelets, and a delayed onset (from 6 to 10 days or more), which is associated, paradoxically, with thromboembolism. This second group has an immune basis and is associated with an immunoglobulin G (IgG) heparin-dependent antibody (Chong *et al.*, 1982). The heparin must be discontinued immediately. A heparin from a different source or a low-molecular-weight heparin may be substituted, but this must be done with caution since cross-reactivity may occur. A change to oral anticoagulation may have to be considered.

Notwithstanding these potential complications, heparin remains the anticoagulant of choice for the prevention and management of venous thromboembolism in pregnancy.

4.3 Management of acute venous thromboembolism

In the UK, the immediate management of acute venous thrombosis or thromboembolism usually includes continuous intravenous infusion of heparin, a bolus of 5000 IU, or up to 10 000 IU in severe pulmonary embolism, being followed by a continuous infusion, commencing with a dose of 1000–2000 IU/hour.

Whenever possible, a platelet count and a coagulation screen should be performed before commencing therapy, and the laboratory response to the infusion should be checked 4–6 hours after its commencement. The heparin dose should be adjusted as necessary, repeating the laboratory monitoring 4–6 hours after any dose adjustment.

Antenatal patients require anticoagulation for the remainder of their pregnancy. This is usually most conveniently and safely achieved by substituting self-administered intermittent subcutaneous heparin after 6–10 days. A preparation of heparin with a concentration of 25 000 IU/ml should be used for subcutaneous administration and the patient taught to use a small-volume syringe to ensure precise dosage. A regimen of 10 000–15 000 IU 12-hourly is usually adequate and safe but should be monitored. Some studies have shown that acute venous thrombosis may be managed from the outset with subcutaneous heparin 15 000 IU 12-hourly, but this remains a less common practice in the UK.

If the patient has delivered, a vitamin K antagonist, usually warfarin, may be started around 3–5 days after heparin has been introduced and overlapped for 3–5 days until full warfarinization is achieved. All patients should remain on anticoagulant therapy until at least 6 weeks after delivery.

The newer low-molecular-weight heparins are more expensive than standard unfractionated heparin but have certain theoretical advantages; for example, they have a longer half-life. There is not enough experience of their use in pregnancy to support their widespread utilization at present, but these agents are evoking much interest and the results of further clinical trials are needed and eagerly awaited.

4.4 Laboratory monitoring of heparin therapy

In the UK, the most commonly used test for monitoring therapy with unfractionated heparin is the APTT. Using the APTT, antithrombotic activity requires a prolongation of 1.5–2.0 times the midpoint of the normal range, and usually the upper 'safe' limit in non-pregnant patients is stated to be 2.5. This test, however, does have some limitations and a specific anti-Xa assay of heparin in plasma should be used in patients where the response to heparin is difficult to predict (e.g. in patients with AT deficiency), aiming to achieve a plasma heparin level of 0.2–0.4 IU/ml which roughly corresponds with the APTT range of 1.5–2.5 (Hirsh, 1991), depending on the APTT reagent used. During pregnancy, high procoagulant levels in plasma, particularly of FVIII and fibrinogen, may result in low APTT values, despite adequate plasma heparin concentrations. This should be borne in mind, particularly when treating patients in the third trimester, when it may be difficult and even dangerous to try to achieve high APTT values. In the situation of apparent heparin resistance, where large doses of heparin fail to prolong the APTT into the therapeutic range, anti-Xa assays may be helpful. If a low-molecular-weight heparin is used, the APTT will not be prolonged and an anti-Xa assay must be used.

The average plasma heparin concentration achieved following sub-cutaneous injection is probably somewhat lower than that achieved by giving the same dose of heparin by intravenous infusion (Andersson *et al.*, 1982). Timing of monitoring relative to heparin injection must be standardized and APTT tests performed at 4–6 hours post injection allow optimum dose control and adjustment.

5 Prophylactic anticoagulation in pregnancy

5.1 Prevention of cardiac/arterial thromboembolism

Patients who are on long-term oral anticoagulants because they have a prosthetic heart valve present a particular problem during pregnancy, as warfarin is known to cause fetal abnormality. It has been shown that substituting low-dose sub-cutaneously administered heparin (5000 IU 12-hourly) for the vitamin K antagonist being taken preconception gives inadequate protection against prosthetic valve thrombosis (Iturbe-Alessio *et al.*, 1986).

Some authors recommend that in these women continuous intravenous heparin in full therapeutic doses is substituted for warfarin therapy during the period when the fetus is considered to be most at risk of teratogenic drug effects (6–12 weeks' gestation) (Iturbe-Alessio *et al.*, 1986). This policy obviously requires careful preconception counselling and easily available facilities for early preg-nancy diagnosis.

Modern pregnancy tests can confirm conception before the first missed menstrual period. After careful pregnancy counselling, women are asked to attend as soon as a pregnancy is suspected. If the pregnancy test is positive, continuous intravenous heparin therapy may be substituted for warfarin until 12 weeks' gestation, when warfarin may be reintroduced. However, early pregnancy tests do not guarantee fetal viability and at this stage of pregnancy miscarriage rates are around 15%. Ultrasound scans at 5–6 weeks' gestation give a more accurate assessment of continuing pregnancy. Because of these problems, many women with prosthetic valves continue on warfarin throughout the first trimester, accepting the risk of teratogenicity.

Careful monitoring of warfarin therapy, using the prothrombin time/inter-national normalized ratio (INR), is required more frequently than in non-pregnant patients because of changing coagulation factor levels and plasma volume. Con-tinuous full-dose therapeutic intravenous heparin must be substituted for oral anticoagulants at around 36 weeks' gestation or 2–3 weeks before the expected delivery. Warfarin may be reintroduced immediately after delivery, either at the previous maintenance dose or at doses of 7 mg, 7 mg and 5 mg respectively on the first 3 days. Heparin must be continued in full doses for at least 3 days until full warfarinization is achieved.

5.2 Prevention of venous thromboembolism

Thrombosis prophylaxis during pregnancy may be considered in two broad groups:
1   Women with a past history of thromboembolism but no known underlying haemostatic abnormality.
2   Women with or without a past history of thrombotic disease who are known to have an inherited 'thrombophilic' abnormality, for example, deficiency of AT, PC or PS, or acquired thrombophilia, due, for example, to the presence in their plasma of antiphospholipid antibodies (e.g. lupus inhibitor and/or anticardiolipin antibodies).

5.2.1 Women with a thrombotic history but no known thrombophilic abnormality

It is very difficult to generalize about the management of these patients, who are the subject of a proposed international collaborative study comparing different management strategies (J.S. Ginsberg, personal communication). Some authors, concerned about the risks of anticoagulation during pregnancy, recommend that patients with a history of a single episode of thromboembolism and no additional thrombosis 'risk factors' are supervised carefully antenatally and given prophylactic anticoagulation intrapartum and for 6 weeks postpartum, statistically the time when thrombosis is most likely to occur (Letsky, 1985). Other authors prefer a policy of heparin prophylaxis throughout pregnancy, using self-administered subcutaneous heparin in doses of 7500–10000 IU 12-hourly (Dahlman *et al.*, 1989).

A policy somewhere between these two extremes may be possible – delaying anticoagulation until the puerperium in those women in whom the past episode occurred postnatally and introducing heparin 4–6 weeks ahead of the stage at which thrombosis occurred in those patients with a past history of thrombosis during pregnancy. Women whose past thrombotic history was not pregnancy-associated may be anticoagulated throughout pregnancy if the past episode was severe but perhaps only during the third trimester or puerperium if the previous episode was less serious. Before 36 weeks, a dose of 7500 IU 12-hourly may be used, increasing to 10000 IU 12-hourly at 36 weeks and decreasing again to 7500 IU 12-hourly postnatally. Monitoring to exclude excessive degrees of anticoagulation and a periodic platelet count are recommended. Warfarin may be introduced immediately after delivery but must be overlapped with or covered with heparin for at least the first 3 days until full warfarinization is achieved. Anticoagulation should be continued at least until 6 weeks postpartum. The management of each of these women and each of their pregnancies must be individually considered.

5.2.2 *Women with known thrombophilic abnormalities*

At present, there is great interest in the management of women who have been shown to have inherited deficiencies of AT, PC or PS or to have acquired anti-phospholipid antibodies, but in many patients it remains extremely difficult to give clear advice (Walker, 1991). The use of prophylactic anticoagulation should not be an automatic consequence of the knowledge that a woman has reduced AT, PC or PS or has antiphospholipid antibodies.

A careful past history and family history must be taken. A previous episode of thrombosis in conjunction with one of these defects would weight a decision in favour of prophylactic anticoagulation. The increased risk of thrombosis associated with AT, PC or PS deficiency in pregnancy and the puerperium is difficult to assess but seems to be greater for AT deficiency than for PC or PS deficiency (Conard *et al.*, 1990). Furthermore, it is quite clear that, at least in non-pregnant patients, the prevalence of thromboembolism associated with AT deficiency is generally less in those in whom functional defects affect only the heparin-binding properties of the molecule than in those in whom there is loss or reduction in function at the active (antithrombin and anti-Xa) site. Characterization of the subtype of inherited AT deficiency may be clinically important in making decisions about the type and timing of intervention in affected women during and after pregnancy, but this requires further study.

In general, women with evidence of significantly reduced antithrombin activity should be anticoagulated with heparin throughout pregnancy and the puerperium, whether or not they have had a previous thrombotic episode and whether or not they are on long-term anticoagulation. Heparin should be self-administered subcutaneously in doses similar to those used for the treatment of venous thrombosis, 10 000–17 500 IU 12-hourly, aiming to achieve an APTT ratio of 1.5–2.0 at 4–6 hours after injection but accepting that, as pregnancy proceeds and FVIII levels rise, this may be impossible to achieve, when an anti-Xa assay may be helpful. Regular monitoring to allow dose adjustment and check the platelet count is essential.

Women who have other inherited thrombophilic abnormalities and who have a past history of thrombosis probably also require anticoagulation during pregnancy and the puerperium. The time when this should be introduced is unclear, but it has been suggested that, if the previous event was in late pregnancy or the puerperium and if there have been no 'spontaneous' events, prophylactic doses of heparin subcutaneously (5000–7500 IU 12-hourly) may suffice during the first and perhaps the second trimester. Full therapeutic doses of heparin, given subcutaneously, should be introduced to cover the third trimester and the puerperium (Haemostasis and Thrombosis Task Force, 1990). At present, it is very difficult to advise on the management of asymptomatic PC- or PS-deficient women in pregnancy, as no ideal regimen exists. Each woman must be considered on an individual basis, but women with a family history of thrombosis probably merit prophylactic anticoagulation, as outlined above, during pregnancy.

Antiphospholipid antibodies are clinically important, since they have been shown to be associated with recurrent fetal loss due to placental insufficiency and, in some women, a tendency to recurrent thrombosis. The management of pregnancy in women with antiphospholipid antibodies is extremely difficult and currently the subject of study. As with inherited thrombophilia, it is at present impossible to identify which women with laboratory evidence of antiphospholipid antibodies (lupus anticoagulant and/or elevated anticardiolipin antibodies) will develop clinical problems. If a woman has antiphospholipid antibodies but no previous history of thromboembolism or pregnancy loss, it would appear of value to treat her with low-dose aspirin (75 mg) daily until 36 weeks' gestation. It is currently recommended that therapy is stopped at 36 weeks because of the potential risk of haematoma formation associated with an epidural injection. This risk is probably overstated and it is hoped that the large multicentre studies on low-dose aspirin in pregnancy will answer the problem. In patients with previous pregnancy loss despite prophylactic aspirin, the role of corticosteroids, intravenous immunoglobulin and heparin remains to be determined.

In general, it is not considered justifiable to put patients without a history of thrombosis on long-term anticoagulants solely on the basis of a laboratory finding of antiphospholipid antibodies. The combination of pregnancy and antiphospholipid antibodies may enhance the risk of thrombosis, but the degree of this potential interaction is not known. Women who are on long-term oral anticoagulants because of recurrent venous thrombosis associated with antiphospholipid antibodies can be managed throughout pregnancy with subcutaneous heparin but must be carefully counselled before conception and, as with other patients on long-term warfarin, advised to seek medical advice as soon as a pregnancy is suspected. Women not on long-term anticoagulants but with a past history of thrombosis should also be considered as candidates for anticoagulation during pregnancy and the puerperium. The question of offering asymptomatic patients, not on long-term anticoagulants, anticoagulant cover during and/or after pregnancy must be individually considered. It is important to realize that, for more than one reason, these are high-risk pregnancies, requiring intensive maternal and fetal monitoring in specialist units. At present, it is suggested that they are best managed in centres with special expertise (Creagh & Greaves, 1991).

6 Preparation for delivery

It is valuable to aim for a planned delivery in patients on anticoagulant therapy. Patients on full therapeutic doses of heparin must reduce their heparin dose on the day of delivery – to a dose of 10 000–15 000 IU/24 hours intravenously (or

5000–7500 IU 12-hourly subcutaneously). Patients on lower prophylactic doses of heparin can continue prophylaxis throughout labour and delivery.

In all patients, the APTT must be checked to ensure it has normalized with reduction or discontinuation of heparin. Pregnant women on subcutaneous heparin may present a management problem at delivery, because they may be at increased risk of bleeding or developing haematomata if a prolonged APTT persists for longer than anticipated, as may happen in patients using heparin subcutaneously over a period of time (Anderson *et al.*, 1991). Replacement of deficient inhibitors with concentrates may be useful at the time of delivery (e.g. AT concentrate (Hellgren *et al.*, 1982)).

Planning the delivery of a patient on warfarin is even more important. Every attempt should be made to change to heparin 2–3 weeks prior to labour or delivery and no later than 36 weeks' gestation. If labour occurs or if delivery is contemplated in a mother still fully anticoagulated using warfarin, caesarean section should be considered to protect the fetus from the possibility of intracranial haemorrhage. If the INR is between 2.0 and 2.5, the risk of maternal bleeding during operation is low, although a result of around 2.0 would be desirable. In patients with an artificial heart valve, it may be dangerous to reduce the INR to below 2.0 in the absence of heparinization. For women whose INR is in the therapeutic range, vitamin K is contraindicated, but vitamin K should be given to the baby intravenously into the cord at delivery. Fresh-frozen plasma (FFP) can be used for bleeding in either mother or baby and 2–3 units should be made available. A suitable dose of FFP is 10 ml/kg for a neonate. Prothrombin complex concentrates may be thrombogenic and should be considered only in life-threatening haemorrhage.

If a patient is anticoagulated at the time of delivery, epidural analgesia is hazardous, as haematoma formation has been reported following both insertion and removal of the cannula. If anticoagulants have been discontinued or if low-dose prophylactic anticoagulants are being administered, providing the coagulation screen is within normal limits, the platelet count greater than $80 \times 10^9/l$ and the bleeding time normal, it is probably safe to introduce an epidural catheter (Letsky, 1991), but no consensus opinion has been achieved. Full discussion and cooperation with the anaesthetist are required in these situations and the relative benefits and risks must be considered on an individual basis.

After delivery, heparin should be reintroduced at a dose of 20 000–30 000 IU/day. Warfarin can be started immediately. If previously on warfarin, patients should be restarted on their prepregnant maintenance dosage. If starting warfarin for the first time, doses of 7 mg, 7 mg and 5 mg should be used respectively on the first 3 days. Heparin must be continued for at least 3 days until full warfarinization is achieved.

7 Breastfeeding

Warfarin has a high degree of protein binding and is not secreted in significant quantity into breast milk (Orme *et al.*, 1977). Mothers may therefore safely breastfeed while taking warfarin. Occasionally, bloodstaining of the milk occurs in anticoagulated mothers. This is usually due to local nipple trauma or mild infection. Neonates may be upset by the presence of this blood and it is often necessary to stop feeding from the affected breast until bleeding stops. Expression of the milk is essential to ensure continued production and patient comfort.

8 Long-term follow-up

It is important that any patient started on anticoagulants during pregnancy or the puerperium is followed up after delivery. A therapeutic plan should be outlined. If the treatment was started because of thromboembolism, further investigation may be necessary for complete diagnosis and anticoagulation can usually be stopped at 6 weeks postpartum. The implications of the diagnosis for future pregnancy and contraception should be outlined. The plan of therapy of subsequent pregnancies should be discussed before any such pregnancy is embarked upon.

9 Note on guidelines

These guidelines should be read in conjunction with *Guidelines on Oral Anticoagulation* (2nd edn, 1990), which was also prepared by the Haemostasis and Thrombosis Task Force.

References

Anderson D.R., Ginsberg J.S., Burrows R. & Brill-Edwards P. (1991) Subcutaneous heparin therapy during pregnancy: a need for concern at the time of delivery. *Thrombosis and Haemostasis* **65**, 248–250.

Andersson G., Fagrell B., Holmgren K., Johnsson H., Wilhelmsson S. & Zetterquist S. (1982) Subcutaneous administration of heparin: a randomised comparison with intravenous administration of heparin to patients with deep vein thrombosis. *Thrombosis Research* **27**, 631–639.

Barnes R.W., Wu K.K. & Hoak J.C. (1975) Fallibility of the clinical diagnosis of venous thrombosis. *Journal of the American Medical Association* **234**, 605–607.

Chong B.H., Pitney W.R. & Castaldi P.A. (1982) Heparin induced thrombocytopenia: association of thrombotic complications with heparin-dependent IgG antibody that induces thromboxane synthesis and platelet aggregation. *Lancet* **ii**, 1246–1249.

Conard J., Horellou M.H., Van Dreden P., Lecompte T. & Samama M. (1990) Thrombosis and pregnancy in congenital deficiencies in ATIII, protein C or protein S: study of 78 women. *Thrombosis and Haemostasis* **63**, 319–320.

Creagh M.D. & Greaves M. (1991) Lupus anticoagulant. *Blood Reviews* **5**, 162–167.

Dahlman T.C., Hellgren M.S.E. & Blomback M. (1989) Thrombosis prophylaxis in pregnancy with use of subcutaneous heparin adjusted by monitoring heparin concentration in plasma. *American Journal of Obstetrics and Gynaecology* **161**, 420–425.

Dahlman T.C., Lindvall N. & Hellgren M. (1990) Osteopenia in pregnancy during longterm heparin treatment: a radiological study post partum. *British Journal of Obstetrics and Gynaecology* **97**, 221–228.

Dauzat M.M., Laroche J.P., Charras C., Blin B., Domingo-Faye M.M., Sainte-Luce P., Domergue A., Lopez F.M. & Janbon C. (1986) Real-time B-mode ultrasonography for better specificity in the noninvasive diagnosis of deep vein thrombosis. *Journal of Ultrasound Medicine* **5**(11), 625–631.

de Swiet M., Dorington Ward P., Fidler J., Horsman A., Katz D., Letsky E.A., Peacock M. & Wise P.H. (1983) Prolonged heparin therapy in pregnancy causes bone demineralisation (heparin induced osteopenia). *British Journal of Obstetrics and Gynaecology* **90**, 1129–1134.

Ginsberg J.S., Hirsh J., Rainbow A.J. & Coates G. (1989a) Risks to the fetus of radiologic procedures used in the diagnosis of maternal venous thromboembolic disease. *Thrombosis and Haemostasis* **61**, 189–196.

Ginsberg J.S., Hirsh J., Turner C., Levine M.N. & Burrows R. (1989b) Risks to the fetus of anticoagulant therapy during pregnancy. *Thrombosis and Haemostasis* **61**, 197–203.

Ginsberg J.S., Kowalchuk G., Hirsh J., Brill-Edwards P., Burrows R., Coates G. & Webster C. (1990) Heparin effect on bone density. *Thrombosis and Haemostasis* **64**, 286–289.

Greer I.A., Barry J., Mackon N. & Allan P.L. (1990) Diagnosis of deep vein thrombosis in pregnancy: a new role for diagnostic ultrasound. *British Journal of Obstetrics and Gynaecology* **97**(1), 53–57.

Haemostasis and Thrombosis Task Force (1990) Guidelines on oral anticoagulation. *Journal of Clinical Pathology* **43**, 177–183.

Haemostasis and Thrombosis Task Force, British Society for Haematology (1990) Guidelines on the investigation and management of thrombophilia. *Journal of Clinical Pathology* **43**, 703–710.

Hall J.A.G., Paul R.M. & Wilson K.M. (1980) Maternal and fetal sequelae of anticoagulation during pregnancy. *American Journal of Medicine* **68**, 122–140.

Hellgren M. & Nygard E.B. (1982) Longterm therapy with subcutaneous heparin during pregnancy. *Gynaecology and Obstetric Investigation* **13**, 76–89.

Hellgren M., Tengborn L. & Abildgaard U. (1982) Pregnancy in women with congenital antithrombin III deficiency: experience of treatment with heparin and antithrombin. *Gynaecologic and Obstetric Investigations* **14**, 127–141.

Hirsh J. (1991) Heparin. *New England Journal of Medicine* **324**, 1565–1574.

Howell R., Fidler J., Letsky E.A. & de Swiet M. (1983) The risks of antenatal subcutaneous heparin prophylaxis: a controlled trial. *British Journal of Obstetrics and Gynaecology* **90**, 1124–1128.

Hull R., Taylor D.W., Hirsh J., Sackett D.L., Powers P., Turpie A.G.G. & Walker I. (1978) Impedance plethysmography: the relationship between venous filling and sensitivity and specificity for proximal vein thrombosis. *Circulation* **58**, 898–902.

Hull R., Hirsh J., Carter C., Jay R., Ockelford P., Buller H., Turpie A.G.G., Powers P., Kinch D., Dodd P., Gill G., Leclerc J. & Gent M. (1985a) Diagnostic efficacy of impedance plethysmography for clinically suspected deep vein thrombosis. *Annals of Internal Medicine* **102**, 21–28.

Hull R., Hirsh J., Carter C., Raskob G.E., Gill E.J., Jay R.M., Leclerc J.R., David M. & Coates G. (1985b) Diagnostic value of ventilation-perfusion lung scanning in patients with suspected pulmonary embolism. *Chest* **88**, 819–828.

Iturbe-Alessio I., Fonesca M.C., Mutchinik O., Santos M.A., Zajarias A. & Salazar E. (1986) Risks of anticoagulant therapy in pregnant women with artificial heart valves. *New England Journal of Medicine* **315**, 1390–1393.

Letsky E.A. (1985) Thromboembolism during pregnancy. *Coagulation Problems in Pregnancy. Current Reviews in Obstetrics and Gynaecology*, Vol. 10, pp. 29–61. Churchill Livingstone, London.

Letsky E.A. (1991) Haemostasis and epidural anaesthesia. *International Journal of Obstetric Anaesthesia* **1**, 51–54.

Letsky E.A. (1992) Thromboembolism. In Calder A.A. & Dunlop W. (eds) *High Risk Pregnancy*, pp. 94–138. Butterworths and Heinemann, Oxford.

Levine M. & Hirsh J. (1986) Non haemorrhagic complications of anticoagulant therapy. *Seminars in Thrombosis and Haemostasis* **12**, 63–65.

Orme L'E.M., Lewis P.J., de Swiet M., Serlin M.J., Sibeon R., Baty J.D. & Brekenridge A.M. (1977) May mothers given warfarin breast feed their infants? *British Medical Journal* **i**, 1564–1565.

Rosner N.H. & Doris P.E. (1988) Diagnosis of femoropopliteal venous thrombosis: comparison of duplex sonography and plethysmography. *American Journal of Roentgenology* **150**(3), 623–627.

Walker I.D. (1991) Management of thrombophilia in pregnancy. *Blood Reviews* **5**, 227–233.

17 Collection, Processing and Storage of Human Bone Marrow and Peripheral Stem Cells for Transplantation*
Prepared by the
Blood Transfusion Task Force

1 Summary

There are no current UK or international guidelines or regulations covering the production, processing and storage of haemopoietic cells such as to allow their engraftment following myeloablative therapy. This chapter seeks to provide such guidelines. It enumerates how quality control and assurance can be applied to this area of transfusion medicine. Procedural steps relating to bone marrow harvest and peripheral-blood stem cell collection are outlined and recommended doses of nucleated cells suggested for both procedures. General specifications for identification, storage and transportation of bone marrow and peripheral-blood stem cells are included, and specific laboratory procedures related to the provision of haemopoietic cells for engraftment are outlined. Umbilical cord blood transplants and long-term bone marrow culture are still in a research phase (Nicol et al., 1994).

2 Introduction

A directive of the Council of European Committees (85/374/EEC) bound member states to introduce product liability by July 1988. In the UK, this became a legal requirement on 1 March 1988 (Consumer Protection Act, 1987, Chapter 43, Part 1).

Human blood and substances prepared from it are products within the terms of the Act, although bone marrow is not specifically mentioned. There are no current UK or international guidelines or regulations covering the production, processing and storage of haemopoietic cells, although experts in the field have dealt with the technique of bone marrow harvesting (Jones & Burnett, 1992) and recommendations and requirements for standardized practice for bone marrow transplantation using volunteer donors (van Rood et al., 1992). The present

---

* Reprinted with permission from *Transfusion Medicine*, 1994, **4**, 165–172.

guidelines are based on the *Guide to Good Manufacturing Practice for Medicinal Products* (Commission of the European Communities, 1989). Marrow donation is on a named-patient basis. The purpose of this chapter is to lay down guidelines for engraftment by the safe collection, sterile processing, documentation and demonstration of reproductive capability of haemopoietic cells, as well as guidelines for long-term storage and culture of these cells. The principle is that the guidelines should enable haemopoietic stem cells to be removed, processed and stored in such a way that they can allow engraftment.

The criteria for collection, processing and storage of haemopoietic cells are very similar to those applied to the handling of blood and elaborated in *Guidelines for the Blood Transfusion Service* (UKBTS/NIBSC Liaison Group, 1993). This includes an aspect of health and safety. Screening of healthy matched unrelated donors should be at least as good as that insisted upon in blood donation (van Rood *et al.*, 1992; UKBTS/NIBSC Liaison Group, 1993). The limited selection of the donor in sibling or autologous transplantation will mean that some of the criteria applied to transfusion donors will have to be omitted. However, these omissions should be as few as possible and viral and other safety factors must be maintained (see Section 7.5).

3 Establishing a quality system for the collection and processing of haemopoietic cells

In order to implement satisfactory quality assurance, it is essential that there should be a structured and organized approach. This is defined as the quality system.

3.1 General principles

Each transplant unit must establish, document and maintain an effective and economical quality system to ensure and demonstrate that adequate and appropriate standards of work are maintained.

The key elements of a quality system include the following:

1 Written defined policies on working practices.

2 Authorized documents (standard operating procedures (SOPs)) detailing for each procedure that is judged to have an effect on the quality of the service or material provided by the unit the approved manner in which that procedure is to be undertaken, written in a manner appropriate to the staff who will undertake that procedure (Roberts, 1991, p. 223, Appendix 1). Such SOPs are to be authorized by the director of the unit prior to their introduction.

3 Test methods for which, unless compendial (*British Pharmacopoeia* (BP), *European Pharmacopoeia* (EurPh) or World Health Organization (WHO)), there is, where relevant, an estimation of uncertainty of measurement.

4 Procedures that have been validated, where practicable and applicable, to show that the results of using that procedure are as intended.

5 Internal audits by individuals not directly concerned with the activities being audited, to ensure compliance with the unit's policies.

6 Staff that have been shown, either by training or from experience, to be competent to undertake their allocated tasks.

7 Control of the purchase of goods or services that have an effect on the quality of the service or material provided by the unit. Such goods or services should comply with an agreed specification.

8 A quality manager, however named, with responsibility for ensuring that the quality policies of the unit are met on a day-to-day basis.

9 The controlled, authorized introduction of any changes to policies and working practices.

Attention is drawn to the *Guide to Good Manufacturing Practice for Medicinal Products* (Commission of the European Communities, 1989), from which advice may be sought.

3.2 Records

Each transplant unit must develop and maintain records that demonstrate that the required quality has been achieved and that the quality system has operated effectively. Records should be kept for 11 years or, in the case of children, until they reach 21, whichever is the longer. Each donation of haemopoietic cells should have a unique number and the harvest procedure be recorded. The date of the processing and the name of the individual(s) performing each collection should be recorded, as well as any major equipment used. The records for each product should be such that the origin of the product can be traced to the donor and the destination and fate of the product identified.

3.3 Documentation

Other aspects of a quality system relating to blood products (listed in UKBTS/ NIBSC Liaison Group, 1993) and standards that apply to blood transfusion should, where appropriate, apply to the quality testing of blood products containing haemopoietic cells.

4 Procedural steps related to bone marrow harvest

4.1 General specifications

The ultimate responsibility for the correct safe procedure for the collection of bone marrow is that of the transplant unit director. It is recommended that the unit should carry out five or more allogeneic transplants per year (Horowitz *et al.*, 1992).

4.2 Donor

Donor suitability must be ensured. The donation may be an autograft or an allograft from a related or unrelated donor. The allogeneic donor should be counselled and a full medical examination carried out to establish that the donor is fit for anaesthesia. Routine haematological, biochemical and virological parameters are checked (see later). A chest X-ray and electrocardiogram (ECG) should be performed. Written informed consent must be obtained from the donor before the recipient commences pretransplant conditioning. It is a cardinal principle that unrelated donors should be anonymous, unpaid and not pregnant. The volunteer donor bone marrow panels recommend that medical assessment, harvest and any necessary medical follow-up of the donor should be at a centre distinct from the transplant centre treating the patient.

The donor is admitted the night before harvest to the transplant centre or hospital experienced in marrow harvests (for definition, see van Rood *et al.*, 1992). The donor receives a unique donor identification number (DIN) and this must be assigned to the marrow, both primary and secondary collection packs and all the sample tubes used (see Section 6.1).

4.3 Marrow collection

Before the start of harvest, the identity of the donor must be checked. Several centres use preservative-free heparin given intravenously to the donor with the premedication (100μ/kg, maximum 5000 units). This is used as a transplant centre option and must be agreed by the donor. Collection should be by aseptic technique into pyrogen-free containers with sufficient anticoagulant for the quantity of marrow to be collected and appropriate for the subsequent processing (see Section 5.2). The container label should state the amount of anticoagulant, the maximum amount of marrow that can be collected and the required storage temperature. The marrow should be anticoagulated with acid citrate dextrose A (ACD-A) unless preservative-free heparin is requested by the transplant centre. In the latter case, marrow should be returned to the patient within 12 hours. The anticoagulant solution must be clear, free from deposit and in date.

Harvest should only be undertaken by trained medical staff. Personnel required are an anaesthetist, operators to harvest marrow, haematology medical laboratory scientific officer, scrub nurse and theatre staff. Harvest lists should be dedicated or at the beginning of the operating list. The volume of marrow withdrawn from the donor must be controlled. The volume taken should be such that a target cell count appropriate to transplant is reached (see Section 4.8).

4.4 Autologous blood transfusion

The harvest centre should aim to collect one or more autologous units from adult allogeneic donors for transfusion to the donor during or after the harvest procedure (see below). Every effort should be made to avoid the use of homologous blood. If homologous blood is given, it should be of known phenotype and cytomegalovirus (CMV) antibody-negative. If transfused during harvest or where the marrow donation may need to be repeated, then the blood should be irradiated to a minimum dose of 2500 cGy.

4.5 Records

A record of the total volume of marrow removed from the donor must be documented in the patient's notes. The most efficient way of measuring the volume in plastic bags is by weight. The mean weight of 1 ml of marrow is 1.06 g; a unit containing 405–495 ml should therefore weigh 430–525 g plus the weight of the container and its anticoagulant.

4.6 Operating procedure

The anaesthetized patient is positioned on the operating table with pelvis supported to make the iliac crests prominent. The choice of harvest needle is one of personal preference and can vary from conventional needles for diagnostic aspiration from iliac crests and sternum through to designed harvest needles with holes along the lateral aspect of the shafts (e.g. Islam). No more than 5 ml of bone marrow should be collected into a 20-ml syringe containing preservative-free heparin and the needle is then repositioned after each aspiration. It is usually possible to take marrow at several different depths from one site. The needle is then withdrawn and resited, samples being taken as widely as possible along the posterior iliac crest. If an inadequate cell count is obtained from the posterior iliac crest, the patient should be turned over and further aspirates taken from the anterior iliac crests and the sternum.

4.7 Peroperative marrow processing

A closed system is preferred where the syringe is emptied directly into 500-ml or 1-l bags containing anticoagulant. Marrow should be filtered in accordance with the harvest centre's routine practice to remove fat, aggregates, clots or bone spicules, if it is not processed further by centrifugation or sedimentation.

Per- and postharvest samples of marrow can be obtained from the bag and a nucleated cell count carried out to ascertain the anticipated volume needed to produce engraftment.

4.8 Estimation of marrow dose at harvest

The present recommended 'dose' of nucleated cells is expressed per kilogram of recipient body weight:

1 Autografts – minimum dose 1.5×10^8 cells/kg.

2 Human leucocyte antigen (HLA)-identical sibling allografts for aplastic anaemia – minimum dose 3×10^8 cells/kg (Storb *et al.*, 1977).

3 Human leucocyte antigen-identical sibling allografts for leukaemia, haemoglobinopathies and inborn errors of metabolism – minimum dose $1.5-2 \times 10^8$ cells/kg.

4 Unrelated donor allograft – minimum dose $2-3 \times 10^8$ nucleated cells/kg.

A minimum number of marrow (nucleated cells) per kilogram recipient body weight should be stated by each transplant unit to permit engraftment. The weight of the recipient must be ascertained.

4.9 Marrow processing postharvest

In allogeneic transplantation, the completed marrow bag is rendered airtight and labelled, and then its contents may be infused intravenously into the recipient where both donor and recipient are ABO-compatible, or cryopreserved. If volume reduction is required, buffy-coat cells can be separated and transferred to a second sterile pack. Where there is major ABO blood group incompatibility between donor and recipient, then a cell fraction known to contain the repopulating stem cells and low in haematocrit should be obtained by density separation (see Section 7.4).

If removal of T cells is required to prevent graft-versus-host disease, the volume of the donation is reduced before incubation with monoclonal antibodies. An appropriate method is to use a blood cell washer or cell separator (Gilmore & Prentice, 1986). Processing may also be modified to collect donor red cells for autologous reinfusion.

Autologous marrow can be similarly separated to leave a buffy coat or further processed to a mononuclear cell fraction, which may be 'purged' before storage. Purging involves incubation of the marrow with, most commonly, the cyclophosphamide antimetabolite 4-hydroxyperoxycyclophosphamide (4-HC) (Kaizer *et al.*, 1985) or with monoclonal antibodies. Monoclonal antibodies may also be used for positive selection of putative progenitor stem cells (e.g. anti-cluster designation 34 (CD34) antibodies). The purged/unpurged marrow is then cryopreserved (see below). Biological methods of purging, such as long-term bone marrow culture, are still experimental.

5 Peripheral-blood stem cell collection

Haemopoietic cells are present at low concentration in steady-state blood. Such cells can be mobilized from the bone marrow into peripheral blood during the recovery phase from myelosuppressive chemotherapy or following administration of haemopoietic growth factors or by a combination of the two. They are collected by leucapheresis on a blood cell separator set to obtain sufficient mononuclear cells for engraftment. A suggested value is 7×10^8 mononuclear cells/kg, but this will vary according to centre and whether myeloablative treatment is given. Some centres use lower values of 2×10^8 mononuclear cells/kg.

Mobilized blood progenitor autografts are usually associated with very rapid haemopoietic reconstitution. Timing of the leucapheresis may be guided by the appearance of CD34-positive cells in the blood or by surrogate markers, such as white blood cell and platelet counts.

During recovery from myelosuppressive therapy, a white count $>1 \times 10^9$/l and platelets $>70 \times 10^9$/l are generally taken as the time to initiate leucapheresis, but absolute counts will vary with the chemotherapy regimen and whether or not growth factors are employed.

Mobilized blood stem cell collections are usually assessed by their content of CD34-positive cells or their ability to grow in tissue culture as colony-forming units–granulocyte macrophage (CFU-GM). 'Threshold doses' need to be determined by each centre, but the recommended minimum number of CFU-GM is usually in the range $5-20 \times 10^4$/kg (Craig *et al.*, 1992). It is usual for the donor to be an autograft recipient and for the material to be stored by cryopreservation.

5.1 Clinical use of blood cell separators

The guidelines for the clinical use of blood cell separators are in Roberts (1991, Chapter 20). This includes clinical management of the cell separator service, donors, drugs and infusion fluids, staff, machine safety, potential complications and guidelines for operators outlining standards of care for donors. A written protocol should be prepared for each apheresis procedure. Instructions should be adhered to and any deviation from the SOP recorded. Full blood counts should be performed on the donor before and at the end of the whole procedure.

5.2 Anticoagulation

This occurs automatically in machine apheresis and a calcium-chelating anticoagulant, such as ACD-A, is recommended. Where purging of the sample is required, using monoclonal antibodies dependent upon complement activation, heparin should be used. However, note that this is anticomplementary where the monoclonal antibodies used are of a rabbit origin.

5.3 Citrate toxicity

Processing of large volumes of blood (usually two to three times the patient's blood volume) may be accompanied by paraesthesiae, due to chelation of calcium. This can be corrected by stopping or slowing the reinfusion rate. Where clinical and electrocardiographic evidence suggests hypocalcaemia, 5 ml of 10% calcium gluconate (proportionally less for children) can be given at 5-minute intervals intravenously until the ECG is normal (see Roberts, 1991, pp. 201, 241).

5.4 Nucleated cell collection

The technique for procurement of the nucleated cell layer rich in stem cells depends on the cell separator machine used. The aim is to collect the buffy coat interface between plasma and red cells. The total nucleated cell volume collected is determined from the total blood volume of the donor, ascertained from his/her height/weight prior to apheresis. It is recommended that, in adults, a volume of 7–15 l is processed. Where the nucleated cell yield is greater than $100 \times 10^9/l$, dilutions in plasma are needed to prevent aggregation during the process of freezing (see Section 6.2).

When the collection is complete, the residual volume of blood is returned to the donor.

6 General specifications for identification, storage and transportation of bone marrow and peripheral-blood stem cells

6.1 Identification

The unit containing stem cells must be labelled with the name of the product, the donor's name and hospital number, unique donation number, date of collection, the presence and type of anticoagulant and additive media if any, ABO and Rh D group and the volume of the product.

6.2 Storage (Rowley & Davis, 1990; Reiman & Sacher, 1991)

6.2.1 Standard operating procedure

An SOP should be written to include the following: a designated storage area; a procedure for quarantine of bone marrow and peripheral-blood stem cells; and a procedure for validating the conditions of storage achieved in any given storage area. This would include temperature control and prevention of microbiological contamination. If as a result of microbiological and virological screening the unit is positive for any of the mandatory microbiological markers (see Table 17.1), then that unit should be stored in isolation to avoid cross contamination with other units.

6.2.2 Storage unfrozen

Unmanipulated bone marrow and peripheral-blood stem cells may be stored unfrozen for up to 72 hours at 4°C ± 2°C. The anticoagulant conventionally used is ACD-A. Heparin is unsuitable. Storage at 4°C will, however, reduce leucocyte viability, and cellular aggregation may occur.

6.2.3 Preparation of frozen bone marrow and peripheral-blood haemopoietic cells

Haemopoietic cells in bone marrow are enriched and concentrated by differential centrifugation into a buffy coat. Further enrichment using a density gradient may be required (see Section 4.9). Peripheral-blood cells are not normally concentrated. The cell concentration frozen should be less than $100 \times 10^9/l$ (Gorin, 1986) (see Section 5.4).

The above products are cryopreserved, using one of the established cryoprotectants, for example 10 or 15% v/v dimethylsulphoxide (DMSO) or 5% v/v DMSO plus 6% w/v hydroxyethyl starch (HES). Dimethylsulphoxide should be added slowly to its diluent to avoid a rise in temperature, since dilution is exothermic. Progenitor cell viability may be improved by preparing a solution in which the desired final concentration of DMSO is isotonic in molar terms. This requires the addition of sufficient compounds that are impermeable to the DMSO. For instance, if autologous plasma or 4.5% human albumin solution (HAS) is used, additional salts or a suitable impermeable sugar are necessary (Pegg, 1984). The diluent is then cooled on ice to 0–4°C, DMSO added and the cryoprotectant mixed with an equal volume of haemopoietic cells.

6.2.4 The freezing process

A feedback-controlled cooling machine (controlled-rate freezer) will provide reproducible, standardized cooling conditions. The cooling programme should be one that has been shown to be effective, such as 2°C/minute to −30°C, followed by 4°C/minute to −70°C, with adequate control of the freezing plateau (Gorin, 1986). Passive cooling methods may also be effective, providing that they produce acceptable cooling profiles (Makino *et al.*, 1991). The bags in which the marrow is cooled should be made from a material that will withstand exposure to liquid nitrogen and should be housed between metal plates to produce a thickness of about 3 mm to facilitate heat transfer. Temperatures should be recorded in a control bag and the data kept with the processing records.

Peripheral-blood cells may be cryopreserved by the same methods.

Once below −70°C, the bone marrow and peripheral-blood stem cells should be transferred for storage. Such deep-frozen material is fragile and container bags may fracture.

6.3 Transportation

The above products should be transported under conditions as similar as possible to the recommended conditions of storage. There are newly designed transport containers where liquid nitrogen is held in an absorbent material (Statebourne Cryogeneic, Washington, UK). Transit times should be minimized and, on receipt, material should be transferred to storage under the recommended conditions, unless for immediate use. Written procedures and documentation of the issue of the products, their transportation, conditions of transport, receipt of the product and its subsequent disposal must be kept.

6.4 Thawing of frozen bone marrow/peripheral-blood cells

1 Contamination of the marrow/peripheral-blood bag with water-bath fluid is to be avoided and it is essential that double bags are used.

2 Thaw in a water-bath at 37–40°C with gentle agitation. Observe carefully for rapid expansion of the bag during thawing, which will suggest that liquid nitrogen has leaked into the bag during storage. If this occurs, release the pressure immediately by puncturing the bag with a sterile needle.

3 Dimethylsulphoxide toxicity is temperature-dependent (Gorin, 1986). It is therefore important to remove the bag from the water-bath as soon as the last ice has melted and not to allow the marrow to reach the water-bath temperature. Keep the thawed marrow cool until administration and infuse within 5 minutes of the completion of thawing. Current practice is not to remove the DMSO before injection into the patient (Rowley & Anderson, 1993). Premedication of the patient with steroid/antihistamine is recommended.

4 Any thawing incidents should be documented and reported to the clinician in charge of the recipient, who will decide whether action is required.

6.5 Testing

Testing of frozen products may be performed utilizing 1- or 2-ml aliquots of material frozen at the same time under conditions that are as close as possible to the bulk product. It should be noted that small ampoules will not cool at the same rate as large bags. Assays may be performed to determine short-term progenitor growth post cryopreservation (see Section 7.6).

7 Specific laboratory procedures related to provision of haemopoietic cells for engraftment

7.1 Serology

The ABO and Rh D blood groups of all donors should be performed. The national specification for the performance of ABO grouping is given in Roberts (1991, p. 150).

7.2 Cell counting

The minimum information required is the total nucleated cell count obtained at stem cell harvest. If counts are corrected for peripheral-blood dilution, this should be clearly indicated to avoid confusion with uncorrected nucleated counts. Such counts should be performed on a cell counting machine by validated methods or manually.

The volume of bone marrow or peripheral-blood harvest is best calculated by weight.

7.3 Cell viability

The quality of frozen cells can be assessed by the trypan blue exclusion test or automated techniques, using a flow cytometer and propidium iodide. These results do not correlate with *in vitro* growth but give an indication of consistency of technique.

7.4 Red cell depletion

Red cell depletion of the donor graft is strongly recommended in ABO-mismatched allogeneic transplants. This can be carried out by HES sedimentation or differential centrifugation (Braine *et al.*, 1982; Ho Winston *et al.*, 1984). An alternative is to plasma-exchange the recipient and/or to give A/B antigen-rich secretor plasma prior to the transplant.

7.5 Microbiology and virology

The sterility of the bone marrow/peripheral-blood product at various stages should be ascertained, using liquid and semisolid culture medium. This is especially important prior to freezing and at the final stage of processing after freezing before the product is infused into the patient. A pilot tube is thawed and cultured. The clinician should be informed if the cultures are positive. Donor bone marrow can transmit infectious diseases (UKTSSA and NIBSC Working Party, 1993). All donors should have the mandatory tests (Table 17.1) carried out and, where possible, the serological tests repeated at not less than 90 days from the first screening sample.

Advisable tests are shown in Table 17.1. Bone marrow from CMV antibody-positive donors may cause serious or life-threatening diseases in CMV antibody-

Table 17.1 Tests for markers of pathogenic organisms in donors, transmitted by bone marrow or peripheral blood

Mandatory
Hepatitis B surface antigen (HBsAg)
Human immunodeficiency virus (HIV) 1 and 2 antibody
Hepatitis C virus antibody
VDRL or equivalent test for syphilis

Advisable
CMV antibody
Toxoplasma gondii antibody

Desirable
Herpes simplex virus (HSV) antibody
Herpes zoster virus (HZV) antibody
Human T-lymphotrophic virus 1 (HTLV-1)

Table 17.2 Individuals in categories at risk of transmitting infectious agents via bone marrow transplantation

Males who have had sex with another male(s) or with prostitutes(s)
Females who have had sex with multiple partners
Intravenous drug users of either sex
Haemophiliacs who have received blood products
People who have lived in or visited countries with high prevalence of HIV and have had sexual contact with persons of the same or opposite sex living in those areas
Sexual partners of people in the above groups
Offspring of people in the above groups
People known or suspected to have clinically active syphilis or tuberculosis
Sufferers of malaria

negative recipients. Consideration should be given to avoiding the situation or providing antiviral prophylaxis for these recipients. Certain HLA-compatible donors may fall into the at-risk category (see Table 17.2) and this may affect their suitability.

7.6 Cell culture
Progenitor cell assay (CFU-GM) is recommended, using a validated technique, with controls where appropriate. Results should be reported as CFU-GM $\times 10^4$/kg recipient body weight. The transplant unit should document the minimum number of progenitor cells acceptable (see above).

7.7 Immunophenotype
Quantitation of CD34-positive cells by immunophenotyping may be used, as well as progenitor cell assays.

8 Umbilical cord blood transplants

A small volume, 70–150 ml, of human umbilical cord blood (HUC) may contain sufficient cells to repopulate ablated adult human bone marrow (Gluckman *et al.*, 1993). Preliminary feasibility studies are in progress by the European Cord Blood Bank Group. There are considerable ethical principles that will need to be clarified. Permission of both mother and biological father will be needed for collection of such material.

References

Braine H.G., Sensenbrenner L.L., Wright S.K., Tutschka P.J., Sasal R. & Santos G. (1982) Bone marrow transplantation with major ABO blood group incompatibility using erythrocyte depletion of marrow prior to infusion. *Blood* **60**(2), 420–425.

Commission of the European Communities (1989) *Rules Governing Medicinal Products in the European Community*, Vol. IV, *Guide to Good Manufacturing Practice for Medicinal Products*. HMSO, London.

Craig J.I.O., Turner M.L. & Parker A.C. (1992) Peripheral blood stem cell transplants. *Blood Reviews* **6**, 59–67.

Gilmore M.M.L. & Prentice H.G. (1986) Standardisation of the processing of human bone marrow for allogeneic transplantation. *Vox Sanguinis* **51**, 202–206.

Gluckman E., Wagner J., Hows J., Kerman N., Bradley B. & Broxmeyer H.E. (1993) Cord blood banking for haematopoietic stem cell transplantation: an international cord blood transplant registry. *Bone Marrow Transplantation* **11**(3), 199–200.

Gorin N.C. (1986) Collection, manipulation and freezing of haemopoietic stem cells. *Clinics in Haematology* **15**(1), 19–48.

Ho Winston G., Champlin R.E., Seig S.A. & Gale R.P. (1984) Transplantation of ABH incompatible bone marrow: gravity sedimentation of donor marrow. *British Journal of Haematology* **57**, 155–162.

Horowitz M.M., Przepiorka D., Champlin R.E., Gale R.P., Gratwohl R.H., Herzig R.H., Prentice G.H., Rimm A.A., Ringden O. & Bortin M.M. (1992) Should HLA identical sibling bone marrow transplants for leukaemia be restricted to large centres? *Blood* **79**(10), 2771–2774.

Jones R. & Burnett A.K. (1992) How to harvest bone marrow for transplantation. *Journal of Clinical Pathology* **45**, 1053–1057.

Kaizer H., Stuart R.K., Brookmeyer R. *et al.* (1985) Autologous bone marrow transplantation in acute leukaemia: a phase 1 study of *in vitro* treatment of marrow with 4-hydroxyperoxycyclophosphamide to purge tumour cells. *Blood* **65**, 1504–1510.

Makino S., Harada M., Akashi K., Taniguchi S., Shibuya T., Inaba S. & Nilo Y. (1991) A simplified method for cryopreservation of peripheral blood stem cells at −80°C without rate-controlled freezing. *Bone Marrow Transplantation* **8**, 239–244.

Nicol A.J., Hows J.M. & Bradley B.A. (1994) Cord blood transplantation: a practical option? *British Journal of Haematology* **87**, 1–5.

Pegg D.E. (1984) Red cell volume in glycerol/sodium chloride/water mixtures. *Cryobiology* **21**, 234–239.

Reiman E.M. & Sacher R.A. (1991) Bone marrow processing for transplantation. *Transplant Medicine Reviews* **5**(3), 214–227.

Roberts B. (ed.) (1991) *Standard Haematology Practice*. Blackwell Scientific Publications, Oxford.

Rowley S.D. & Davis J.M. (1990) Standards for bone marrow processing laboratories. *Transfusion* **30**(6), 571–572.

Rowley S.D. & Anderson G.L. (1993) Effect of DMSO exposure without cryopreservation on haemopoietic progenitor cells. *Bone Marrow Transplantation* **11**, 390–393.

Storb R., Prentice R.L. & Thomas E.D. (1977) Marrow transplantation for treatment of aplastic anaemia: analysis of factors associated with graft rejection. *New England Journal of Medicine* **296**, 621–626.

UKBTS/NIBSC Liaison Group (1993) *Guidelines for the Blood Transfusion Service*, 2nd edn. HMSO, London.

UKTSSA and NIBSC Working Party (1993) *Promoting the Safety of Transplantation of Human Tissues and Organs: an Advisory Note Prepared by an Informal Working Party Convened Jointly by UKTSSA and NIBSC*. Department of Health, London (in press).

van Rood J., Goldman J.M. & Brutoco R. (1992) Bone marrow transplants using volunteer donors – recommendations and requirements for a standardised practice throughout the world. *Bone Marrow Transplantation* **10**, 287–291.

18 Transfusion of Infants and Neonates*
Prepared by the
Blood Transfusion Task Force

1 Introduction

Although the transfusion needs of infants command a relatively small proportion of routine blood bank workload, it is important to bear in mind that babies in special care units are now amongst the most intensively transfused of all hospital patients. Despite such a high volume of activity, this area of transfusion practice is beset with uncertainties. Many widely accepted practices are not based on secure scientific foundations and could benefit from controlled investigation.

These guidelines seek to identify those practices which, by broad agreement, seem to be most firmly justified. The clinical indications for transfusion sometimes differ from those for adults, and neonates are more susceptible than adults to some of the various harmful effects of transfusion. As a consequence of the frequency of transfusion, the associated hazards are correspondingly increased. In practice, selection of blood products, compatibility testing and their administration also require separate consideration.

Detailed discussion of the clinical indications for transfusion of individual blood products are beyond the scope of the present guidelines and readers are referred to specialist publications. For the purpose of these guidelines, neonates are considered to be babies within 4 weeks past their normal gestational age. Unless explicitly stated as applying to neonates, other recommendations have been considered in the context of transfusions within the first year of infant life.

2 Red cell transfusion

For practical purposes, red cell transfusion is categorized according to the volumes administered, as this has practical relevance to the specifications of product required. Most are small volumes given to replace the blood losses of investigative sampling or to alleviate the anaemia of prematurity. Larger transfusions will also

* Reprinted with permission from *Transfusion Medicine*, 1994, **4**, 63–69.

be needed for replacement of surgical or pathological blood loss, in common with adult transfusion practice. At the other extreme are exchanges or equivalent massive transfusions (e.g. during extracorporeal membrane oxygenation (ECMO), or cardiac bypass) during which an amount in excess of the entire blood volume may be transfused.

It must be appreciated that the metabolic concerns governing the choice of blood only apply if substantial volumes of blood are to be given and are not relevant to top-up transfusions. Similarly, the freshness of blood, in terms of its haemostatic qualities, is of no relevance when only small volumes are given.

2.1 Source of blood for transfusion

Transfusion specialists in the UK agree that blood donated by unpaid volunteers selected and tested according to national guidelines (Department of Health, 1992) fully meets safety requirements. Walking donor programmes, schemes entailing collection of small volumes of transfusable blood as and when required from special panels of donors, are vulnerable to both serological and viral transmission mishaps and can no longer be condoned. In addition, Medicines Control Agency regulations and product liability requirements mandate stringent standards for record-keeping, blood grouping and microbiological screening, which prove difficult to meet under the pressures of providing acute clinical services. Directed donations (including donations from relatives) cannot be assumed to be safer than microbiologically screened volunteer donations (see Table 18.1), and their use is not advocated. On rare occasions, the use of maternal blood may be permissible; however, fatal graft-versus-host disease (GVHD) has occurred in this situation and prior irradiation of blood is necessary (Vogelsang, 1990).

2.2 Pretransfusion testing (for neonates and infants within the first 4 months) (Table 18.2)

Samples from mother and neonate should be obtained and the ABO and Rh D groups determined. The maternal serum should be screened for the presence of atypical antibodies and a direct antiglobulin test (DAT) done on the neonate's red cells.

If maternal blood is unavailable, a neonatal sample should be screened to

Table 18.1 Microbiological screening of volunteer donor blood collected in the UK

Hepatitis B (HBsAg)
Hepatitis C (anti-HCV)
Human immunodeficiency virus types 1 and 2 (anti-HIV 1/2)
Syphilis
Cytomegalovirus (anti-CMV) for selected recipients

Table 18.2 Pretransfusion testing of blood within the first 4 months

Maternal samples ABO and Rh D group Antibody screen
Infant samples ABO and Rh D group Direct antiglobulin test Antibody screen (if maternal sample unavailable)

exclude atypical antibodies. The presence of these in either the maternal or the neonatal serum or a positive DAT on neonatal red cells may reflect the presence of haemolytic disease of the newborn. In such cases, special serological procedures will be necessary to determine the infant's blood group and allow selection of appropriate blood for transfusion. Note that the baby's ABO group is determined from the red cells alone, since the corresponding antibodies will be weak or absent in the serum. The serum may contain passively transferred maternal antibodies.

2.2.1 Choice of the ABO blood group

Blood selected should be compatible with the maternal ABO antibodies.

The choice is between the following:

1 Use of the infant's own ABO group or, if necessary, an alternative compatible ABO group, provided the above requirement is met.

2 If the mother's blood group is unknown, blood should be cross-matched, using the indirect antiglobulin test against the baby's serum to ensure ABO compatibility.

3 Group O blood donations are generally suitable, but, if used for massive transfusion to non-group O recipients, these must be screened to exclude donations with high anti-A/B titres.

Note that, in the absence of a direct matching policy for each transfusion episode (see Section 2.2.2), the use of donations other than group O requires total assurance in the systems for ABO designation of the intended recipient.

In practice, because of the other requirements of blood for neonatal use (described below), transfusion centres may specifically designate a supply a low anti-A/B titre group O Rh D-negative blood for use in neonatal transfusions (see Appendix 18.1).

2.2.2 The need for conventional 'cross-matching'

Provided that there are no atypical antibodies demonstrable in maternal or infant's serum and the DAT on the infant's red cells is negative, a conventional cross-match is unnecessary. The transfusion centre may, however, recommend that the ABO/

Rh D group be confirmed on all blood transfused without direct cross-matching.

Small-volume replacement transfusions can be given repeatedly during the first 4 months of life without further serological testing. The formation of allo-antibodies has been shown to be exceptionally rare during this period and appears to be related to repeated massive transfusions and the use of relatively fresh blood. It is only, therefore, under these circumstances that repeat antibody screening of the recipient is required (De Palma, 1992).

Historically, the practice had been to perform conventional cross-matching using maternal serum or, if unavailable, the infant's serum prior to each transfusion. This practice and, in particular, neonatal sampling for routine transfusions is now regarded as unnecessary.

If the antibody screen and/or DAT are positive, serological investigation and full compatibility testing will be necessary.

After the first 4 months of life, compatibility testing should conform to the requirements for adults, as described in the British Committee for Standards in Haematology (BCSH) guidelines (BCSH, 1991).

2.3 Presentation of red cell products
2.3.1 Small-volume transfusions
Primary packs containing either whole blood or red cells (haematocrit 0.55–0.75), with multiple aseptically sealable satellites, are ideal. These enable transfusion of several small aliquots from a single donation.

Despite the extremely low risks of virus transmission by transfused blood in the UK, every effort should be made to minimize the number of donor exposures to which any infant is exposed. This can be done by dedication of a single donation for each patient, as well as by ensuring that an adequate transfusion volume is administered on each occasion.

2.3.2 Exchange transfusions
Plasma-reduced red cells (within a haematocrit range of 0.50–0.60) are the most generally acceptable products for exchange transfusion. Where these are not routinely available, whole-blood donations can be used, but partial concentration by removal of around 120 ml of plasma into a sterile transfer pack may be necessary to provide an acceptable haematocrit. Red cells as conventionally provided concentrates (haematocrit 0.55–0.75) may be less satisfactory in that those packs with the highest haematocrit levels may require simultaneous administration of a plasma expansion material. This can be achieved with saline or 4.5% albumin. Fresh-frozen plasma (FFP) has often been used for this purpose but it doubles the donor exposure risk and is therefore not recommended unless indicated as a product in its own right. For smaller transfusions, saline will normally be entirely satisfactory as a resuspension material.

Despite initial reservations regarding their suitability, red cells in optimal additive solutions, e.g. saline adenine glucose mannitol (see Appendix 18.2), are increasingly used for top-up transfusion. There is so far no agreement regarding their suitability for exchange transfusions, but there is concern that their use could lead to risks of metabolic, haemostatic and oncotic pressure problems.

2.4 Age of blood for transfusion

The age of blood does not matter for small-volume top-up transfusions and blood can be used at any time throughout its approved storage life.

It is a common misconception that fresh blood is necessary for all neonatal transfusions. In practice, the needs for the separate attributes of fresh blood require individual consideration, bearing in mind the volume to be transfused. Supernatant plasma potassium can reach concentrations of up to 30 mmol/l in 5-week-old blood and this is the most important reason for limiting the age of red cells for neonatal transfusions. For this reason, blood used for exchanges and other large transfusions should ideally be within 5 days from collection, i.e. 120 hours from midnight of the day of collection (see Table 18.3). If this is not available, the red cell pack may be concentrated by removal of the supernatant plasma and the transfusion volume restored with 4.5% albumin. The content of potassium is small in top-up transfusions in relation to daily needs and practice has shown that blood of any storage age is perfectly safe.

Storage-related depletion of 2,3-diphosphoglycerate (2,3-DPG) and the resulting high oxygen affinity is a theoretical disadvantage of aged blood, but there is no evidence that this constitutes a clinical problem. For top-up transfusions, the dilution effect renders the 2,3-DPG content of the donor blood immaterial. A number of studies show reasonable retention of 2,3-DPG levels (>70%) and

Table 18.3 Blood for neonatal exchange transfusion: considerations for selection

Product	Plasma-reduced red cells (Hct 0.55–0.60)
Age	Within 5 days from collection
Blood group	ABO group of neonate, or an alternative provided that it is compatible with maternal ABO antibodies. Otherwise use designated group O Rh D negative compatible units
Antibody screen	Exclude high anti-A/B titres (group O donations) and other significant irregular blood group antibodies
Compatibility selection	Compatible with any maternal irregular antibodies
Anti-CMV status	Negative if used for vulnerable recipients (see Section 7.6)
Haemoglobin S screen	Negative*

*This is advised unless the regional transfusion centre recommends that screening is unnecessary.
Hct, haematocrit.

oxygen affinity during the first 5 days of storage; the most profound deterioration occurs after this time. 2,3-Diphosphoglycerate also regenerates rapidly following transfusion. It seems reasonable, however, for exchange and other massive transfusions in the most critically ill neonates, to use blood as close to the collection date as is conveniently possible, provided that all microbiological testing requirements have been met.

The use of close-to-collection-date (24–48 hours) donations for prevention of haemostatic problems during massive transfusion of high-risk neonates has re-emerged as a contentious issue. In the presence of some supportive evidence (Manno *et al.*, 1991), a permissive policy seems reasonable for these rather uncommon transfusions, pending availability of more conclusive evidence.

The use of absolutely 'fresh' blood (e.g. prior to required testing and release procedures), with the aim of contributing haemostatic and anti-infective factors, is not acceptable. Diagnosis of the specific haemostatic lesion and appropriate therapy, e.g. platelet concentrates, cryoprecipitate or FFP, should be instituted.

2.5 Indications for top-up transfusions

As for any red cell transfusion, reduction of the red cell mass and its oxygen transport capacity to the extent that it prejudices cardiorespiratory function constitutes the fundamental indication for transfusion. Haemoglobin estimation alone permits an imperfect assessment, particularly within the neonatal period and is in any case complicated by the gestational age and prematurity-associated changes. Haemoglobin reduction, coupled with symptoms that are presumed consequences of anaemia at this time, for example feeding difficulties, lethargy and failure to thrive, is generally agreed to support a need for transfusion. It must be admitted, however, that controlled studies have not so far provided clear evidence of clinical benefit following transfusion under these circumstances. Nevertheless, haemoglobin concentrations provide the only practical guide in the absence of more sophisticated physiologically validated assessments of red cell mass or oxygen availability.

It is suggested that transfusion should be considered for any symptomatic neonate whose haemoglobin concentration is less than 10.5 g/dl. It is generally accepted that neonates requiring supplemental oxygen should be maintained at a higher value. For example, target haemoglobin values of 13.0 g/dl have been suggested in the presence of severe pulmonary or cardiac disease.

When transfusion is given for the anaemia of prematurity, the volume transfused should be sufficient to increase the haemoglobin level to within the range of that found in full-term babies.

Blood sampling for investigation purposes is well recognized to contribute to neonatal anaemia, and replacement of these losses by transfusion is considered to be fully justified. This is the most frequent indication for transfusion in preterm infants, although there is no common agreement about the frequency and volume of replacements required.

2.6 Rates and volumes for transfusion

Because of the risk of bacterial proliferation in non-refrigerated blood, transfusions from each blood pack should not exceed 6 hours' duration. Neonates are particularly vulnerable to circulatory overload; transfusion rates must therefore be carefully controlled. Volumes of around 5 ml/kg/hour are regarded as safe; infusion rates will need to be increased in the presence of active haemorrhage. Lower rates of transfusion should be selected when there is a risk of cardiac failure. If large volumes are transfused in a short space of time, diuretics should also be considered. Transfusions are most conveniently given via syringe pumps (provided a pressure warning device is incorporated). The syringe can be preloaded with blood from the pack, filling the syringe through a filter assembly. Larger volumes are best administered via standard blood administration sets incorporating a calibrated burette reservoir. The routine use of microaggregate filters during neonatal top-up transfusions has not been shown to be necessary. A reasonable approach which parallels their use in adult medicine would be to recommend filter use for massive transfusions (>1 blood volume/24 hours) or where respiratory distress is present, although their benefits in these situations are still unproved.

2.7 Blood warmers

These should be used during rapid blood replacement, for example during exchange transfusions. Only approved and regularly maintained blood warming equipment should be used. Both fatal haemolytic transfusion reactions and bacteriological contamination have followed use of inappropriate blood warming procedures.

3 Treatment of hypovolaemic shock/plasma volume expanders

Albumin solutions, usually 4.5% in isotonic saline, are the preferred plasma volume expansion agents. Container volumes of 100 ml (4.5%) are available for paediatric use. Fresh-frozen plasma should not be used in these situations unless there are co-existing coagulation abnormalities.

Albumin solutions can be rapidly available as first-line treatment for unexpected hypotensive shock when the cause is unknown.

3.1 Exchange transfusion for polycythaemia

Hyperviscosity arising from polycythaemia (e.g. where the central venous haematocrit exceeds 0.65) can be associated with significant morbidity. Serious pathology (e.g. renal vein thrombosis) can occur without warning symptoms. Partial exchange can be employed to reduce the haematocrit to 0.55 (Letsky, 1991). Human albumin 4.5% solution exchanged in 10-ml aliquots is the preferred material, unless coagulation abnormalities indicate a need for FFP.

4 Fresh-frozen plasma

General recommendations for the use of this material are available (BCSH, 1992a).

Disseminated intravascular coagulation (DIC) is one of the commonest coagulation problems. This may require FFP, supplemented by cryoprecipitate if there is evidence of a severe consumptive state with fibrinogen depletion.

5 Platelet therapy

General recommendations for the use of platelet products are available in the recently published guidelines (BCSH, 1992b). However, thrombocytopenia is believed to be more hazardous in neonates, and prophylactic therapy is probably justified at counts below $30 \times 10^9/l$ or, in the case of the very sick and premature, when counts fall below $50 \times 10^9/l$. Thrombocytopenia may result from sepsis or DIC and may also be a complication of a variety of neonatal infective problems. Generally, one platelet concentrate will constitute a single dose; it will also contribute approximately 50 ml of 'fresh' plasma. If volume overload is a particular concern, the dose may be concentrated even further by arrangement with the regional blood transfusion centre. It is then necessary to allow the platelet packs to stand for about 1 hour without disturbance before resuspension is possible. Platelets concentrated in this way must be administered within 12 hours, as prolonged storage in this reduced volume is unsatisfactory.

5.1 Neonatal alloimmune thrombocytopenia

Specialist advice should be sought for the management of this rare condition. Emergency treatment of unexpected and symptomatic cases can usually be provided by transfusion of a unit of washed maternal platelets.

6 Granulocyte therapy

The benefit of granulocytes in the management of neonatal sepsis has not been conclusively confirmed and treatment is best reserved for those serious cases in which antibiotic therapy alone appears insufficient. Treatment should not be contemplated without proved or strongly suspected bacterial sepsis, co-existing with low blood neutrophil counts. A dose contributing around $0.5-1.0 \times 10^9/$ granulocytes/kg is probably adequate. Trëtment may be required twice daily for several days in succession. Granulocytes may be obtained by leucapheresis or from random donor buffy coats. Unless red cells are removed from buffy coats, compatibility selection must be as for red cell administration. Granulocyte concentrates carry a risk of cytomegalovirus (CMV) transmission, and CMV-seronegative donations should be used where appropriate (see Section 7.6). Granulocyte concentrates must be irradiated where recipients are judged to be vulnerable to GVHD (see Section 7.5).

7 Special hazards of transfusion in the neonatal period

These problems are mainly confined to exchange transfusions or other circumstances of massive blood replacement.

7.1 Hypocalcaemia

Neonates are more likely than adults to develop hypocalcaemia (total serum calcium <1.5 mmol/l, ionized calcium <0.8 mmol/l), although the clinical effects may be less pronounced. This complication is now rare, following the use of citrate phosphate dextrose in place of acid citrate dextrose as an anticoagulant, but it can follow rapid transfusion, as, for example, during exchanges. Blood should be warmed to minimize the effect and, if clinical suspicion of hypocalcaemia is confirmed biochemically, calcium gluconate should be administered.

7.2 Citrate toxicity

This can be a problem for premature infants and shows as an alkalosis with increased plasma bicarbonate.

7.3 Rebound hypoglycaemia

This can be induced by the high glucose levels of blood transfusion anticoagulants. Blood glucose levels should be monitored during and following exchange transfusions.

7.4 Thrombocytopenia

This can be a problem following exchange transfusion and may reflect either a dilution effect or an underlying process of DIC.

7.5 Graft-versus-host disease

This has been an exceptionally rare problem of intrauterine transfusions and neonatal transfusions. The actual level of risk is unknown and there is controversy over the need for prophylactic irradiation of cellular blood components. Infants with congenital cellular immune deficiency should certainly be given blood components which have been irradiated. For other patients, the most persuasive evidence supports the use of irradiation for intrauterine transfusion, for any subsequent exchanges such babies may receive and for exchanges given to very-low-birthweight babies (<1500 g). Irradiation is also necessary for directed blood donations from first-degree relatives, in view of the propensity for shared-haplotype transfusions to induce GVHD. Doses of 25 Gy are used. Because of the accelerated K^+ leak, irradiated red cells should be used within 4 days for top-up transfusions and 24 hours for exchange transfusions*.

7.6 Cytomegalovirus infection
Anti-CMV-negative cellular components should be given to very-low-birthweight babies (<1500 g), as it is only in this category that significant morbidity occurs. If these are unavailable, leucocyte depletion of blood components by filtration is believed to be effective.

7.7 Transfusion overload
Neonates are particularly susceptible to volume overload and accordingly need careful monitoring.

7.8 Haemolytic transfusion reactions in necrotizing enterocolitis
These rare but serious events are due to destruction of T-activated autologous red cells by the natural anti-T in transfused plasma. The transfusion laboratory should be notified to enable the diagnosis of T activation to be investigated if this condition is suspected in infants who require transfusion. If confirmed, transfusion of any product containing plasma must be avoided.

Appendix 18.1: Additional serological screening of blood for neonatal use

These recommendations pertain to blood likely to be used for massive/exchange transfusions.

1 Exclusion of group O donations with high levels of anti-A/B
In the UK, it is not mandatory to screen all group O donations for the presence of high levels of anti-A/B. However, additional testing is recommended on group O donations used for massive/exchange transfusion of neonates to exclude blood containing high-titre anti-A/B. This policy will ensure protection for non-group O neonates receiving large-volume group O transfusions.

There is no general agreement on measures for routine screening for significant titres of haemolysins or agglutinins. Exclusion of donations with saline titres of >32 or examination

---

* This recommendation will be reviewed during preparation of the BCSH Guidelines on the use of irradiated blood products.

of a 1:50 dilution of donor plasma against A1 and B cells by indirect antiglobulin test are acceptable approaches.

2 Screening for irregular blood group antibodies

Donation screening protocols for irregular blood group antibodies acceptable for routine adult transfusion purposes may not be adequate for massive neonatal transfusions.

Under these circumstances, it is recommended that donor plasma be screened fully for all common clinically significant antibodies as is customary for transfusion recipients. The same caution applies when equivalent volumes of FFP are transfused to neonates.

Appendix 18.2: Composition of saline adenine glucose mannitol (Baxter) optimal additive solution

Constituent	Quantity	Estimated toxic level for neonates*
Volume	100 ml	
Sodium chloride	877 mg (150 meq/l)	
Dextrose	818 mg	240 mg/kg/day
Mannitol	525 mg	360 mg/kg/day
Adenine	16.9 mg	15 mg/kg/dose

* Source: Luban *et al.*, 1991.

This optimal additive solution is in common use within the UK.

Other formulations of optimal additive solutions are available, some of which contain substantially greater dextrose concentrations to enable better red cell preservation, and these cannot be assumed to be equally suitable for neonatal use without individual verification.

References

BCSH (1991) Compatibility testing in hospital blood banks. In Roberts B.E. (ed.) *Standard Haematology Practice*, pp. 150–163. Blackwell Scientific Publications, Oxford.

BCSH (1992a) Guidelines for the use of fresh frozen plasma. *Transfusion Medicine* **2**, 57–63.

BCSH (1992b) Guidelines for platelet transfusions. *Transfusion Medicine* **2**, 311–318.

De Palma L. (1992) Review: red cell alloantibody formation in the neonate and infant: considerations for current immunohaematological practice. *Immunohaematology* **8**, 33–37.

Department of Health (1992) *Guidelines for the Blood Transfusion Services in the United Kingdom.* HMSO, London.

Letsky E.A. (1991) Polycythaemia in the newborn infant. In Hann I.M., Gibson B.E.S. & Letsky E.A. (eds) *Fetal and Neonatal Haematology*, pp. 95–121. Baillière Tindall, London.

Luban N.L.C., Strauss R.G. & Hume H.A. (1991) Commentary on the safety of red cells preserved in extended-storage media for neonatal transfusions. *Transfusion* **31**, 229–235.

Manno C.S., Hedbery K.W., Kim H.C. *et al.* (1991) Comparison of the hemostatic effects of fresh whole blood, stored whole blood, and components after open heart surgery in children. *Blood* **77**, 930–936.

Vogelsang G.B. (1990) Transfusion-associated graft-versus-host disease in nonimmunocompromised hosts. *Transfusion* **30**, 101–103.

Further reading

Anon. (1991) Guidelines for auditing paediatric blood transfusion practices. *American Journal of Diseases of Childhood* **45**, 787–796.

Brubaker D.B. (1986) Transfusion associated graft versus host disease. *Human Pathology* **17**, 1085–1088.

Cairo M.S. (1991) The role of granulocyte transfusions as adjuvant therapy in the treatment of neonatal sepsis. *Transfusion Science* **12**, 247–256.

Judd W.J., Luban N.L.C., Ness P.M., Silberstein L.E., Stroup M. & Widmann F.K. (1990) Prenatal and perinatal immunohematology: recommendations for serologic management of the fetus, newborn infant, and obstetric patient. *Transfusion* **30**, 175–183.

Luban N.L.C. (1991) A review: controversies in blood component use in newborns. *Immunohematology* **7**, 1–7.

Strauss R.G. (1991) Transfusion therapy in neonates. *American Journal of Diseases of Childhood* **145**, 904–911.

Strauss R.G., Saucher R.A., Blazina J.F. *et al.* (1990) Commentary on small volume transfusions for neonatal patients. *Transfusion* **30**, 565–570.

Tegtmeier G.E. (1988) The use of cytomegalovirus-screened blood in neonates. *Transfusion* **28**, 201–203.

Wardrop C.A.F., Jones J.G. & Holland B.M. (1991) Detection, correction and ultimate prevention of anemias in the preterm infant. *Transfusion Science* **12**, 121–135.

19 The Use of Fresh-Frozen Plasma*
Prepared by the
Blood Transfusion Task Force

1 Introduction

Studies of the use of fresh-frozen plasma (FFP) have shown that it is often misused (NIH Consensus Conference, 1985; Snyder *et al.*, 1986). This is largely due to the misconceptions regarding its haemostatic effectiveness and inadequate knowledge of the situations in which its use is inappropriate.

In the UK, the number of units of FFP transfused during the past 15 years has increased greater than 10-fold. Although FFP has been used in an increasingly wide range of clinical situations, in many instances there is no rational basis for its administration.

The purpose of these guidelines is to specify the circumstances in which FFP is the treatment of choice and those in which its use cannot be justified.

2 Properties of fresh-frozen plasma

Fresh-frozen plasma is prepared from anticoagulated whole blood by separating and freezing the plasma to a core temperature of −30°C or below, within 6 hours of blood collection. Fresh-frozen plasma can be stored at this temperature for a maximum period of 12 months. The volume of a typical unit is approximately 200 ml (Department of Health, 1989).

Prior to use, FFP must be thawed according to the manufacturer's instructions detailed on the package. It is recommended that a second heat-sealed bag is used for added protection when thawing in a water-bath. An alternative option for the future may include the use of a microwave oven to replace the standard 37°C water-bath. The thawed plasma should be administered with a minimum delay (i.e. not more than 2 hours) to avoid loss of potency of the coagulation factors.

Under these conditions of processing, FFP will have high levels of all coagulation proteins, including the labile factors V and VIII. The guidelines of the

---

* Reprinted with permission from *Transfusion Medicine*, 1992, **2**, 57–63.

Council of Europe specify that the minimum level of factor VIII in FFP is 0.7 IU/ml. A typical unit also includes:

- sodium 170 mmol/l;
- potassium 4.0 mmol/l;
- glucose 22 mmol/l;
- citrate 20 mmol/l;
- lactate 3.0 mmol/l;
- pH 7.2–7.4.

The dosage of FFP depends upon the clinical situation and underlying disorder, but 12–15 ml/kg is a generally accepted starting dose. It is important to monitor the response, both clinically and with measurement of prothrombin time (PT), partial thromboplastin time (PTT) or specific factor assays.

Fresh-frozen plasma units are labelled with the donor ABO and Rh D group. ABO-compatible FFP should be used, but compatibility testing is not required. Group O FFP should only be given to group O recipients. On the other hand, group A or B FFP can be given to group O recipients. Because of its scarcity, group AB FFP should be reserved for group AB recipients and rarely for emergencies when the blood group of a patient is unknown.

The small amount of red cell stroma present in FFP is capable of inducing Rh immunization and can boost anti-D levels in subjects with preformed anti-D. It is therefore advisable to give Rh D-compatible FFP to females of child-bearing age; when this is not possible, anti-D immunoglobulin should be given at a dose of 50 IU per unit of FFP transfused.

2.1 Adverse effects

1 Allergic reactions may occur. Urticaria has been reported in 1–3% of patients. The incidence of life-threatening anaphylactic reactions is unknown but has been reported to be as high as 1:20 000 transfusions (Bjerrum & Jersild, 1971).

2 Infectious complications. The risk of infection with human immunodeficiency virus (HIV), hepatitis B, hepatitis non-A non-B and parvovirus following transfusion of FFP is similar to that following the transfusion of whole blood. However, agents transmitted by cellular components are not transmitted by FFP (e.g. herpes viruses, malaria). There have been no reported cases of cytomegalovirus (CMV) transmission (Bowden & Sayers, 1990) or graft-versus-host disease following transfusion of FFP and therefore irradiation of FFP or the provision of CMV-negative FFP is not required.

3 Haemolysis. If ABO-incompatible plasma is infused, potent anti-A or anti-B, which may be present, can cause lysis of the recipient's red cells. Plasma infusion has also been associated with intravascular haemolysis in neonatal patients with necrotizing enterocolitis and associated T activation.

4 Fluid overload. Treatment of severe factor deficiencies is often limited by the

patient's ability to tolerate the infused volume of plasma without developing fluid overload. Specific factor concentrates are preferred when available.

5 Very rarely, potent antibodies against the patient's granulocytes may be present in donor plasma. They can cause leucocyte aggregation in pulmonary vessels and acute pulmonary injury, a syndrome known as transfusion-related acute lung injury (TRALI) (Nordhagen *et al.*, 1986).

6 Recent reports have suggested that plasma infusion may cause immune suppression (Blumberg & Heal, 1988; Hermanek *et al.*, 1989).

3 Clinical indications for the use of fresh-frozen plasma

There are few well-documented and universally accepted indications for the use of FFP (Braunstein & Oberman, 1984; NIH Consensus Conference, 1985). They are limited to the treatment of bleeding episodes or preparation for surgery in patients with factor deficiencies where specific factor concentrates are unavailable. There are a number of clinical situations in which the use of FFP has been advocated but has not been shown to be of benefit.

4 Definite indications for the use of fresh-frozen plasma

4.1 Replacement of single factor deficiencies

More specific factor concentrates are becoming available for clinical use and FFP is only required when specific or combined factor concentrates are unavailable. The dose will depend upon the specific factor being replaced, as both the half-life

Table 19.1 Coagulation factors in plasma (adapted from AABB, 1989)

Coagulation factor	Plasma concentration required for haemostasis	Half-life of transfused factor	Stability in plasma and whole blood (4°C storage)	Specific concentrate available
I (fibrinogen)	1 g/l	4–6 days	Stable	No*
II (prothrombin)	0.4 IU/ml	2–3 days	Stable	No*
V	0.1–0.15 IU/ml	12 hours	Unstable†	No
VII	0.05–0.1 IU/ml	2–6 hours	Stable	Yes
VIII	0.1–0.4 IU/ml	8–12 hours	Unstable‡	Yes
IX	0.1–0.4 IU/ml	18–24 hours	Stable	Yes
X	0.1–0.15 IU/ml	2 days	Stable	No*
XI	0.3 IU/ml	3 days	Stable	Yes
XII	–	–	Stable	No*
XIII	0.01–0.05 IU/ml	6–10 days	Stable	Yes

* See text for comment.
† Fifty per cent remains at 14 days in blood or plasma stored at 4°C.
‡ Twenty-five per cent remains at 24 hours in blood or plasma stored at 4°C.

and the plasma concentration required for haemostasis vary for individual factors (Table 19.1). For dosage calculations, 1 ml of FFP contains approximately one unit of coagulation factor activity.

Although specific factor II and X concentrates are unavailable, replacement therapy with a concentrate of combined factors II, IX and X (prothrombin complex concentrate (PCC)), not FFP, is recommended in deficiency states. Cryoprecipitate, which contains fibrinogen, fibronectin and factor VIII, should be used as the replacement therapy in patients with a deficiency of fibrinogen (factor I). There is rarely a need for replacement therapy in factor XII deficiency, as its clinical complications, if any, are those of thrombosis (Ratnoff & Saito, 1979).

Deficiency of von Willebrand factor (vWf) should not be corrected with FFP, as alternative therapy is available. This includes 1-desamino-8-D-arginine vasopressin (DDAVP) and some intermediate-purity factor VIII concentrates. Specific vWf concentrates have now been developed, so that cryoprecipitate should rarely be needed in this condition.

4.2 Immediate reversal of warfarin effect
Patients taking oral anticoagulant therapy have a deficiency of functionally active vitamin K-dependent proteins (i.e. the procoagulant factors II, VII, IX and X and anticoagulant factors proteins C and S). This functional deficiency can be reversed by the parenteral administration of vitamin K; 4–6 hours should be allowed for adequate clinical response in the average patient. Recommendations for the reversal of anticoagulant therapy are outlined in Table 19.2. In patients who are grossly overdosed and who have developed serious life-threatening bleeding

Table 19.2 Recommendations for reversal of oral anticoagulant treatment (BCSH, 1990)

Life-threatening haemorrhage
Immediately give 5 mg vitamin K by slow intravenous infusion and a concentrate of factor II, IX and X with factor VII concentrate (if available)
The dose of concentrate should be calculated based on 50 IU factor IX/kg body weight
If no concentrate is available, FFP should be infused (about 1 l for an adult), but this may not be as effective

Less severe haemorrhage such as haematuria and epistaxis
Withhold warfarin for 1 or more days and consider giving vitamin K, 0.5–2.0 mg IV

INR of >4.5 without haemorrhage
Withdraw warfarin for 1 or 2 days; then review

Unexpected bleeding at therapeutic levels
Investigate possibility of underlying cause, such as unsuspected renal or alimentary tract disease

INR, International Normalized Ratio.

episodes, immediate reversal of anticoagulant therapy is required. The recommended approach is to use a concentrate of factors II, IX and X (PCC) with factor VII concentrate (if available). If these are not available, then FFP should be infused. It must be noted, though, that the use of PCC and factor VII concentrate for reversal of anticoagulation or liver disease has not been approved by the Licensing Authority and can therefore only be undertaken by a doctor on his/her own responsibility. Clinical trials which address the safety and efficacy of the use of factor concentrates in these specific clinical situations are currently in progress. If it is necessary to treat patients with minor bleeding episodes, such as epistaxis or extensive skin bruising, FFP infusions of between two and six units will partially correct the anticoagulant effect.

4.3 Vitamin K deficiency

Haemorrhagic disease of the newborn and conditions which may impair vitamin K absorption, such as biliary duct obstruction, are associated with a coagulation abnormality similar to that described with oral anticoagulant therapy. If bleeding results, a similar treatment regimen should be employed.

4.4 Acute disseminated intravascular coagulation

Disseminated intravascular coagulation (DIC), which can be associated with shock, trauma and sepsis, results in variable deficiencies of factors V and VIII, fibrinogen, fibronectin and platelets due to activation of the coagulation and fibrinolytic systems. The spectrum of presentation is wide, ranging from a compensated state, with abnormalities of coagulation demonstrable only in the laboratory, to a fulminant form, with major bleeding and thrombotic complications.

The treatment of all patients must first be directed at the cause of the DIC. There is no evidence that any supportive or replacement therapy is of benefit unless it is possible to correct the underlying condition (Mount & King, 1979).

Replacement therapy is indicated in acute DIC, where there is haemorrhage and abnormality of coagulation. The infusion of FFP, cryoprecipitate and platelet concentrates forms the basis of initial therapy. The response should be closely monitored by repeated laboratory tests and clinical assessment and further replacement judged by both.

In chronic DIC, or in the absence of haemorrhage, there is no indication to give component therapy in an attempt to normalize laboratory results.

4.5 Thrombotic thrombocytopenic purpura

Fresh-frozen plasma is the accepted form of treatment for thrombotic thrombocytopenic purpura (TTP), often in conjunction with plasma exchange (Machin, 1984). At least 3 l/day are generally given.

4.6 Inherited deficiencies of inhibitors of coagulation

Fresh-frozen plasma has been used as a source of antithrombin (AT), protein C and protein S in patients with inherited deficiencies of these inhibitors who are undergoing surgery or who require heparin for treatment of spontaneous thrombosis. Antithrombin preparations are now widely available and have been used in the management of patients with inherited deficiencies. Protein C and protein S preparations are becoming available. Several clinical studies are in progress to determine the efficacy of AT preparations as a prophylactic and therapeutic agent in the management of acquired AT deficiency, especially shock and DIC (Vinazzer, 1987). These specific preparations will obviate the need for FFP.

4.7 C1 esterase inhibitor deficiency

Fresh-frozen plasma infusion can be used to treat patients with C1 esterase inhibitor deficiency who develop severe angio-oedema. However, specific preparations of C1 esterase inhibitor are becoming increasingly available.

5 Conditional uses: fresh-frozen plasma is only indicated in the presence of bleeding and disturbed coagulation

5.1 Massive transfusion

'Massive transfusion' is defined as the replacement of the patient's total blood volume with stored blood in less than 24 hours. The occurrence of clotting disorders in patients who receive large-volume transfusions is more closely associated with the duration of volume deficit than with the volume of blood transfused (Harke & Rahman, 1980). Early adequate resuscitation from shock is therefore the most important factor in preventing the development of coagulopathy in massively transfused patients. 'Dilution' of clotting factors with stored blood is not commonly the cause of haemostatic disturbance. More important causes include the consumption of platelets and clotting factors and the possible development of DIC in patients who are hypotensive or septic or have pre-existing liver disease (BCSH, 1988; Hewitt & Machin, 1990).

There is no evidence to suggest that prophylactic replacement regimens with FFP or platelet concentrates, which have often been advocated, either prevent the onset of abnormal bleeding or reduce transfusion requirements (Mannucci *et al.*, 1982).

To prevent the indiscriminate use of blood components in patients receiving massive transfusion, early laboratory assessment is needed to determine the precise nature of any disorders of coagulation which may be present. These patients may develop microvascular bleeding with oozing from the mucosae, raw wounds and puncture sites as a result of thrombocytopenia (platelet count <50 × 10^9/l) when one-and-a-half to twice their blood volume has been replaced

(Ciavarella *et al.*, 1987). Initial treatment to control bleeding should therefore be with platelet concentrates. Plasma fibrinogen, PT and PTT should be monitored as a guide to additional replacement therapy. If the fibrinogen level is less than 0.8 g/l, then cryoprecipitate is indicated. If either the PT or PTT is prolonged to more than one-and-a-half times the control value but the fibrinogen level is greater than 0.8 g/l, then significant deficiency of factors V and VIII is likely to be present and FFP is recommended. The volume of FFP that will usually promote coagulation in an adult is at least 4 units (Braunstein & Oberman, 1984).

5.2 Liver disease

A variety of abnormalities of coagulation are seen in patients with liver disease. Bleeding, however, seldom occurs as the result of a haemostatic defect alone, but usually has a precipitating cause, such as surgery, including liver biopsy, or the rupture of oesophageal varices. In practice, FFP is indicated either if bleeding has taken place, or may confidently be expected because surgery is proposed (Spector *et al.*, 1966; Mannucci *et al.*, 1976). However, because of the large volumes of FFP required by patients who already have an expanded plasma volume due to ascites and oedema and because of the short biological half-life of some of the factors, complete correlation is virtually never possible. If an FFP infusion of 6 to 8 units fails to control bleeding or provide adequate correction of the PT to allow essential surgery, a trial infusion of PCC may be considered.

Studies in patients with liver disease have shown sufficient correction of coagulation after the infusion of factor VII-rich PCC to permit the performance of liver biopsies without haemorrhagic complications (Green *et al.*, 1975). However, better haemostatic control was achieved with the use of a combination of FFP and PCC than with FFP alone (Mannucci *et al.*, 1976). Nevertheless, PCCs contain variable amounts of activated coagulation factors (IIa, IXa, Xa and VIIa) and their widespread use has not become the accepted practice because of the risk of inducing thromboembolic disease or DIC. In advanced liver disease, in which there is impaired hepatic clearance of activated clotting factors and reduced AT levels, the risk will be greater. Factor concentrates should therefore only be used after carefully balancing these risks against the expected haemostatic advantages.

There is no agreement as to the levels of coagulation factors which are 'safe' for patients with liver disease prior to surgery or intervention. A PT of 1.6–1.8 times the control value is probably realistic. Platelet concentrates may be needed to correct the thrombocytopenia and platelet function defects which are often also present.

5.3 Cardiopulmonary bypass surgery

The majority of patients undergoing cardiopulmonary bypass surgery do not have major coagulation abnormalities (McCarthy *et al.*, 1988). On the other hand, there are changes in the haemostatic mechanism during cardiopulmonary bypass. In most studies, non-surgical bleeding has been attributed to platelet dysfunction rather than to a deficiency of plasma coagulation factors (Woodman & Harker, 1990). Normally the platelet dysfunction reverses within 1 hour after completion of bypass. However, bleeding due to a persistent functional platelet defect may sometimes occur.

In the presence of microvascular bleeding or postoperative bleeding that is not surgically correctable, the initial management should be with platelet concentrates. Fresh-frozen plasma should only be used in those patients in whom bleeding is associated with proved abnormalities of coagulation other than residual heparin effect. Such patients have usually been massively transfused and may have developed consumptive coagulopathy. The routine perioperative use of FFP for cardiopulmonary bypass surgery exposes the patient to unnecessary risk and provides no known benefit (Trimble *et al.*, 1964).

The wider use of pharmacological agents to reduce non-surgical perioperative bleeding is just beginning. From the data available, aprotinin therapy offers the potential for a major reduction in perioperative blood loss and transfusion requirements in cardiac surgery, and probably in other surgery as well (Hunt, 1991). Further studies are needed to understand the mechanism of action of aprotinin in this situation and to determine its most appropriate dose.

5.4 Special paediatric indications
In paediatric patients with severe sepsis, including sepsis in the newborn, therapy with FFP and cryoprecipitate has been advocated. Fresh-frozen plasma is often clinically indicated for the supportive treatment of DIC, which may be a complication in these patients. However, even in the absence of DIC, the use of FFP has been advocated, as it provides not only clotting factors but also a source of complement, fibronectin and protease inhibitors, which may be deficient in these infants. No evidence confirming the efficacy of this use of FFP is yet available. Note, however, that, in neonates with necrotizing enterocolitis and associated erythrocyte T-antigen activation, infusion of plasma may cause intravascular haemolysis.

Paediatric FFP, containing smaller volumes than the standard FFP for adults, is available from most transfusion centres.

6 No justification for the use of fresh-frozen plasma

6.1 Hypovolaemia
There is no place for FFP in the management of hypovolaemia. Crystalloids, synthetic colloids or 4.5% human albumin solution are safer, cheaper and more readily available.

6.2 Plasma exchange procedures

Intensive plasma exchange using coagulation factor-free replacement fluids results in progressive reduction in plasma coagulation factors and platelets. Despite marked abnormalities of coagulation, haemorrhagic episodes are rare and, when present, are usually due to thrombocytopenia (Keller *et al.*, 1979). Fresh-frozen plasma therapy should only be used to correct the coagulation abnormality when abnormal bleeding occurs. Immunoglobulins, complement (Keller & Urbaniak, 1978) and fibronectin (Norfolk *et al.*, 1985) are also depleted by intensive plasma exchange. As there is no evidence that this leads to infections or immune deficiencies, however, replacement with FFP is not indicated.

6.3 'Formula' replacement

There is no indication for the use of FFP according to predetermined replacement schedules (e.g. 1 unit of FFP following each 4–6 units of blood). Such a policy cannot be justified, as it exposes the patient to unnecessary risk and is of no proved benefit.

6.4 Nutritional support and protein-losing states

There is no justification for the administration of FFP for nutritional purposes, for chronic cases of cirrhosis with ascites and nephrosis, for cases of protein-losing enteropathy or for chronic thoracic duct drainage.

6.5 Treatment of immunodeficiency states

In the past, FFP has been used as a source of immunoglobulins in the treatment of inherited immunodeficiency states. Purified intravenous immunoglobulin is now available and has replaced the need for FFP in these patients.

7 Control of issue and transfusion

As with blood and other blood components, transfusion of FFP should be fully documented in the patient's notes. This documentation requires a signed medical order for the precribed units of FFP. The persons administering each unit must sign the plasma issue slip and fluid chart to confirm that they have identified that the unit and patient are matched. An entry should also be made on the patient's notes stating clearly the reasons for prescribing FFP.

8 Conclusions

Education programmes which outline the benefits and complications of blood component therapy have achieved a reduction in both the amount of FFP transfused and the number of patients transfused for inappropriate reasons (Barnette *et al.*, 1990). Hospital transfusion committees should examine the current use of FFP and other blood components and a programme of education should be implemented to promote the appropriate use of blood and blood components.

References

AABB (1989) *Blood Transfusion Therapy: a Physician's Handbook*, 3rd edn. American Association of Blood Banks, Arlington, VA.

Barnette R.E., Fish D.J. & Eisenstaedt R.S. (1990) Modification of fresh-frozen plasma transfusion practices through educational intervention. *Transfusion* 30, 253–257.

BCSH (1988) BCSH guidelines for transfusion for massive blood loss. *Clinical and Laboratory Haematology* 10, 265–273.

BCSH (1990) BCSH guidelines on oral anticoagulation: second edition. *Journal of Clinical Pathology* 43, 177–183.

Bjerrum O.S. & Jersild C. (1971) Class specific anti-IgA associated with severe anaphylactic transfusion reactions in a patient with pernicious anaemia. *Vox Sanguinis* 21, 411–424.

Blumberg N. & Heal J.M. (1988) Evidence for plasma-mediated immunomodulation – transfusions of plasma-rich blood components are associated with a greater risk of acquired immunodeficiency. *Transplantation Proceedings* 206, 1138–1142.

Bowden R. & Sayers M. (1990) The risk of transmitting cytomegalovirus by FFP. *Transfusion* 8, 762–763.

Braunstein A.H. & Oberman H.A. (1984) Transfusion of plasma components. *Transfusion* 24, 281–286.

Ciavarella D., Reed R.L., Counts R.B., Baron L., Pavlin E., Heimbach D.M. & Carrico C.J. (1987) Clotting factor levels and the risk of diffuse microvascular bleeding in the massively transfused patient. *British Journal of Haematology* 67, 365–368.

Department of Health (1989) Fresh frozen plasma. In *Guidelines for the Blood Transfusion Services in the United Kingdom*, Vol. 1, Section 8.19, p. 50. HMSO, London.

Green G., Dymock I.W., Poller L. & Thomson J.M. (1975) Use of factor VII-rich prothrombin complex concentrate in liver disease. *Lancet* i, 1311–1314.

Harke H. & Rahman S. (1980) Haemostatic disorders in massive transfusion. *Biblioteca Haematologica* 46, 179–188.

Hermanek P., Guggenmoos-Holzmann I., Schricker K.T., Resch T., Freudenberger K., Neidhardt P. & Gall F.P. (1989) Der Einfluss der Transfusion von Blut und Haemoderivaten auf die Prognose des colorectalen Carcinoms. *Langenbecks Archiv für Chirurgie* 374, 118–124.

Hewitt P.E. & Machin S.J. (1990) Massive blood transfusion. *British Medical Journal* 300, 107–109.

Hunt B.J. (1991) Modifying perioperative blood loss. *Blood Reviews* 5, 168–176.

Keller A.J. & Urbaniak S.J. (1978) Intensive plasma exchange on the cell separator: effects on serum immunoglobulins and complement components. *British Journal of Haematology* 38, 531–540.

Keller A.J., Churnside A. & Urbaniak S.J. (1979) Coagulation abnormalities produced by plasma exchange on the cell separator with special reference to fibrinogen and platelet levels. *British Journal of Haematology* 42, 593–603.

McCarthy P.M., Popovsky M.A., Schaff H.V., Orszulak T.A., Williamson K.R., Taswell H.F. & Ilstrup D.M. (1988) Effect of blood conservation efforts in cardiac operations at the Mayo Clinic. *Mayo Clinic Proceedings* 63, 225–229.

Machin S.J. (1984) Thrombotic thrombocytopenic purpura. *British Journal of Haematology* 56, 191–197.

Mannucci P.M., Franchi F. & Dioguardi N. (1976) Correction of abnormal coagulation in chronic liver disease by combined use of fresh frozen plasma and prothrombin complex concentrates. *Lancet* 2, 542–545.

Mannucci P.M., Federici A.B. & Sirchia G. (1982) Haemostasis testing during massive blood replacement: a study of 172 cases. *Vox Sanguinis* **42**, 113–123.

Mount M.J. & King E.G. (1979) Severe, acute disseminated intravascular coagulation: a reappraisal of its pathophysiology, clinical significance and therapy based on 47 patients. *American Journal of Medicine* **67**, 557–563.

NIH Consensus Conference (1985) Fresh frozen plasma: indications and risks. *Journal of the American Medical Association* **253**, 551–553.

Nordhagen R., Conradi M. & Dromtorp S.M. (1986) Pulmonary reaction associated with transfusion of plasma containing anti-5b. *Vox Sanguinis* **51**, 102–108.

Norfolk D.R., Bowen M., Cooper E.H. & Robinson E.A.E. (1985) Changes in plasma fibronectin during donor apheresis and therapeutic plasma exchange. *British Journal of Haematology* **61**, 641–647.

Ratnoff N. & Saito M. (1979) Surface-mediated reactions. In Piomelli S. & Yachnin S. (eds) *Current Topics in Haematology*, Vol. 2, pp. 1–57. A.R. Liss, New York.

Snyder A.J., Gottschall J.L. & Menitove J.E. (1986) Why is fresh-frozen plasma transfused? *Transfusion* **26**, 107–112.

Spector I., Corn M. & Ticktin H.E. (1966) Effect of plasma transfusion on the prothrombin time and clotting factors in liver disease. *New England Journal of Medicine* **275**, 1032–1037.

Trimble A.G., Osborn J.J., Kerthwood G. & Gerbode F. (1964) The prophylactic use of fresh frozen plasma after extracorporeal circulation. *Journal of Thoracic and Cardiovascular Surgery* **48**, 314–316.

Vinazzer H. (1987) Clinical use of antithrombin III concentrates. *Vox Sanguinis* **53**, 193–198.

Woodman R.C. & Harker L.A. (1990) Bleeding complications associated with cardiopulmonary bypass. *Blood* **76**, 1680–1697.

20 Platelet Transfusions*

Prepared by the
Blood Transfusion Task Force

1 Introduction

The use of platelet transfusions has risen considerably in recent years, mainly as a consequence of the increasingly intensive treatment of patients with haematological malignancies.

The purpose of this chapter is to give guidance about platelet transfusion therapy, including the appropriate indications for platelet transfusions, the handling and administration of platelet concentrates, the assessment of reponses to platelet transfusions and the management of refractory patients and reactions after platelet transfusions. It also gives recommendations for the transfusion support of patients likely to require repeated transfusions.

Guidelines for the selection of donors and preparation of platelet concentrates are described in the *Guidelines for the Blood Transfusion Service* (UKBTS/NIBSC Liaison Group, 1993) and will not be addressed in detail in this chapter.

2 Indications for platelet transfusions

Platelet transfusions are indicated for the prevention and treatment of haemorrhage in patients with thrombocytopenia or platelet function defects. Clinically, this may involve one or more transfusions for the treatment of a single incident or repeated transfusions over a period of time.

In general, the cause of the thrombocytopenia should be established before a decision about the use of platelet transfusions is made because the role of platelet transfusions depends on the underlying disorder.

2.1 Bone marrow failure
2.1.1 Platelet transfusions for patients who are bleeding
Platelet transfusions are established as effective treatment for patients with

* Reprinted with permission from *Transfusion Medicine*, 1992, **2**, 311–318.

thrombocytopenic bleeding associated with bone marrow failure caused by disease, cytotoxic therapy or irradiation. Serious spontaneous haemorrhage due to thrombocytopenia alone is unlikely to occur at platelet counts above $10–20 \times 10^9/l$ (Slichter, 1980). Minor bleeding, such as purpura and epistaxis, may occur at platelet counts below $50 \times 10^9/l$.

2.1.2 Prophylactic platelet transfusions

Prophylactic platelet transfusions have been shown to decrease morbidity, although not mortality, in patients with thrombocytopenia due to bone marrow failure (Roy *et al.*, 1973; Higby *et al.*, 1974).

The use of platelet transfusions to keep the platelet count above $10 \times 10^9/l$ reduces the risk of haemorrhage as effectively as keeping it above any higher level (Slichter, 1980; Consensus Conference, 1987). A recent study showed that a further reduction in the threshold for prophylactic platelet transfusions may be possible (Gmur *et al.*, 1991). However, if factors associated with bleeding in thrombocytopenic patients are present, such as fever and infection, concurrent coagulopathy or a rapid fall in platelet count, or if there are potential bleeding sites as a result of surgery, the use of prophylactic platelet transfusions might be considered to keep the platelet count above $20 \times 10^9/l$. An optimal policy for prophylactic platelet transfusions has not been defined (Schiffer, 1992) and the threshold platelet count should be based on an audit of local clinical practice.

Long-term prophylactic platelet transfusions are not usually indicated for patients with chronic failure of platelet production due to aplastic anaemia or myelodysplasia, although some patients may need regular prophylactic transfusions to prevent recurrent haemorrhage, particularly during unstable periods associated with infection.

2.2 Platelet function disorders

Patients with platelet function disorders rarely need platelet transfusions to prevent haemorrhage unless they are undergoing surgical procedures. An attempt should be made to correct a prolonged bleeding time prior to surgery. This may be achieved by:

1 withdrawal of any drug which may have anti-platelet activity;
2 correcting the underlying condition, if possible;
3 correcting the haematocrit to greater than 0.30 in patients with uraemia, by either the use of erythropoietin or the transfusion of red cell concentrates;
4 considering the use of 1-deamino-8-D-arginine vasopressin (DDAVP) or cryoprecipitate in patients with uraemia, if correction of the haematocrit is ineffective;
5 platelet transfusions where the above measures are not appropriate or are ineffective.

2.3 Massive blood transfusion

Clinically significant dilutional thrombocytopenia only occurs with transfusion of more than 1.5 times the blood volume of the recipient. The platelet count should be maintained above $50 \times 10^9/l$ in patients receiving massive transfusions (BCSH, 1988).

2.4 Cardiopulmonary bypass surgery

Platelet function defects and some degree of thrombocytopenia frequently occur after cardiac bypass surgery (Slichter, 1980). Platelet transfusions should be reserved for patients with bleeding not due to surgically correctable causes.

Prophylactic platelet transfusions are not required for patients undergoing bypass procedures.

2.5 Disseminated intravascular coagulation

In acute disseminated intravascular coagulation (DIC), where there is bleeding associated with thrombocytopenia, platelet transfusions should be given in addition to coagulation factor replacement (BCSH, 1992).

In chronic DIC, or in the absence of bleeding, platelet transfusions have no clinical benefit and should not be given merely to correct abnormal laboratory results.

2.6 Thrombotic thrombocytopenic purpura

Platelet transfusions should not be given to patients with thrombotic thrombocytopenic purpura (TTP). There are reports of rapid deterioration and death associated with platelet transfusions in patients with TTP (Harkness *et al.*, 1981).

2.7 Immune thrombocytopenias
2.7.1 Autoimmune thrombocytopenia

Platelet transfusions should be reserved for patients with major haemorrhage. A large number of platelet concentrates may be required to achieve haemostasis due to the effect of platelet autoantibodies on the survival of the transfused platelets.

2.7.2 Post-transfusion purpura

Platelet transfusions are ineffective in patients with post-transfusion purpura (PTP), even if they are prepared from donors who are negative for the appropriate human platelet alloantigen (HPA) (Mueller-Eckhardt, 1986). The optimal treatment is currently considered to be a combination of steroids and high-dose intravenous immunoglobulin (Mueller-Eckhardt, 1986; Waters, 1989).

2.7.3 Neonatal alloimmune thrombocytopenia

Platelet concentrates prepared from donors known to be negative for the appropriate HPA should be used to treat neonates with severe thrombocytopenia. If donors with the appropriate HPA type are not available or if the specificity of the antibody responsible for neonatal alloimmune thrombocytopenia (NAIT) is unknown, the mother should be used as the donor.

Platelet concentrates for intrauterine fetal transfusions should be prepared in as small a volume as possible and should be γ-irradiated to prevent transfusion-associated graft-versus-host disease (GVHD) (Waters *et al.*, 1991). In addition to standard donor testing, donors other than the mother should be seronegative for cytomegalovirus (CMV).

2.8 Prophylaxis for surgery

Bone marrow aspiration and biopsy may be performed even in patients with severe thrombocytopenia without platelet supportive therapy, provided that adequate surface pressure is applied.

For lumbar puncture, epidural anaesthesia, insertion of indwelling lines, transbronchial biopsy, liver biopsy, laparotomy or similar procedures, the platelet count should be raised to at least $50 \times 10^9/l$.

For operations in critical sites, such as the brain or eyes, the platelet count should be raised to $100 \times 10^9/l$.

3 Blood bank documentation and procedures

The documentation of platelet transfusions should comply with the BCSH guidelines for hospital blood bank documentation and procedures (BCSH, 1990).

3.1 Generation of the request

The request for a platelet transfusion should come from the clinician to the consultant haematologist in charge of the hospital blood bank. If there is agreement that a platelet transfusion is indicated, the haematologist or his/her nominee will arrange for platelet concentrate(s) to be provided.

3.2 Labelling and documentation

Labels should be attached to each platelet concentrate, as for red cell concentrates, as follows:

3.2.1 Product label

The product label (UKBTS/NIBSC Liaison Group, 1993) should include the following:
- platelets and the nominal volume;
- the producer's name;
- the donation number;

- the ABO group;
- the Rh D group stated as positive or negative;
- the composition and volume of any additive solution;
- the date of collection and expiry date;
- the temperature of storage and a comment that continuous gentle agitation throughout storage is recommended;
- a statement that the component must be administered through a suitable transfusion set, incorporating a 170 μm filter;
- a statement that the component may transmit infection.

Notes

1 If pooled, the donation number of all contributing platelet components, or a unique batch or pool number, must appear on the component label.

2 The expiry time must be included on the label for platelet concentrates which have been pooled and/or filtered or prepared by apheresis.

3.2.2 Patient identification label

The patient identification label should include the following (BCSH, 1990):

- surname;
- forename(s);
- date of birth;
- hospital number;
- ABO group;
- Rh D group;
- unique donor number of the pack;
- date blood required.

3.3 Storage and shelf-life

Platelet concentrates should be kept at $22 \pm 2°C$ during the period of storage to ensure maximum viability. The storage period depends on the nature of the container and on whether an open or closed system is used for the preparation of the concentrates. Plastics in current use allow for storage for up to 5 days in a closed system (UKBTS/NIBSC Liaison Group, 1993).

Care should be taken to ensure that platelet concentrates are not refrigerated during transport. Containers for transport should be equilibrated at room temperature before use. During transportation, the temperature of platelets must be kept as close as possible to the recommended storage temperature and, on receipt, unless intended for immediate therapeutic use, they should be transferred to storage at $22 \pm 2°C$ (UKBTS/NIBSC Liaison Group, 1993).

It is recommended that platelet concentrates are agitated continuously during the storage period (UKBTS/NIBSC Liaison Group, 1993).

3.4 Gamma-irradiation

Patients at significant risk from transfusion-associated GVHD include bone marrow transplant recipients, fetuses receiving intrauterine transfusions, patients with congenital immunodeficiency syndromes, patients with Hodgkin's disease and patients receiving transfusions from first-degree relatives (Anderson *et al.*, 1991). Platelet concentrates for these patients should be γ-irradiated with a minimum of 25 Gy (UKBTS/NIBSC Liaison Group, 1993).

3.5 Calculation of dose of platelets

The dose of platelets may be calculated, using the formula shown below, from the desired platelet increment $\times 10^9/l$ (*PI*), calculated from the pre- and post-transfusion platelet counts, the patient's blood volume (*BV*) in litres (estimated by multiplying the body surface area in square metres by 2.5), and a correction or recovery factor (*F*) of 0.67 to allow for pooling of approximately 33% of platelets in a normal spleen.

$$\text{Dose} = PI \times BV \times F^{-1}$$

For example, if a platelet increment of $40 \times 10^9/l$ is required for a patient with a blood volume of 5 l, a dose of 300×10^9 platelets will be required. This is approximately equivalent to 6 units of platelet concentrates prepared from units of whole blood, each platelet concentrate containing 55×10^9 platelets.

The average number of platelets in platelet concentrates prepared from whole-blood donations or by platelet apheresis should be provided by the producer as part of quality control.

3.6 ABO compatibility

Platelet concentrates from donors of the same ABO group as the patient should be used as far as possible (Anon., 1990). The survival of ABO-incompatible platelets may be impaired and acute haemolytic events have occasionally occurred in group A and B patients due to transfusion of high-titre anti-A or anti-B in the plasma of the platelet concentrate. This is most likely to occur with platelet concentrates prepared by apheresis from group O donors.

If group O donors are used for group A, B or AB patients, it is important to ensure that the donors do not have high-titre anti-A or anti-B. It is the responsibility of the producer to establish this and to label any high-titre concentrates detected.

3.7 Rh D incompatibility

Rh D incompatibility has no effect on platelet survival, but the extent of red cell contamination in platelet concentrates may be sufficient to immunize Rh D negative patients receiving Rh D positive platelet concentrates.

Rh D negative platelet concentrates should be given to Rh D negative patients, particularly to females who have not reached the menopause.

If Rh D positive platelets are given to Rh D negative females who have not reached the menopause, 250 international units (IU) anti-D immunoglobulin should be given to prevent primary immunization with each dose of platelets, typically five or six platelet concentrates. If the dose exceeds 10 platelet concentrates, 500 IU anti-D should be given. To prevent immunization after transfusion of each platelet concentrate prepared by apheresis, using modern technology, such as the Haemonetics PCS Plus and Cobe Spectra cell separators, 250 IU anti-D is sufficient. If the platelet concentrate has been prepared using other apheresis techniques, where red cell contamination of the concentrate may be higher, advice should be obtained from the appropriate Regional Transfusion Centre about the dose of anti-D.

Anti-D immunoglobulin for intramuscular use should be given subcutaneously in thrombocytopenic patients.

4 Administration of platelet concentrates

Before being issued from the hospital blood bank, platelet concentrates may be pooled into a single bag and/or filtered to remove leucocytes. If pooling and/or filtering is by an open system, platelet concentrates should be transfused as soon as possible and no longer than 6 hours after the procedure (UKBTS/NIBSC Liaison Group, 1993). When a sterile connecting device is used, the system can be regarded as closed (UKBTS/NIBSC Liaison Group, 1993).

Platelet concentrates should be transfused as soon as possible after reaching the ward. Standard blood transfusion sets, with 170 μm filters, or special platelet transfusion sets may be used; the only advantage of a platelet transfusion set is a decrease in the loss of platelets if the residual concentrate in the giving set is not rinsed through at the end of the transfusion. Platelets should not be transfused through transfusion sets which have already been used for blood.

The time over which platelets are transfused is not critical but the transfusion should normally be completed within 30 minutes. Observations during a platelet transfusion should include pulse and temperature before the transfusion, after 30 minutes, at 1 hour and later, if indicated.

5 Response to platelet transfusions

5.1 Expected response to therapeutic and prophylactic transfusions

It is important to monitor the response to platelet transfusions, as this will serve as a guide to further platelet supportive care.

If the patient is bleeding, the clinical response is an important indication of the effectiveness of the transfusion. The response to a prophylactic platelet transfusion is assessed by measuring the increase in platelet count following the transfusion. Various formulae have been used to correct for the variation in response depending on the patient's size and the number of platelets transfused (Daly, 1980; Waters *et al.*, 1981). Two such formulae are listed below:

1 *Platelet recovery.* The percentage platelet recovery (*R*) is calculated from the platelet increment $\times 10^9/l$ (*PI*), the blood volume (*BV*) in litres and the platelet dose (*PD*) transfused ($\times 10^9$):

$$R(\%) = PI \times BV \times PD^{-1} \times 100$$

2 *Corrected platelet increment.* The corrected increment $\times 10^9/l$ (*CI*) is calculated from the platelet increment (*PI*), the body surface area in square metres (*BSA*) of the patient and the number of platelet concentrates (*n*) prepared from whole blood:

$$CI = PI \times BSA \times n^{-1}$$

Although a successful tranfusion may produce a platelet recovery of 67% in a stable patient, the minimum standard for a successful transfusion may be considered as a platelet recovery of greater than 30% at 1 hour post-transfusion and greater than 20% after 20 hours, or a corrected increment of greater than 7.5 $\times$ $10^9/l$ at 1 hour post-transfusion and greater than 4.5 $\times$ $10^9/l$ after 20 hours. In practice, however, an increase in the patient's platelet count of less than 20 $\times$ $10^9/l$ at 20–24 hours after the transfusion is often used as a measure of a poor response.

Poor responses to platelet transfusions may be due to immune or non-immune causes. The main immune cause is the presence of human leucocyte antigen (HLA) alloimmunization. The non-immune causes include infection, including its treatment with antibiotics and amphotericin, DIC and splenomegaly (Bishop *et al.*, 1988).

6 Refractoriness to platelet transfusions

Refractoriness is the repeated failure to obtain satisfactory responses to platelet transfusions. It is not usually a problem in patients requiring a small number of transfusions associated with an isolated clinical episode. However, it may occur in approximately 50% of patients receiving repeated platelet transfusions (Murphy & Waters, 1990).

There are two approaches to the problem of 'immune' refractoriness: (i) to reduce HLA alloimmunization to minimize refractoriness by using leucocyte depletion of blood components; or (ii) to take no preventive measures and manage refractoriness if it occurs.

Both approaches have advantages and disadvantages (Murphy & Waters, 1991; Schiffer, 1991); further studies are required to determine which is the best approach. The debate mainly concerns the possible clinical benefits of prevention of refractoriness balanced against the cost of leucocyte-depletion. Some of this cost may be offset against savings made from: (i) a decrease in the number of platelet transfusions required to support patients with bone marrow failure through periods of thrombocytopenia; (ii) a reduced requirement for HLA-matched donors; and (iii) the replacement of CMV screening of blood components by leucocyte-depletion, although further studies are required to confirm that leucocyte-depletion is an effective alternative.

6.1 Consideration of methods to prevent alloimmunization

Primary HLA alloimmunization associated with transfusion therapy is dependent on the presence of cells such as lymphocytes and antigen-presenting cells which express HLA class II antigens.

Leucocyte-depletion of blood components (usually by filtration of both red cell and platelet concentrates) is effective in reducing the incidence of HLA allo-immunization and platelet refractoriness. Transfusions with fewer than 5×10^6 leucocytes have been found to induce primary HLA alloimmunization in only a small number of patients (Murphy & Waters, 1991). The prevention of alloim-munization by irradiation of platelet concentrates with ultraviolet light is still in the experimental stage.

6.2 Investigation of refractoriness

If refractoriness to random-donor platelet transfusions occurs, a clinical assessment should first be made for factors likely to be associated with non-immune platelet consumption, such as splenomegaly, DIC or septicaemia. If there is no obvious cause for non-immune platelet consumption, an immune mechanism should be suspected and the patient's serum should be tested for HLA antibodies. It may be helpful to test patients receiving repeated platelet transfusions at regular intervals.

It is often not possible to determine the specificity of HLA antibodies in multitransfused patients. However, if the specificity can be identified, this will assist in the selection of compatible donors when fully matched donors are unavailable.

If HLA antibodies are not detected in a patient where an immune mechanism seems to be the most likely cause of refractoriness, the patient's serum should be tested for HPA antibodies.

6.3 Management of refractoriness
6.3.1 Use of HLA-matched donors
Patients who are likely to receive repeated platelet transfusions should be typed

for HLA-A and B antigens at the beginning of platelet supportive care. HLA-matched platelet donors are matched for the HLA-A and B antigens of the recipients.

Platelet transfusions from HLA-matched donors should be used for patients who are refractory to platelet transfusions from random donors and who have HLA antibodies. HLA-matched platelet transfusions are not indicated for refractory patients where HLA antibodies have not been detected.

6.3.2 HLA-typed donor panels

These should be available in each region. The size of the panels varies; most contain more than 2500 donors. The polymorphic nature of the HLA system makes it difficult to provide sufficient numbers of compatible donors for patients with unusual HLA types, whatever the size of the HLA-typed donor panel.

6.3.3 Poor responses to HLA-matched platelet transfusions

Poor responses to HLA-matched platelet transfusions occur in about 30% of alloimmunized refractory patients. The reason for poor responses should be sought and platelet cross-matching (Murphy & Waters, 1990; von dem Borne *et al.*, 1990) may be helpful to determine the cause and identify compatible donors for future transfusions.

The differentiation of HLA and HPA antibodies as the cause of a positive platelet cross-match may be difficult but may be achieved using the chloroquine modification of the platelet immunofluorescence test or a solid-phase technique using monoclonal antibody immobilization of platelet antigens.

It is important to continue to bear in mind that non-immune consumption of platelets may be responsible for the refractoriness (Murphy & Waters, 1990; von dem Borne *et al.*, 1990).

It is frequently impossible to identify compatible donors for some patients who are refractory to platelet transfusions because of alloimmunization, despite using the methods described above. The management of such patients during periods of severe thrombocytopenia is often very difficult. Attempts to provide prophylactic platelet support should be discontinued. If bleeding occurs, platelet transfusions from random donors, although incompatible, may reduce the severity of haemorrhage; larger doses of platelets may be required.

7 Reactions after platelet transfusions

A number of reactions may follow platelet transfusions. They are the same as those which can occur after the transfusion of red cell concentrates.

7.1 Febrile reactions

These are a frequent adverse effect after platelet transfusions. They are often due to the presence of leucocyte antibodies against donor leucocytes but may be an indication of other complications, such as bacterial contamination of the donor unit or haemolysis due to incompatible high-titre anti-A or anti-B in the donor plasma. Fever may also be unrelated to the transfusion and due to coincidental infection in the patient.

The following course of action is suggested for the management of patients with febrile reactions.

1 If a febrile reaction (rise in temperature of >1°C) occurs, the transfusion may be completed unless the patient is distressed.

2 Paracetamol rather than aspirin should be used to reduce the fever in patients with thrombocytopenia. In patients with severe symptoms, the transfusion should be stopped, 100 mg hydrocortisone intravenously (IV) given and the cause investigated.

3 If there are repeated febrile reactions, the use of leucocyte-depleted platelet concentrates should be considered if they are not being used already. Detailed serological investigations, including tests for HLA, granulocyte-specific and platelet-specific antibodies, should be carried out if there are reactions after the transfusion of leucocyte-depleted platelet concentrates.

Note that the cause of the febrile reactions may be HLA alloimmunization and, if so, platelet refractoriness may also develop in the same patient.

Premedication with hydrocortisone and/or antihistamines should not be given routinely before platelet transfusions in an attempt to suppress reactions; if reactions occur they should be managed as above.

7.2 Urticarial reactions

These are often attributed to plasma protein incompatibility, although in most cases the cause is not found. Urticarial reactions are often mild and usually respond to interrupting the transfusion and giving intravenous antihistamines, such as 10 mg chlorpheniramine; it is often possible to complete the transfusion after an interval of about 1 hour.

Antihistamines may be useful as prophylaxis in patients with recurrent urticarial reactions.

7.3 Anaphylactic reactions

These may be severe but occur rarely. They should be treated by stopping the transfusion and giving 0.5–1.0 mg adrenaline subcutaneously (SC) and 100–200 mg hydrocortisone IV.

The possibility of immunoglobulin A (IgA) deficiency should be considered in patients with severe reactions, and it may be necessary to remove the donor plasma by washing or to use platelet concentrates prepared from IgA-deficient donors to prevent further severe reactions.

8 Recommendations for patients requiring repeated platelet transfusions

The following procedure should be followed for the optimal transfusion support of patients likely to receive repeated platelet transfusions:

1 determine policy for prophylactic platelet support, and select the platelet count below which platelet transfusions will be used;

2 consider using leucocyte-depletion of red cell and platelet concentrates to prevent HLA alloimmunization from the outset;

3 type patients for HLA-A and B antigens at an early stage;

4 use random donor platelet concentrates for initial platelet support (either single or multiple donor, depending on availability);

5 if refractoriness occurs, determine whether clinical factors, which may be associated with non-immune consumption of platelets, are present and test the patient's serum for HLA antibodies;

6 use HLA-matched platelet transfusions if HLA alloimmunization is the most likely cause of refractoriness;

7 if there is no improvement with HLA-matched transfusions, platelet cross-matching may identify the cause of the problem and help with the selection of compatible donors;

8 discontinue prophylactic platelet support if a compatible donor cannot be found. Use platelet transfusions from random donors to control bleeding and increase the dose, if necessary.

9 Implementation of the guidelines

It is the responsibility of the consultant haematologist in charge of blood transfusion to implement these guidelines in their hospital(s). This might be most easily accomplished through discussion with clinicians who use large numbers of platelet transfusions.

10 Audit

These guidelines are presented as a standard against which platelet transfusion practice in hospitals could be audited. The audit measures might include the indications for and the effectiveness of platelet transfusions, and the incidence of platelet refractoriness. Adequate documentation of the transfusion should be included in the audit.

References

Anderson K.C., Goodnough L.T., Sayers M., Pisciotto P.T., Kurtz S.R., Lane T.A., Anderson C.S. & Silberstein L.E. (1991) Variation in blood component irradiation practice: implications for prevention of transfusion-associated graft-versus-host disease. *Blood* **77**, 2096–2102.

Anon. (1990) ABO incompatibility and platelet transfusion. *Lancet* **335**, 142–143.

BCSH (1988) Guidelines for transfusion for massive blood loss. *Clinical and Laboratory Haematology* **10**, 265–273.

BCSH (1990) Guidelines for hospital blood bank documentation and procedures. *Clinical and Laboratory Haematology* **12**, 209–220.

BCSH (1992) Guidelines for the use of fresh frozen plasma. *Transfusion Medicine* **2**, 57–63.

Bishop J.F., McGrath K., Wolf M.M., Matthews J.P., De Luise T., Holdsworth R., Yuen K., Veale M., Whiteside M.G., Cooper A. & Szer J. (1988) Clinical factors influencing the efficacy of pooled platelet transfusions. *Blood* **71**, 383–387.

Consensus Conference (1987) Platelet transfusion therapy. *Journal of the American Medical Association* **257**, 1777–1780.

Daly P.A. (1980) Platelet transfusion – clinical applications in the oncology setting. *American Journal of Medical Sciences* **280**, 130–142.

Gmur J., Burger J., Schanz U., Fehr J. & Schaffner A. (1991) Safety of stringent prophylactic platelet transfusion policy for patients with acute leukaemia. *Lancet* **338**, 1223–1226.

Harkness D.R., Byrnes J.J., Lian E.C.Y., Williams W.D. & Hensley G.T. (1981) Hazard of platelet transfusion in thrombotic thrombocytopenic purpura. *Journal of the American Medical Association* **246**, 1931–1933.

Higby D.J., Cohen E., Holland J.F. & Sinks L. (1974) The prophylactic treatment of thrombocytopenic leukaemic patients with platelets: a double blind study. *Transfusion* **14**, 440–446.

Mueller-Eckhardt C. (1986) Post-transfusion purpura. *British Journal of Haematology* **64**, 419–424.

Murphy M.F. & Waters A.H. (1990) Platelet transfusions: the problem of refractoriness. *Blood Reviews* **4**, 16–24.

Murphy M.F. & Waters A.H. (1991) Leukocyte depletion of red cell and platelet concentrates. In Harris J.R. (ed.) *Blood Separation and Plasma Fractionation*, pp. 155–182. Wiley-Liss, New York.

Roy A.J., Jaffe N. & Djerassi I. (1973) Prophylactic platelet transfusions in children with acute leukaemia. *Transfusion* **13**, 283–290.

Schiffer C.A. (1991) Prevention of alloimmunization against platelets. *Blood* **77**, 1–4.

Schiffer C.A. (1992) Prophylactic platelet transfusion. *Transfusion* **32**, 295–298.

Slichter S.J. (1980) Controversies in platelet transfusion therapy. *Annual Reviews of Medicine* **31**, 509–540.

UKBTS/NIBSC Liaison Group (1993) *Guidelines for the Blood Transfusion Service*, 2nd edn. HMSO, London.

von dem Borne A.E.G.Kr., Ouwehand W.H. & Kuijpers R.W.A.M. (1990) Theoretical and practical aspects of platelet crossmatching. *Transfusion Medicine Review* **4**, 265–278.

Waters A.H. (1989) Post-transfusion purpura. *Blood Reviews* **3**, 83–87.

Waters A.H., Minchinton R.M., Bell R., Ford J.M. & Lister T.A. (1981) A crossmatching procedure for the selection of donors for alloimmunized patients. *British Journal of Haematology* **48**, 59–68.

Waters A., Murphy M., Hambley H. & Nicolaides K. (1991) Management of alloimmune thrombocytopenia in the fetus and neonate. In Nance S.J. (ed.) *Clinical and Basic Science Aspects of Immunohaematology*, pp. 155–177. American Association of Blood Banks, Arlington, VA.

21 Autologous Transfusion*

Prepared by the
Autologous Transfusion Working Party of the
National Blood Transfusion Service for the
Blood Transfusion Task Force

1 Introduction

Guidelines for preoperative autologous donation (autologous predeposit) were
published by the British Committee for Standards in Haematology Blood Transfusion Task Force in 1988 (BCSH, 1988). Since then, experience with autologous
transfusion has grown and this has encouraged a revision of the guidelines. The
term 'autologous transfusion' has tended in the past to be linked particularly with
autologous predeposit but is now generally used in a wider context to include
predeposit, acute normovolaemic haemodilution (ANH) and red cell salvage.
These procedures complement each other, and this revised guideline for autologous transfusion will deal with predeposit.

While these guidelines seek to deal with situations likely to be met in current
clinical practice, it is recognized that exceptional circumstances may arise and that
the final decision regarding the use of autologous predeposit rests with the doctor
who undertakes the procedure.

2 General considerations

Preoperative autologous donation can provide an alternative to blood from
volunteer donors for transfusion to some patients during elective surgical procedures, avoiding the possibilities of alloimmunization and immunosuppression
and of acquiring transfusion-transmitted infection.

These guidelines relate to blood which is stored at 4°C in CPD-A1 for
up to 35 days or in an optimal additive solution for up to 42 days. Predeposit of blood to be stored frozen for longer periods is not considered in
detail.

Autologous predeposit will only be appropriate for a minority of patients
requiring transfusion. Apart from eligibility on medical grounds, other factors,

* Reprinted with permission from *Transfusion Medicine*, 1993, **3**, 307–316.

such as reliable dates for elective surgery and adequate venous access, are essential considerations.

Directed blood donation, that is, donations from relatives or motivated friends of the patient, is not considered and should be actively discouraged, since there is no evidence that directed donations are safer than blood provided by the transfusion services. One has to consider that a relative who is in a risk group and under pressure to donate may find it difficult or impossible to avoid doing so. An exception may be made for the use of maternal blood for a neonate under special circumstances; indeed, maternal platelets may be the only suitable platelets for the management of neonatal alloimmune thrombocytopenia. However, the increased risk of graft-versus-host disease should be seriously considered, in view of the shared human leucocyte antigen (HLA) haplotypes. Maternal blood or blood components should therefore be irradiated if given to her newborn child.

The risks of viral transmission by allogeneic transfusion in the UK are very small. Whilst the avoidance of these risks undoubtedly adds to the patient's safety, it should be remembered that other hazards of blood transfusion remain, particularly those associated with documentation. These may be more likely to occur during an unfamiliar predeposit procedure. It is also the case that one or more venesections over a period of weeks may result in morbidity, which needs to be balanced against the potential risks of receiving blood from volunteer donors, given the local prevalence of transfusion-transmitted viruses in the donor population.

Careful selection of appropriate patients is an important part of a safe and successful autologous predeposit programme. No less important is a clear understanding by all those involved of their responsibilities at the various stages of the procedure, from the first consideration of eligibility through to the final checks before transfusion. A standard operating procedure incorporating details of local arrangements and specifying these responsibilities is essential.

Predeposited blood should be transfused using similar clinical indications to those for allogeneic transfusion; it should not be transfused simply because it is available.

Autologous predeposit may reduce or avoid the need for transfusion of allogeneic blood. Attention is drawn to other factors which assist with this aim, particularly the use of haematinics rather than transfusion to raise the haemoglobin, where appropriate, and the use of aprotinin to reduce blood loss during cardiac surgery. Other forms of autologous transfusion should also be considered.

3 Selection of patients

Preoperative autologous donation should only be considered for those elective surgical procedures with a reasonable expectation that blood will be transfused.

Hospitals should have a maximum surgical blood-ordering schedule (BCSH, 1990) before they embark on a programme of predeposit. Autologous predeposit should only be available for those patients who would normally have blood available for the procedure to be undertaken. Patients who would normally have a 'group and screen' should not be considered.

Selection of patients and consideration of their fitness for the procedure and of the other criteria in this section should be undertaken by the doctor with clinical responsibility for the patient. He/she should discuss with the patient the relative merits of autologous and allogeneic transfusion, together with the possibility that, even if an autologous transfusion programme is undertaken, it may be necessary to transfuse allogeneic blood. Referral of suitable patients who wish to predeposit should be made in a standard format signed by the clinician who has discussed predeposit with the patient (Appendix 21.1).

The final responsibility for ensuring that the patient's health is satisfactory to allow donation of the required number of units rests with the doctor who undertakes the predeposit procedure. This doctor should also obtain written consent to the procedure (Appendix 21.2).

Patients with virological markers which indicate infectivity for hepatitis B virus (HBV), human immunodeficiency virus (HIV) or hepatitis C virus (HCV) should not be considered for autologous predeposit.

Active bacterial infection is a clear contraindication to predeposit, because of the possibility of bacteraemia and subsequent bacterial proliferation during storage of the blood.

The patient's haemoglobin should normally be greater than 11 g/dl in both men and women and never less than 10 g/dl. In pregnancy, the haemoglobin should exceed 10 g/dl. The place of epoetin to encourage haemopoiesis in patients donating several units remains unclear and its general use is not recommended. It may be justified in patients with rheumatoid arthritis awaiting orthopaedic surgery or for patients with multiple or difficult alloantibodies where surgery is urgent. It should be noted that, currently, epoetin is not licensed for this application.

It is now recognized that most elderly patients can predeposit safely, provided that a careful assessment of their general health is made, with particular reference to cardiovascular and cerebrovascular fitness.

Predeposit in children under 25 kg is technically difficult and rarely justified. Children between the ages of 8 and 16 with no unstable cardiovascular or pulmonary problems can be considered for predeposit. The major indications are orthopaedic surgery (e.g. spinal fusion) and extensive plastic surgery. Predeposit is also indicated for paediatric bone marrow donors, a situation in which it has been used successfully for some years. An important requirement is that the child is able to comprehend and willing to cooperate with the procedure. Parental consent is mandatory. The donations should be collected in a hospital in close collaboration with a paediatrician.

Adult patients under 50 kg need special consideration, and care should be taken that the volume drawn does not exceed 12% of the estimated blood volume (see Section 4, p. 254).

There are few indications for predeposit in pregnancy. Although the procedure appears to be without significant hazard for the mother, there is still insufficient information about possible harmful effects to the fetus. Where there is a specific indication for predeposit, e.g. multiple or difficult alloantibodies, it is preferable, where possible, to collect blood from the patient early in pregnancy and store it frozen. Autologous predeposit is contraindicated in pregnancies complicated by any condition associated with impaired placental blood flow and/or intrauterine growth retardation, including hypertension, pre-eclampsia, diabetes mellitus or any severe pre-existing medical condition. (See also Appendix 21.4.)

Subject to assessment by the referring cardiologist, some patients with cardiac disease can predeposit safely. Predeposit should not be offered to patients with significant aortic stenosis, prolonged and/or frequent angina, significant narrowing of the left main coronary artery and cyanotic heart disease. The value of isovolaemic replacement with crystalloid has not been subjected to proper clinical trials, but it seems reasonable to believe that maintenance of the blood volume will minimize the hazardous sequelae which may follow a reduction in blood volume. Volume replacement should be considered for patients on treatment with β-blockers and/or angiotensin-converting enzyme (ACE) inhibitors, since their ability to respond to a reduction of blood volume may be compromised by their treatment. The blood-pressure should be monitored following donation to confirm a return to the baseline figure. Patients with uncontrolled hypertension should not be bled.

Patients with a history of epilepsy should not be considered, as withdrawal of blood may precipitate a fit. Patients who have been blood donors and sustained a delayed faint, i.e. weakness or loss of consciousness several hours after donation, should not be considered.

4 Practical aspects of collection, storage and transfusion

Collection and storage of predeposited blood should be under medical supervision. The doctor must obtain the patient's written informed consent to the procedure (Appendix 21.2) advising the patient about possible complications, particularly the possibility of needing allogeneic blood in addition to any blood prepared for autologous transfusion. The medical officer should be immediately available during donation.

Blood collection procedures may differ in detail between regional transfusion centres and hospitals. Important points of procedure can be found in Appendix 21.4. Consultation with the regional transfusion centre may also be appropriate.

Blood should not be drawn more often than once a week, with the last donation at least 4 days (preferably a week) before surgery; this will normally allow up to 4 or 5 units to be collected. Exceptionally, e.g. where surgery is postponed, it may be possible to use a 'leap-frog' technique, returning the oldest unit(s) to the patient to allow another (others) to be withdrawn.

The haemogloblin should be determined before each donation, and blood should normally only be drawn where the haemoglobin is greater than 11 g/dl. Blood should never be taken from patients whose haemoglobin is 10 g/dl or lower.

For paediatric patients and for adults <50 kg, blood should be drawn into packs for paediatric use, which contain 35 ml of anticoagulant and are suitable for the collection of up to 250 ml of blood. For children <30 kg, the volume collected should not exceed 12% of the estimated blood volume. Pedipacks with needles of appropriate gauge for phlebotomy in children should be used, when available. Preoperative ANH should be considered for paediatric patients, especially when phlebotomy would be difficult or preoperative donation is contraindicated.

For all patients who predeposit, oral iron should be prescribed before the first donation and continued until surgery.

The label for the blood pack should include the information listed in Appendix 21.3. The patient (or, in the case of a child, the parent) should sign the label to validate this information and should do so immediately before donation, i.e. when the patient is on the couch. The label should be affixed during donation. The label should have a suitable adhesive for refrigerated storage.

Labelled blood bags or sample tubes should not be placed on a shared table or trolley between two adjacent donors. Any risk of transposition must be avoided.

Blood collected into CPD-A1 may be stored for up to 35 days. Red cells suspended in optimal additive solutions have an extended shelf-life of 42 days. Where several units are being predeposited, it may be advantageous to collect the first two into packs which will allow separation of the red cells and their resuspension in optimal additive solution.

Blood which has been predeposited for autologous transfusion should be stored, securely and segregated, in a blood bank refrigerator at a controlled temperature of 4 ± 2°C, which should be equipped with a recorder and an alarm.

The following tests should be carried out on the patient's blood:

1   ABO and Rh D grouping, the results to be displayed on the pack label.

2   At the first donation, serological screening for atypical red cell antibodies, in case allogeneic blood is required.

3   On the first and last donation (as a minimum), tests for hepatitis B surface antigen (HBsAg), anti-HIV 1 and 2, and anti-HCV which conform to current UK

Blood Transfusion Service (UKBTS) guidelines and specifications. These are essential both to establish the patient's status for these markers and because current practices are such that donations which are positive for any of these tests would not be issued for use, and the same criteria should apply for autologous transfusion. A test for syphilis should also be carried out. Advice for the patient about the significance of a positive result in any of these tests should be available and must be in the case of HIV.

Where an autologous donor's blood is found to be reactive in screening test(s) for a virological marker(s) (see above) which, on confirmatory testing, does not indicate infectivity, i.e. false positive results, there is no contraindication to predeposit. However, practical problems arise. The planned predeposit programme is likely to be delayed while confirmatory tests are performed and reported; in many regional transfusion centres, release procedures will not allow such donations to be issued.

Where the results of reference tests show that an autologous donor's blood has a virological marker indicating infectivity for HBV, HIV or HCV, any donation(s) which have been collected should be discarded, with appropriate precautions, and the autologous programme for the patient should be abandoned.

In those cases where the virological screening tests are repeatably reactive and the results of confirmatory tests are awaited from the reference laboratory, any donation(s) must be quarantined securely until the results of these tests indicate whether the donation is infectious.

5 Pretransfusion tests

A blood sample should be obtained from the patient for compatibility testing when he/she is admitted for surgery.

Pretransfusion testing should be carried out in accordance with the guidelines for compatibility testing (BCSH, 1987).

Each donation should carry the same type of compatibility label as that used routinely in the hospital to facilitate checking in theatre and at the bedside. The design of the autologous transfusion label should allow the compatibility label to be overstuck, leaving the information about the blood group and expiry date readily visible.

6 Disposal of unused blood

Blood collected for autologous transfusion which is not required for the donating patient should not be transfused to another patient. It may be used for laboratory purposes, provided that tests for HBsAg, anti-HIV and anti-HCV have been performed and found negative. Otherwise, unused blood must be discarded.

Plasma from unused blood should not be included in pools for fractionation. The fate of autologous blood should be fully documented to ensure that each unit can be accounted for (Department of Health, circular HC/84(7)).

7 Records

Records of all predeposit procedures should be retained in a similar way to those for allogeneic blood.

8 Quality control and audit

Where autologous transfusion programmes are carried out in the form of pre-operative collection, storage and retransfusion of donated blood, the procedures should be subjected to periodic medical and quality audits.

9 Product liability

Although such a situation has not yet been tested in the courts, it appears inevitable that, where an autologous donation becomes defective at any stage between collection and transfusion, there would be product liability under the Consumer Protection Act 1987 in the same way as with an allogeneic donation.

Appendix 21.1: Referral letter for autologous predeposit

This should be addressed to the doctor in charge of the predeposit programme.

Dear

This patient has requested autologous predeposit for his/her operation. I have discussed this with the patient, with appropriate reference to guidelines for preoperative autologous donation and am of the opinion that he/she is medically suitable for the procedure.

I would be grateful if you could see him/her with a view to making the necessary arrangements.

Patient's name (Mr/Mrs/Ms): ....

Patient's address: ....

....

Patient's date of birth: ....

Ward: ....

Hospital: ....

Hospital number: ....

Date of admission: ....

Date of operation: ....

Planned procedure: ....

Underlying pathology: ....

Requested number of donations (maximum is 5): ....

Haemoglobin (g/dl): ....

Additional comments: ....

....

Signature of referring consultant clinician: ....

Name of referring consultant clinician (BLOCK LETTERS): ....

Date: ....

Appendix 21.2: Consent to autologous transfusion

This consent form is intended for adults and will need to be adapted in the case of children.

The purpose of autologous transfusion has been explained to me by Dr .... who has also explained its possible complications and hazards.

I agree to my blood being withdrawn and stored for autologous transfusion.

I understand that it may not be possible for technical reasons to return to me all or any of the units which I donate.

I understand that it may be necessary to supplement my autologous transfusion with blood from volunteer donors from the transfusion services.

I agree to my blood being tested for HBsAg (one of the viruses causing hepatitis), for anti-HCV (another virus causing hepatitis), for anti-HIV and for syphilis. In the event of a positive result in any of these tests, I agree to the clinician in charge of my case being informed.

Signed: ....

Dated: ....

Witnessed: ....

Appendix 21.3: Blood pack label

Blood for autologous transfusion should be identified with an overstick label* which includes the following information:

Blood for autologous transfusion only

Surname: ....

First names: ....

Date of birth: ....

Hospital number: ....

Date of collection: ....

Date of expiry: ....

ABO and Rh D groups: ....

Laboratory reference number: ....

Patient's signature: ....
(Parent or guardian in the case of a child)

The patient signs the pack to confirm that the details on the label (apart from the ABO and Rh D group, which may not be entered when the first unit is drawn) are correct. The signature can also be compared, as part of a pretransfusion checking procedure, with the signature on the consent form, which by then will be in the patient's notes.

*This label should not occlude the information given on the manufacturer's standard pack label.

Appendix 21.4: Blood collection

The advice in this appendix may assist those other than regional transfusion centres collecting autologous donations.

The following points are of importance in collecting a blood donation:

1 Check the patient's blood-pressure.

2 Blood may be collected into a single pack with CPD-A1 anticoagulant, giving a shelf-life of 35 days. Where it is planned to take several units, the first two may be collected into a multiple pack system, allowing subsequent processing and resuspension of the red cells in optimal additive solution, giving a shelf-life of 42 days.

3 Use a balance to measure the volume of blood drawn.

4 The skin should be cleaned thoroughly, using chlorhexidine (in alcohol) or equivalent.

5 The use of local anaesthetic is recommended.

6 The donor tubing should be clamped, for example with 'non-toothed' Spencer Wells forceps, before the guard is removed from the needle. This will prevent air entering the bag and possibly contaminating the donation. The clamp should remain in place until after the venepuncture.

7 A donation from an adult should normally be approximately 450 ml, but a smaller

volume may be appropriate from small adults or children. Packs for the collection of 250 ml are available.

8 The pack should be agitated gently throughout collection to mix the blood with the anticoagulant.

9 Samples for laboratory tests can be taken at the end of the donation before the needle is withdrawn by clamping the donor tube in two places and cutting the tube between the clamps.

10 Attention to haemostasis after withdrawal of the needle will be particularly important if several donations need to be collected from the vein.

11 It is important to use a technique which will evacuate the blood from the donor tube and allow it to be replaced with anticoagulated blood from the pack.

12 The donor tube should be sealed, both at its cut end and close to the pack.

Note: pregnant patients

In the latter part of pregnancy, the weight of the uterus in the dorsal position impedes venous return. Because of this, these patients are more likely to react adversely to venesection, and donations should therefore be collected with the patient lying in the lateral position.

Appendix 21.5: Fact sheet

This fact sheet provides information for patients. Additions or amendments, taking account of local practices, may be needed.

Facts about autologous blood transfusion
What is autologous blood?

Autologous blood is blood from an individual to be given back to that individual should the need for transfusion arise. Blood can be stored for up to 42 days between collection and use.

What are the advantages of autologous blood?

Autologous blood has the advantage over blood from other individuals in that it is incapable of stimulating antibodies to red cells, white cells, platelets and plasma proteins. It also carries no risk of transmitting infections such as hepatitis or HIV. However, the very small risk of bacterial contamination at the time of collection is the same as for any blood donation.

What are the disadvantages of autologous blood?

In general, donation for autologous transfusion has the same minimal risk as any blood donation. Because of the need to collect several units of blood within a period of a few weeks, it will be necessary for the patient to take an iron supplement. There is also a minimal risk, as with any transfusion, that blood other than one's own may be transfused accidentally.

Who may donate for autologous transfusion?

Patients whose general health is good can be considered for autologous transfusion for some planned surgical and obstretric procedures. Some children may also be able to take part in an autologous programme. The consultant in charge of your case will decide if you are suitable for autologous transfusion.

How many units of autologous blood may be donated?
The exact number would be determined by your consultant. As many as 4 or 5 units may be taken at approximately weekly intervals before the planned date for surgery.

Where is blood donated?
The donations will be taken at your local hospital or regional transfusion centre. The request is made by your consultant to the consultant haematologist, who will arrange to collect and store your donations.

How long does the procedure take?
Collecting a donation takes about 30 minutes each time, after which you will be asked to rest for 15 minutes before leaving. You can drive a car afterwards if you feel perfectly well, but it may be advisable to have a friend who is willing to drive on the first visit. If you feel unwell or if you are in any doubt, you should inform the doctor. Some occupations involve some personal risks or include responsibility for the safety of others. If such hazards are a normal part of your work, ask the doctor how long you should wait before resuming your activities.

Points to note after the donation

1 Most people feel fine after donating; however, if you do feel light-headed, it may mean that your system has not had enough time to adjust. You should restrict your activities and, if necessary, lie down and rest until you feel better.

2 Drinking extra fluid helps to replace some of the liquid portion of the blood you have donated. You will normally be offered a drink following donation.

3 If your arm starts to bleed, do not be alarmed. Simply raise the arm above your head and apply gentle continuous pressure immediately to the venepuncture for 10 or 15 minutes until bleeding stops.

4 Occasionally the area may appear bruised. This discoloration will disappear within a few days and should cause you no concern.

5 Usually the venepuncture heals without difficulty. However, if the site should become reddened and painful, you should contact the doctor who took your blood or your general practitioner.

References

BCSH (1987) Guidelines for compatibility testing in hospital blood banks. *Clinical and Laboratory Haematology* 9, 333–341.

BCSH (1988) Guidelines for autologous transfusion. *Clinical and Laboratory Haematology* 10, 193–201.

BCSH (1990) Guidelines for implementation of a maximum surgical blood order schedule. *Clinical and Laboratory Haematology* 12, 321–327.

22 Medical Audit: Notes for Haematologists
Prepared by the Clinical Haematology Task Force

1 Introduction

Medical audit is becoming widely accepted by the medical profession and its informal use by individuals and small groups is gradually evolving, so that almost all clinicians now need to use audit as a routine part of their practice.

For those coming new to audit, there are a number of publications available, mostly from the Royal Colleges, which give a general viewpoint. However, in addition to these guidelines, haematologists will need more specific advice on unique aspects of their subject. These notes are the result of meetings of an informal group of haematologists under the patronage of the British Committee for Standards in Haematology (BCSH). It is hoped that they will provide a useful guide.

2 What is medical audit?

The government's White Paper *Working for Patients* (HMSO C150 2/89) defines medical audit as 'the systematic, critical analysis of the quality of medical care, including the procedures used for diagnosis and treatment, the use of resources, and the resulting outcome and quality of life for the patient'. It is important that those new to medical audit appreciate that, as defined by the White Paper, it does not include audit of the finances of health care, which is a separate issue. Data could be used to influence the allocation of resources.

The three main categories of clinical care can be measured and are interrelated:
1 *Structure*. This includes the quantity and type of resources available and is usually relatively easy to measure, set standards for and change.
2 *Process*. This is what is done to the patient. A review of process can be done quickly and cheaply. It includes consideration of medications prescribed, the adequacy of notes and compliance with consensus policies, such as use of the hospital formulary.
3 *Outcome*. This is the result of clinical intervention and is the most relevant

indicator of the quality of patient care. It can be measured, for example, by studies of patient mortality, residual disability and patient satisfaction. Frequently, outcome cannot be assessed until some time after the clinical event.

3 Why is audit needed?

Medical audit requires peer review, and therefore a forum must be created for the presentation and critical discussion of audit data. This requires the participation of senior staff, who may act as meeting chairperson in rotation. However, all grades of staff must act as presenters. When senior staff are presenters, it is important to have an independent chairperson to avoid the presenter dominating proceedings. Conversely, an independent chairperson will protect junior presenters from misplaced or unjustified criticism.

Where appropriate, nursing staff should be invited to attend and participate in medical audit. Other non-medical staff may be invited, as occasions arise. In hospitals where medical students are taught, they should be invited to attend audit meetings.

Occasionally, it will be beneficial to hold a joint audit with one or more specialist groups. Some examples are:

1 general physicians – anticoagulants;
2 surgeons – Hickman lines, splenectomy, lymph node biopsy;
3 radiotherapists – management of lymphoma;
4 histopathologists – post-mortem;
5 microbiologists – infection policy;
6 various clinicians – blood product usage.

Meetings should take place regularly – weekly or monthly, depending on local

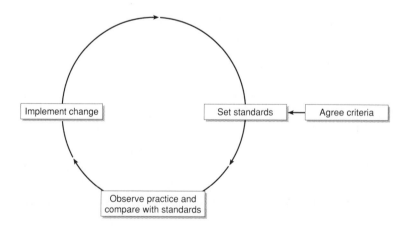

Fig. 22.1 The audit cycle.

circumstances. A suggested pattern is weekly for 30 minutes or monthly for 1 or 2 hours.

Attendance should be explicitly encouraged and an attendance register must be kept.

4 Action

Audit is of less value if action does not result, and this is likely to be the most difficult step. It requires agreement to be reached and conclusions or recommendations to be implemented. Action may be implemented by medical or non-medical staff or by management to ensure better clinical practice. Discussion alone, without clear lines of action, is unsatisfactory, and it is good practice to reaudit topics from time to time to check that recommendations have resulted in a change in clinical practice.

5 Techniques

Medical audit must be unselected. Consequently, when case audit is done, it must be random and confidential; grand rounds or departmental meetings which examine interesting patients are not audit meetings and must not substitute for them.

Furthermore, medical audit implies the critical evaluation of quality (and sometimes the quantity of care where relevant to the quality), but must not be confused with activity analysis.

Analysis of specific aspects of clinical practice (criteria) leads to the setting of standards against which future practice can be measured and evaluated. Any criticism which flows from this process may result in change. This is the audit cycle (Fig. 22.1).

It is important when setting standards to be able to measure current practice, as this is the baseline from which changes can be audited. One method of achieving this is by the use of questionnaires, which all participants in the audit meeting are asked to complete prior to the meeting. Examples of such a questionnaire are given in Appendices 22.1 and 22.2. Questions within a questionnaire can be open (easier to complete, more difficult to analyse, e.g. the clinical audit for haemophilia centres in Appendix 22.3) or closed (simple yes or no, more difficult to complete but easier to analyse, e.g. the physicians' questionnaire in Appendix 22.1).

A number of techniques may be used to examine current practice and each technique might form the basis of an audit meeting. The techniques can be alternated to give a varied pattern to a series of audit meetings, thus heightening interest among the participants.

5.1 Review of deaths or disasters

This is one of the oldest types of audit. A review of deaths can be varied by having a post-mortem audit with histopathology colleagues. Audit of 'disasters' will hopefully be infrequent, but examples might include blood transfusion practice, intravenous chemotherapy, septic shock, etc.

5.2 Audit of randomly selected case records

This requires the least preparation and initially is the most revealing form of audit. It can be done on at least two levels: first, examining clerical standards (e.g. the format of the notes, filing of reports, typing of discharge letters) and, second, audit of the quality of the medical case notes. The latter lends itself to the type of analysis used at the Central Middlesex Hospital (Appendix 22.1), to which we have added a few additional questions of particular relevance to the haematologist (Appendix 22.2).

5.3 Topic-related (or criterion-based) audit

This is the most time-consuming but probably the most educational type of audit. A topic is chosen, which might be purely clinical (e.g. management of polycythaemia, anticoagulant usage, care of intravenous lines) or more managerial (e.g. reasons for out-of-hours laboratory tests, reasons for follow-up visits in the outpatients department (OPD), waiting times for outpatients receiving blood products). Ideally, and especially for the purely clinical topic audit, guidelines should be agreed which can then be put into practice. Reappraisal of the standards set can then occur after a suitable interval, resulting in modification to future practice.

5.4 Prospective analysis of outcome

Once a database has been established, this will be the easiest method of analysis. Information on diagnosis, investigation, treatment and outcome can be routinely collected and regularly analysed. In order to practice this type of audit, it is essential to store and analyse data on computer (see below).

6 Outcome of audit meetings

Documentation of outcome is essential, with dissemination of the conclusions reached to appropriate health care personnel and in an appropriate format (e.g. clinical management protocol). Members of other disciplines (e.g. nursing, secretarial, clerical, managerial) must be notified and consulted as appropriate. Any discussion or consultation which the reviewer generates after the meeting must be reported to the next meeting for approval of the group.

7 Resources

Audit is time-consuming, expensive and often difficult to implement. However, good audit leads directly to better clinical practice so that the effort expended becomes worthwhile.

There must be recognition by management of the time devoted to audit meetings, which, if properly attended, may interfere with other duties. Proper preparation and implementation of decisions takes time and support from all grades of staff, and, almost certainly, to audit effectively you will need additional clerical or secretarial help. Money intended for this purpose has been allocated by the Department of Health to regions (letter from the DHSS to Regional General Managers, 19.12.89 Ref: EL (89) MB/224). This money is intended to cover the expenditure required for computers and computer software, for help with handling data (e.g. computer operator, audit assistant) and for secretarial or clerical help.

8 Haematology audit

8.1 Process

The simplest form of audit is the most appropriate first step for haematology. This is the audit of current practice, using an analysis of data which may be obtained by questionnaire or by computer analysis. Examples are the practice of using fresh-frozen plasma, platelet concentrates or whole blood, the treatment of venous thromboembolism and the treatment of megaloblastic anaemia in the elderly. The review findings can be tabulated or presented as a short report. One outcome of this exercise is usually a clear identification of points of difference, allowing a further discussion before the criteria for the next step in auditing are set. Points of difference emerging from the review may be, for example, in the management of iron deficiency, in the decision to investigate the gastrointestinal (GI) tract in women of reproductive age and in the diagnostic procedures for idiopathic thrombocytopenic purpura (ITP).

Guidelines can be produced on the basis of a review of current practice. It is important that the criteria are not perceived as immutable and that different approaches are considered and included. For example, in one department, fresh-frozen plasma is only issued if the coagulation screening tests show a haemostatic abnormality. In another, fresh-frozen plasma is issued automatically if a patient receives 8 or more units of blood in 48 hours. The criteria should not judge which approach is better if both practices are used locally, but should attempt to audit in a manner where both can be accommodated. However, subsequent audit may determine which of the practices is better in terms of effectiveness and efficiency.

A topic may be audited against published professional guidelines. For example, BCSH guidelines for the investigation and management of thrombophilia (Roberts,

1991) can be used as a standard for comparing local practices in dealing with young people with thrombosis; BCSH guidelines for the use of fresh-frozen plasma (see Chapter 19) could be used for comparing the management of patients receiving large-volume blood transfusion.

8.2 Outcome

Recommendations and guidelines resulting from a haematology audit can be of two kinds, local and general.

8.2.1 Local recommendations

The haematology audit may provide local recommendations on how to manage certain common and important haematological situations, such as neutropenic fever, suspected malaria, severe sickle-cell (SC) chest syndrome, overdose of oral anticoagulants, etc. Such recommendations are usually simple, short and directive. They should be regularly reviewed and updated, with a clear statement of the last review date on each copy. They are usually made available to all medical staff.

8.2.2 General recommendations

Topic-related guidelines may be prepared by a group of haematologists on the state of the art for a given topic as relevant locally. Examples of this are the investigation of the diagnosis and management of myelodysplasia, the use of intravenous immunoglobulin in adults with ITP, the management of SC disease in pregnancy and non-blood product treatment and blood product usage in haemostatic disorders. Such guidelines must be relevant to the local situation and deal openly with contentious issues. They may be used to identify or emphasize local strengths and weaknesses (the presence of a specialist unit, unclear funding of specialist services, lack of facilities, etc.). Clearly, this type of audit requires several haematologists and could be done on a hospital, district or regional basis, depending on circumstances.

Haematologists should also be involved in at least two specialist audit activities of particular importance: the hospital or district transfusion committee and the review of the usage of cytotoxic drugs.

Hospital transfusion committees are being established on the recommendations of the Department of Health and the National Blood Transfusion Service. Such committees should be haematology-led and organized by the consultant in charge of transfusion medicine. Their brief is to review current practices, produce local recommendations and implement them in order to achieve the safest and most efficient transfusion practice locally.

Cytotoxic drugs contribute significantly to the pharmacy bill. In some centres with active 'malignant' haematology, haematologists are the main users of cytotoxics and their practices are likely to require monitoring and scrutiny. An audit of current practices should be instituted as early as possible to establish the pattern of usage and identify the areas requiring guidelines or recommendations.

9 Interdepartmental audit

Examples of shared topics would include anaemias and especially the anaemia of pregnancy (obstetricians) and anticoagulant management (general physicians), in addition to the other examples indicated in Section 3. Shared topics would usually be audited on a hospital-by-hospital basis.

Examples of topics exclusively managed by haematologists would include haemophilia (on a regional or supraregional basis, as shown in Appendix 22.3) and the leukaemias. Generally, these topics are best audited on a district or regional basis to achieve the critical mass required for effective audit.

Appendix 22.1: Physicians' audit of patients' notes*

Audit no. ....

CONFIDENTIAL
PHYSICIANS' AUDIT OF PATIENTS' NOTES

Patient's sex: Male 1   Female 2

Date of admission: ....   Date of discharge: ....

Date of birth: ....   Date audited: ....

Consultant in charge: ....

Diagnosis on discharge: ....

PLEASE RING ANSWERS TO *ALL* QUESTIONS. Note the time (see question 23).

1 Is the presenting complaint identified clearly?   Yes   1
                                                                          No   2

2 Does the history of the presenting complaint include:
  (a) Some indication of duration?   Yes   1
                                                                          No   2

  (b) Some indication of severity?   Yes   1
                                                                          No   2

  (c) Some indication of how well the patient could function before   Yes   1
      this episode?   No   2

continued

---

*The Clinical Haematology Task Force is grateful to the Central Middlesex Physicians' Group for permission to reprint this questionnaire.

Appendix 22.1 *Continued*

3 Does the social history include a note on each of the following?

   (a) Occupation?   Yes 1
                                                                   No   2

   (b) With whom they live (or some other clear indication   Yes 1
       of potential need for home or social services)?   No   2

   (c) Alcohol intake?   Yes with amount and frequency OR states 'none'   1
                       Includes some note but no details   2
                       No notes included   3

   (d) Smoking?   Yes with amount and frequency OR states 'none'   1
                 Includes some note but no details   2
                 No notes included   3

4 Is the patient's ethnic origin documented?   Yes 1
                                                              No   2

5 Is the patient's medication on admission clearly documented?
  ('Fully' = with dose and frequency or states 'no medication')

                                                  Yes fully   1
                                              Yes but not fully 2
                                            Nothing recorded 3

6 Are known allergic responses or abnormal drug reactions
either documented on the front of the notes or placed under the drug
section of the admitting history?   In correct place   1
                                          Present elsewhere 2
                                          Not found   3

7 Does the baseline information in the systems review include the items below? ('Others' = aspects of the system not included in the list given, e.g. 'orthopnoea' OR 'palpitations'. Please circle '3' if there is more than one 'other')

			Yes	No	
(a)	CVS	Chest pain	1	2	
(b)		Breathlessness	1	2	
(c)		Claudication	1	2	
(d)		Ankle oedema	1	2	
(e)		Others	1	2	3 (for more than 1)
(f)	RS	Cough	1	2	
(g)		Sputum	1	2	
(h)		Wheeze	1	2	
(i)		Others	1	2	3 (for more than 1)
(j)	GI	Weight	1	2	
(k)		Bowel habits	1	2	
(l)		Abdominal pain	1	2	
(m)		Others	1	2	3 (for more than 1)

continued

Appendix 22.1 *Continued*

(n) GU		Haematuria	1	2	
(o)		Dysuria	1	2	
(p)		Frequency	1	2	
(q)		Periods/menopause	1	2	8 (male patient)
(r)		Others	1	2	3 (for more than 1)
(s) CNS		Headaches	1	2	
(t)		Visual disturbances	1	2	
(u)		Syncope	1	2	
(v)		Others	1	2	3 (for more than 1)
(w) Locomotor system			1	2	3 (for more than 1)

8 Does the physical examination include remarks on each of the following?

		Number of remarks	
(a) General examination	None	One	2–4	5+
(b) CVS	None	One	2–4	5+
(c) Respiratory system	None	One	2–4	5+
(d) Abdomen	None	One	2–4	5+
(e) CNS	None	One	2–4	5+
(f) Locomotor system	None	One	2–4	5+

9 Does the information in the notes include each of the following? (N/A = not applicable)

	Yes	No	N/A
(a) Blood pressure recorded by a doctor	1	2	
(b) Peripheral pulses recorded by a doctor	1	2	
(c) Weight of patient recorded anywhere	1	2	
(d) Urinalysis result recorded anywhere	1	2	
(e) Peak flow where applicable*	1	2	8
(f) PR where applicable†	1	2	8

* Asthma; COAD; URTI with wheeze; unexplained breathlessness; patient on bronchial dilators.

†GI bleed; abdominal pain; constipation; bowel habit change; DVT; prostatism; urinary retention; weight loss; low back pain/sciatica.

10 Is there a statement in the notes as to whether the patient or relative	Yes	1
has been informed of the diagnosis, prognosis, or treatment?	No	2

11 Is there a treatment plan present following the admission?	Yes	1
	No	2
	N/A	8

12 Is there an investigation plan present following the admission?	Yes	1
	No	2
	N/A	8

continued

Appendix 22.1 *Continued*

---

13 Is there a note that the following investigations were requested?

   (a) Chest X-ray   Yes   1
                                                             No   2

   (b) Electrocardiogram (ECG)   Yes   1
                                                             No   2

       (If No to both 13a and 13b please go to question 15.)

14 Were comments written by the doctor in the notes on the results
of the investigations below?

   (a) Chest X-ray   Yes   1
                                                             No   2
                                                        N/A   8

   (b) ECG   Yes   1
                                                            No   2
                                                        N/A   8

15 How many of the first 25 and last 25 words of the entire notes
for this admission are NOT legible?

                                       No. illegible . . . .

16 (a) How many separate entries are there in the doctors' notes? . . . .

   (b) How many of those entries are NOT signed? . . . .

17 (a) What is the maximum number of consecutive days when
no doctors' notes have been written? (e.g. if written on the
6th then on the 10th, please score 3) . . . .

   (b) How many noteless periods of 2 days are there in total?
(e.g. one 6-day break and one 2-day break = 3 + 1 = 4) . . . .

18 Is the final diagnosis clearly written at the *end of the inpatient notes*?   Yes   1
                                                                No   2

19 Was the standard discharge pro forma or equivalent (i.e. discharge summary sent in 3 days)
present in the notes?

                                      Yes copy or equivalent in notes   1
                                      No copy in notes   2
                                      3 copies present (i.e. assumed not sent)   3

   (If No please go straight to question 21.)

20 (a) What is the date on the standard discharge pro forma or equivalent? . . . .

   On the standard discharge pro forma or equivalent:

   (b) Was diagnosis stated?   Yes   1
                                        No   2

   (c) Were drugs to take away stated?   Yes fully   1
                                        Yes but not fully   2
                                        No   3
                                        N/A   8

continued

Appendix 22.1 *Continued*

21 Was a discharge summary present in the notes?	Yes	1
	No	2
(If No please go to question 23.)		

22 (a) What is the date of the discharge summary? ....

Did the discharge summary include:

(b) Main diagnosis?	Yes	1
	No	2
(c) Subdiagnoses?	Yes, all subdiagnoses	1
	Yes, but not all	2
	No	3
	N/A	8
(d) Date of admission?	Yes	1
	No	2
(e) Date of discharge?	Yes	1
	No	2
(f) Drugs to take away?	Yes fully	1
	Yes but not fully	2
	No	3
	N/A	8
(g) Follow-up arrangements?	Yes	1
	No	2
	N/A	8

23 Before you continue, please note how long it has taken you
to fill in this form so far. .... minutes

CONFIDENTIAL
PHYSICIANS' AUDIT OF PATIENT MANAGEMENT

For doctors only:

Name of doctor doing audit: ....

Please ring: Cons = 1   SR = 2   Reg = 3   SHO = 4   HO = 5

24 Is there any cause for concern over the clinical management of the patient in the following
areas?

	Yes	No	Cannot judge
(a) Admission	1	2	3
(b) Investigations	1	2	3
(c) Treatment	1	2	3
(d) Other aspects of management in hospital	1	2	3
(e) Follow-up arrangements	1	2	3
(f) Other	1	2	3

continued

Appendix 22.1 *Continued*

	Yes	No	Cannot judge
25 In your opinion does this case merit further discussion?	1	2	3

If you have answered Yes for any of the above questions, please write a brief explanation below, and overleaf if necessary. If you 'can't judge', please say what additional information you would require to make a judgement.

Appendix 22.2: Haematology questions to be added to the audit of patients' notes

1 Do the medical notes make clear if this is a first admission with this haematological diagnosis or a re-admission?	Yes No	1 2
2 Do the notes indicate if the patient was in a haematology bed or elsewhere in the hospital?	Yes No	1 2
3 Do the medical and nursing notes indicate if the patient received the following: (a) Red cell transfusion	Yes No	1 2
(b) Platelet transfusion	Yes No	1 2
(c) Other blood products	Yes No	1 2
If blood products were given, do the medical or nursing notes, the nursing chart or the laboratory forms indicate the number of units? (a) Red cell transfusion	Yes No	1 2
(b) Platelet transfusion	Yes No	1 2
(c) Other blood products	Yes No	1 2

Appendix 22.3: Audit protocol – UK haemophilia centres 1992*

1 Patients' comments on centre

The auditor should select at random up to 20 moderate-to-severely affected haemophiliacs from the confidential list provided by the audited haemophilia centre director, and mail the enclosed questionnaire (Fig. A22.1) with a covering letter and stamped addressed envelope, asking for a reply within 2 weeks. The list should then be destroyed. The auditors should incorporate patient comments in their report.

2 Visit to centre

The auditor should agree a date for this visit as soon as possible with the director of the audited centre, who should be available on this day. A full day will be required.

2.1 Inspection of coagulation laboratory

The auditor should record:

1 The ability of the laboratory to carry out all tests necessary for definitive diagnosis of haemophilias, including the identification and assay of specific haemostatic factors, platelet function abnormalities and inhibitors of haemostasis (where appropriate, in conjunction with other haemophilia centres).
2 Out-of-hours availability of assays.
3 Quality control assurance – external (National External Quality Assessment Scheme (NEQAS)) participation and internal.

2.2 Inspection of clinical service and hospital records

The auditor should record:

1 The clinical service cover provided (24-hour) and the experience of staff involved.
2 The facilities available for treatment and advice of patients and relatives.
3 The adequacy of documentation in hospital records (random selection of up to seven records of moderate or severe haemophiliacs, which should be available in the haemophilia centre on the day of audit):
  (a) family type of disorder and level of relevant factor;
  (b) family tree;
  (c) outpatient clinic reviews: (i) adequate documentation? (ii) screening for inhibitors, hepatitis and human immunodeficiency virus (HIV)?
  (d) hospital admissions – use the Royal College of Physicians (RCP) of London form (Fig. A22.2) to audit one or two recent admissions;
  (e) treatment given – amount and type of therapeutic products given in previous year (Oxford returns) and current year.

3 Report

The auditor should write a signed report (two to four A4 pages, plus RCP forms) on his/her findings as outlined in the above protocol, including constructive comments as to how the service might be improved. The report should be sent in confidence to the audited centre director, and the auditor should keep one copy in confidence.

* The Clinical Haematology Task Force is grateful to the United Kingdom Haemophilia Centre Directors' Organisation for permission to publish this audit protocol.

AUDIT QUESTIONNAIRE – HAEMOPHILIA CENTRE

Dear

Thank you for agreeing to help us with the auditing of haemophilia care at your local haemophilia centre. Please return this questionnaire to me in the enclosed stamped addressed envelope. All your answers and comments will be treated in total confidence, and your name will not be divulged to any of your doctors. Please feel free to make any comments you wish.

Do you attend your haemophilia centre regularly? ....

How satisfied are you with the following aspects of haemophilia care at your centre?

1 Treatment of bleeds: ....

....

2 Reviews at clinics: ....

....

3 Treatment of chronic joint and muscle problems, for example by physiotherapy:

....

4 Counselling and answering your questions on haemophilia: ....

....

5 Counselling and answering your questions on complications, such as HIV infection or hepatitis: ....

....

6 Dentistry and other surgery: ....

....

7 Arrangements for home treatment (if applicable): ....

....

8 Counselling and advice on employment, insurance, social work, school: ....

....

What improvements in care of haemophilia would you like to see at your centre?

....

....

....

What other comments would you like to make? ....

....

....

....

Thank you for your help. Please return the questionnaire to me in the next two weeks if possible.

Yours sincerely

Fig. A22.1 Audit questionnaire to ascertain patients' comments on haemophilia centres.

Consultant: ....   Date: ....

Auditor: ....

> **Patient's name and details are NOT to be included
> in order to maintain strict confidentiality**

Final diagnosis: ....

....

....

A *Details of admission*

1 Source of admission:

   (a) Emergency take ....   Bed bureau ....

   (b) Waiting list of OP ....   GP ....

   (c) Other ....

2 Is there evidence to suggest a delay in admission? Yes/No

   If so, at what stage? ....

   ....

3 Do the notes indicate what drugs the patient was taking on admission? Yes/No

   ....

B *Documentation of illness*

1 Were initial medical notes adequate? Yes/No

....

2 Were the clinical problems clearly set out? Yes/No

....

3 Was the subsequent course of the illness well documented? Yes/No

....

4 Were notes signed and dated? Yes/No

....

continued

Fig. A22.2 Royal College of Physicians of London form. This form is suggested for use when visiting and auditing case notes. GP, general practitioner. OP, outpatient.

C *Patient education and welfare*

1 Is it clear from the notes what discussions took place and what information was given to:

(a) Patients? Yes/No

....

(b) Relatives? Yes/No

....

2 Is it clear whether the GP was consulted about admission, management or discharge? Yes/No

....

D *Discharge*

1 **House physician's letter**

How many days after discharge was it sent?

Does it contain adequate information about:
(a) Diagnosis? Yes/No

....

(b) Discharge medication? Yes/No

....

(c) Patient information? Yes/No

....

(d) Follow-up arrangements? Yes/No

....

(e) Request for domiciliary services, if appropriate? Yes/No

....

2 **Case notes summary**

How many days after discharge was it sent?

Was documentation of admission adequate? Yes/No

....

Was drug therapy clearly stated? Yes/No

....

Was it clear what information was given to patient and relatives? Yes/No

....

Are follow-up plans clearly stated and appropriate? Yes/No

....

continued

Fig. A22.2 *Continued*

E *General comments*

....

....

....

....

Fig. A22.2 *Continued*

Further reading

Department of Health (1990) *The Quality of Medical Care*. Report of the Standing Medical Advisory
    Committee. HMSO, London.
Hopkins A. (ed.) (1989) *Appropriate Investigation and Treatment in Clinical Practice*. Royal College of
    Physicians, London.
Hopkins A. (ed.) (1990) *Measuring the Quality of Medical Care*. Royal College of Physicians, London.
Hopkins A. & Costain D. (eds) (1990) *Measuring the Outcomes of Medical Care*. Royal College of
    Physicians, London.
Roberts B.E. (ed.) (1991) *Standard Haematology Practice*, pp. 112–127. Blackwell Scientific
    Publications, Oxford.
Royal College of Physicians (1989) *Medical Audit*. Royal College of Physicians, London.
Royal Society of Medicine (1990) *Computers in Medical Audit*. A guide for hospital consultants to
    personal computer (PC)-based medical audit systems. Anderson Consulting, New York.

Appendix: Guidelines on the Control of Near-Patient Tests and Procedures Performed on Patients by Non-Pathology Staff*
Prepared by the Joint Working Group on Quality Assurance

1 Investigations should be performed in clinical laboratories or other suitable environments by laboratory staff whenever possible. Under certain circumstances, and provided that appropriate equipment is available, it may be advantageous for a limited range of tests and procedures to be performed outside laboratories by properly trained and supervised non-pathology staff.

Laboratory staff should take responsibility for the near-patient service in a manner agreed between the heads of the appropriate laboratory and clinical services or directorates.

2 In the case of hospitals and clinics, whether in the public or private sector, managers of pathology and clinical services must jointly develop and enforce a policy consistent with the Health and Safety at Work Act (1974), the Consumer Protection Act (1987), the Control of Substances Hazardous to Health Regulations (1988) and their subsequent amendments and associated Approved Code of Practice, Safe Working and the Prevention of Infections in Clinical Laboratories (1991) and its associated Model Rules for Staff and Visitors (1991). The following criteria should be made when developing and managing the service:

(a) Equipment must be ordered in collaboration with the professional head of the appropriate laboratory department to ensure satisfactory standards of performance and safety.

(b) Each instrument must have a log book in which details of maintenance, faults, repairs and corrective action taken are recorded by a named individual.

(c) Before using the equipment in service, staff must be trained by members

---

* These guidelines on the control of near-patient tests were drawn up by the Joint Working Group on Quality Assurance and are included here by kind permission of Professor Dame Rosalinde Hurley, Chairperson of the Joint Working Group. Professional organizations represented on the Joint Working Group include the Royal College of Pathologists, the Association of Clinical Biochemists, the Institute of Medical Laboratory Sciences, the Association of Clinical Pathologists, the Association of Clinical Cytogeneticists, the Pathological Society of Great Britain and Northern Ireland, the Association of Medical Microbiologists, the British Society for Haematology, the British Society for Immunology and the British Society for Clinical Cytology.

of the appropriate pathology department. Once competence has been assured, individuals thus trained may be placed on a list of 'authorised users'. This is usually delegated to a senior MLSO, who has been appointed by the professional head to train the users, issue and monitor quality control (QC) material and authorize the use of the equipment.

(d) Arrangements made for training will include instruction in safe working practices, recording of results, the use and recording of QC materials and regular assessment of the competence of staff certified as authorized users by the professional head of the appropriate laboratory department.

(e) Tests and procedures on patients may only be performed by those who have been trained to an appropriate level of competence and are certified as such.

(f) The unit providing the training must be registered with relevant external quality assessment schemes. Full written instructions on internal QC procedures, including limits of acceptability, must be available to staff who perform tests and procedures.

3 Similar arrangements must also be made where diagnostic instruments are used in general practices and elsewhere, e.g. industrial medical centres, pharmacies, etc. Your local hospital pathology directorate will be able to advise.

4 When instruments are issued to (or bought by) patients for self-monitoring, the consultant or family doctor responsible for care should ensure that patients are properly trained in use and maintenance of the instrument(s), know when and how to perform tests and know how to record and act on results. This can be and is usually done by specialized and highly trained nurses appointed by the consultant or family doctor.

5 If reserve equipment is not available in the case of breakdown, the service should be resumed by the responsible laboratory.

Index

Page numbers in *italic* indicate an illustration appearing away from its text; page numbers in **bold** indicate a table.